NURSING CARE PLANNING GUIDES FOR CHILDREN

NURSING CARE PLANNING GUIDES FOR CHILDREN

Edited by

CINDY SMITH GREENBERG, RN, MS, CPNP

Assistant Professor
Maternal-Child Nursing
California State University, Long Beach
Long Beach, California

WILLIAMS & WILKINS
Baltimore • Hong Kong • London • Sydney

Editor: Rose Mary Carroll-Johnson
Associate Editor: Linda Napora
Copy Editor: Catherine Chambers
Design: JoAnne Janowiak
Production: Raymond E. Reter
Cover Design: A. Marshall Licht

Portions of the material on which this book is based were originally published in Neal, Cohen, and Cooper: *Nursing Care Planning Guides for Maternity and Pediatric Care*, copyright © 1982 to 1984, Margo Creighton Neal; copyright © 1985, Williams & Wilkins

Printed in the United States of America

Library of Congress Cataloging-in-Publication Data

Nursing care planning guides for children.

  Bibliography: p.
  Includes index.
  1. Pediatric intensive care. 2. Nursing care plans.
I. Greenberg, Cindy Smith. [DNLM: 1. Critical Care—in infancy & childhood—nurses' instruction.
2. Nursing Process. 3. Patient Care Planning.
4. Pediatric Nursing. WY 159 N97394]
RJ370.N874 1988   610.73'62   87-13347
ISBN 0-683-09571-4

88 89 90 91
10 9 8 7 6 5 4 3 2 1

Foreword

Today's pediatric nurses face a tremendous challenge to provide optimal family-oriented comprehensive care. The pediatric acute care setting has changed as a result of the increased use of one-day surgery units and outpatient care. Hospitalized children are frequently in for short periods of time, are much more critically ill than the average pediatric patient of the past, or are facing the challenge of living with a chronic illness. These changes, along with technical advances and the rapidly changing knowledge base for practice, make it difficult for the nurse to confidently provide care based on current state-of-the-art knowledge. Decisions must be made quickly. Teaching and care that once could be extended over time must now be condensed and modified. This book presents both the beginning and experienced nurse with knowledge necessary to utilize the nursing process and nursing diagnosis in an effective and efficient manner to meet this challenge.

The authors provide an in-depth discussion of the nursing process as it is applied to common medical and surgical problems of the acute pediatric patient. The patient as a pediatric client is considered at each stage of the nursing process, recognizing the unique adaptations for care that must be made because of the developmental and physiologic status of the ever-changing child. The child is viewed from a holistic perspective; psychosocial and developmental aspects of providing care are addressed throughout. The content for each medical problem includes a discussion of the condition, assessment criteria and guidelines, appropriate nursing diagnoses with their rationale, interventions based on each of the nursing diagnoses, and evaluative criteria. Information is provided to enable the nurse to care for these patients and their families from the time of entrance into the acute care setting to discharge. Teaching and learning needs and requirements are emphasized throughout.

Nursing Care Planning Guides for Children is an excellent resource for nurses providing care to acute pediatric patients in a variety of settings. With this wealth of information, the nurse can individualize patient care, utilizing those aspects of the content that are pertinent to a given patient. Thus, rather than providing a cookbook approach, this book encourages creative, individualized, and yet comprehensive patient care.

Cindy Smith Greenberg has provided a tool that can potentially reduce clinical errors as well as frustration on the part of the nurse, and enhance the provision of care that is knowledge based. Thus, nurses can be more confident they are providing quality care to the diverse number of patients that comprise today's typical pediatric caseload.

Bobbie Crew Nelms, PhD, RN, CPNP
Professor of Nursing
California State University, Long Beach
Long Beach, California

Preface

As a nursing educator and practicing clinician, I share the concerns of my colleagues that "standardized" care plans do the work for students and nurses and overlook patient/family specific problems. This book is intended to serve as a starting point for the user who needs to individualize nursing problems according to patient specific behaviors culled from the assessment. Students may find them helpful in providing guidelines for safe care when learning opportunities unexpectedly present themselves in the clinical area; nurses in clinical practice can use them to master the terminology of nursing diagnosis and to aid in creating comprehensive, individualized care plans. The guides are intended to be used in conjunction with textbooks, periodicals, and other supplemental resources.

The nursing process was used as a framework for developing the care planning guides. Each guide includes assessment data; long-term goals; nursing diagnoses with rationale; short-term goals for each nursing diagnosis; nursing actions that address the independent, interdependent, and dependent domains of nursing care; and evaluation criteria/desired outcomes. When using the guides in specific patient situations, they need to be tailored to fit the situation. Include only those diagnoses that are validated by assessed data. Inherent throughout should be an awareness of where that child and family are developmentally and how they are coping with the experience; specific interventions should be written accordingly. Material from several guides can be combined to individualize care even further.

Acknowledgments

A finished manuscript is the product of hours of work and collaboration by many individuals. This process was infinitely aided by the expert editorial guidance, patience, and calm manner of Rose Mary Carroll-Johnson of Williams & Wilkins. Recognition should also go to the many children, students, and staff whom I have cared for and cared with over the years, teaching me about pediatric care as I have taught them.

Special gratitude goes to my parents, William R. and Barbara K. Smith, who provided such a strong foundation of love to grow up on and who are excellent role models for child and family nurturance; to my husband Jay who always gave loving support and shares with me the demands and wonders of parenting and experiencing life through the eyes of a child; and to Erin and Jordan who patiently chewed on and scattered papers as Mommy worked, provided many distractions, and who are of the generation all this is for—the children.

Contributors

Rachel E. Bressler, RN, MN
Nephrology Clinical Nurse Specialist
Transplant Coordinator
Childrens Hospital of Los Angeles
Los Angeles, CA

Marjorie Buck, RN, MN
Clinical Nurse Specialist
A Child's Garden Preschool
Albuquerque, NM

Patricia McKay Bufalino, RN, MN
Assistant Professor of Nursing
Riverside Community College
Riverside, CA

Nancy Jo Bush, RN, MN
Oncology Clinical Nurse Specialist
Valley Presbyterian Hospital
Van Nuys, CA

Randy Marion Caine, RN, MS, CCRN
Associate Professor of Nursing
California State University, Long Beach
Long Beach, CA

JoAnn Chasteen, RN, MN
Dean of Nursing Education
Riverside Community College
Riverside, CA

Sharon J. Evans, RN, MSN
Associate Professor of Nursing
Riverside Community College
Riverside, CA

Susan B. Fowler, RN, MS, CCRN
Critical Care/Neuroscience Clinical Nurse Specialist
Luther Hospital
Eau Claire, WI

Cindy Smith Greenberg, RN, MS, CPNP
Assistant Professor, Maternal-Child Nursing
California State University, Long Beach
Long Beach, CA

Susan Warren Horelick, RN, MSN
St. John's Lutheran Hospital
Libby, MT

Retha Vornholt Keenan, RN, MSN, NP
Instructor, Mental Health Nursing

Los Angeles Community College
Los Angeles, CA
El Camino Community College
Torrance, CA

Jennifer L. Kozakowski, RN, MN
Graduate Student
UCLA School of Public Health
Los Angeles, CA

Carolyn Sue Kross, RN, MSN
Associate Professor of Nursing
Riverside Community College
Riverside, CA

Mary Lou Mackus, RN, MN
Lecturer, School of Nursing
University of Wisconsin, Milwaukee
Milwaukee, WI

Deborah Jean Nash, RN, MS
Visiting Lecturer
University of California
Los Angeles, CA

Kathleen Simons Piggott, RNC, MS
Pediatric Nursing Consultant
Seattle, WA

Patti Roberts, RN, BSN, CPNP, MSN Candidate
Pediatric Nurse Practitioner
CIGNA Healthplans
Long Beach, CA

Lynn Rogers, RN, MN
Clinical Nurse Specialist
Childrens Hospital of Orange County
Orange, CA

Sarah Rothery, RN, MS
Clinical Nurse Specialist
Child Development Service
University of Massachusetts Medical Center
Worcester, MA

Cheryl K. Seaman, RN, MSN
Staff Development Coordinator
Newborn Intensive Care
Indiana University Hospital
J. W. Riley Hospital for Children
Indianapolis, IN

Brenda Hanson Smith, RN, MSN
Assistant Professor of Nursing
California State University, Long Beach
Long Beach, CA

Kathleen Templin, RN, MN, CCRN
Assistant Professor of Nursing
California State University, Long Beach
Long Beach, CA

Mary Tennies-Moseley, RN, MN
Assistant Professor of Nursing
Riverside Community College
Riverside, CA

Linda Tirabassi, RN, MN
Clinical Nurse Specialist
Memorial Medical Center Long Beach
Childrens Hospital
Long Beach, CA

Bethany K. Worgess, RN, BSN, ANP
Graduate Student in Nursing
California State University, Long Beach
Emergency Room Staff Nurse
Memorial Medical Center
Long Beach, CA

Contents

Introduction

Nursing process is the method by which the professional nurse acts to improve the health status of patients. It is applied in the context of the patient's medical diagnosis but leads the nurse to develop strategies individual to the particular patient's needs.

There are five steps to the process
1. Assessment
2. Analysis
3. Plan
4. Implementation
5. Evaluation

The guides developed in this book detail each of these steps for commonly encountered medical conditions. By extrapolating from each section the information pertinent to the particular client and by adapting the nursing plan in light of the patient's needs and the physician's orders, the reader can arrive at a plan of care designed to enhance the patient's chances of attaining maximum health.

Each part of the nursing process builds on and grows out of the preceding step. In addition, the process is cyclical and ongoing. In this context, then, specific information is presented for specific kinds of patient problems.

Assessment, the organized, systematic, and purposeful gathering of information about a patient's current or future health, is essential to permit grouping or clustering of data for analysis leading to identification of nursing concerns or nursing diagnosis. Assessment data are compiled from the patient record, through physical examination, and by interviews with the patient, family members, or other health care professionals; however, the most important source of information is the patient.

To assist the nurse in clustering data, four components of a nursing assessment have been identified. They are *pertinent history, physical findings, psychosocial concerns and developmental factors,* and *patient and family knowledge* about the condition and its treatment.

Pertinent history includes the precipitating events and/or illnesses leading to the patient's current condition. This information may already be documented in the patient record or the nurse may have to structure the nursing interview to ensure gathering of meaningful data. Knowing the patient's history enables the nurse to better interpret other aspects of the nursing assessment, leading to more valid nursing diagnoses and appropriate selection of specific strategies likely to be effective in assisting the patient in achieving desired goals.

The nursing physical examination, routinely performed on patients at the time of admission, provides a physical overview of the patient from head to toe. In the physical findings section of each nursing care planning guide, you will find key physical assessment data especially significant for the condition under discussion. Sometimes this will be specific manifestations or abnormalities you may expect to find. In other cases it was more appropriate to list specific parameters needing assessment. Additionally, many guides include laboratory findings that aid the physician in making a diagnosis and that the nurse can expect to monitor while caring for a patient with that specific condition.

Understanding the ways in which a person has been influenced by society, cultural heritage, and the expected developmental tasks for a person of a given age are helpful in predicting patient responses and in planning specific nursing interventions to achieve desired goals. Information about previous coping strategies and existing functional support systems provides clues to identifying psychosocial nursing diagnoses. Additionally, certain patient conditions are more likely to be manifested in specific ethnic or age groups. For these reasons, the psychosocial concerns and developmental variations likely to be associated with the condition described in the nursing care planning guide are highlighted.

In current nursing practice, it is imperative that discharge planning begin at the time of admission to the health care agency. To help the nurse assess the learning needs of patients and families, important aspects of the condition and treatment plan that the patient needs to promote compliance after discharge are listed. Each nursing care planning guide includes the nursing diagnosis "Knowledge deficit." The nurse's choice to use the suggested diagnosis, to adapt it to the specific learning needs of the patient/family, or identify a more relevant diagnosis depends upon the interpretation of the assessment data obtained concerning the patient's and family's baseline knowledge.

Just as nursing diagnosis provides a framework for nursing practice, an organized nursing assessment is essential to identifying valid nursing diagnoses for a particular patient. An incomplete or incorrect database will interfere with the identification of actual or potential problems. Therefore, by systematically reviewing or obtaining information about the patient's pertinent history, physical findings, psychosocial concerns and developmental variations, and the patient's and family's knowledge of the condition and treatment, the nurse ensures that a complete database is collected. The stage is set for competent analysis leading to identification of pertinent nursing diagnoses as a framework for providing care.

A **nursing diagnosis** is a statement of a nursing problem based on a critical appraisal and analysis of the assessment data. It represents those activities the nurse performs that acknowledge her/his independent functioning. Nursing diagnosis is an ongoing process, not restricted only to the written nursing care plan.

Within the scope of individual state nurse practice law there are important aspects of both dependent and independent functions. The dependent dimensions of nursing practice describe those interventions the nurse cannot legally prescribe. For example, the nurse cannot prescribe nitroglycerin to a patient admitted with acute chest pain. The nurse requires an order from the physician prior to the administration of that medication. This represents the dependent domain of nursing. The independent dimension of nursing practice on the other hand describes those interventions the nurse can legally prescribe. An example of this is a patient in traction who complains of boredom and frustration because of confinement to bed. The nurse may in this situation prescribe diversional activities such as television or referral to volunteer services to obtain books or magazines.

The important aspect to consider when identifying nursing diagnoses is that the diagnostic statement describes an actual or potential problem that nurses, because of their education and experience, are licensed and legally responsible and accountable to treat. Therefore, nursing diagnoses are different from other patient-related problems that are the responsibility of other health care providers.

The nursing diagnosis is written as a two-part statement, the nursing diagnostic statement and the etiology/contributing factors. For example

Ineffective individual coping related to chronicity of disease condition, effect on usual roles and responsibilities, inadequate support system

The **nursing diagnosis** directs the nurse in terms of her/his goals and interventions. Nursing diagnoses may apply to either individuals or groups. That is, not all diagnostic statements refer only to the patient. The family member or significant other may also require nursing actions in order to ensure a successful patient outcome.

Nursing diagnoses utilized in this book have been established and approved by the North American Nursing Diagnosis Association. A complete list can be found in Appendix II.

Planning is the third step in the nursing process and follows patient-specific assessment and diagnosis of nursing problems. Planning allows nursing care to be delivered in a logical, organized, goal-directed, patient-centered manner and directs the implementation and evaluation of nursing care. Planning always occurs prior to implementation of nursing actions. In emergency situations planning may occur simultaneously with implementation because of the acuity of the situation.

Planning involves
- prioritizing patient problems
- establishing patient-centered goals
- stating specific nursing actions/interventions for each problem

The changing environment of the health care setting necessitates that the nurse set priorities to allow for appropriate delivery of care to the patient in a time-efficient, cost-effective manner, thus enabling one to address the patient's biopsychosocial needs more completely. Prioritization is influenced by patient status, the degree of urgency with which the patient views the problem, the treatment plan, and potential complications. The nursing care section of each care plan has been organized in order of decreasing priority to assist the reader in this process.

When establishing goals, the nurse collaborates with the patient, when possible. Mutually agreed-upon goals foster patient compliance and motivation. The best goals reflect the prior nursing assessment and diagnosis. Included in each plan are both short- and long-term goals to promote optimal wellness. Goals need to reflect observable behaviors so that the nurse can measure progress toward the goal or lack thereof.

Implementation is the fourth step in the nursing process. It is during this step that the plan of care is put into action through ongoing assessment, actual performance of bedside nursing actions, appropriate charting of nursing care that has been given, and communication with other health team members. Nursing actions need to be individualized for each patient. They are developed to meet the established goals and should direct care to answer the questions who, where, what, when, how, and how often. The need for assessment of changing patient status is invaluable in providing current and relevant information to maintain a plan of care. As the client moves along the health-illness continuum, the nursing role increasingly focuses on patient/family education and maximizing self-care abilities. The need for quality care and equally good documentation is essential to maintain a care plan reflective of the patient's changing status.

Evaluation, the last step of the nursing process, includes observing the patient's response to the nursing actions; determining the patient's progress towards the goals, objectives, expected outcomes; and revising or modifying the written care plan accordingly.

The patient's estimation of progress towards the goal and degree of satisfaction with the outcome is an essential part of the evaluation process. In addition, family or significant others, the chart, and appropriate health team members are also consulted. Data from each source should confirm and validate the data from other sources; inconsistent findings require further investigation to determine reasons for discrepancies.

When the patient's response to the nursing actions and progress towards the goals are evaluated, a number of outcomes are possible. If the goal has been achieved and the identified need/problem has been resolved, the nurse determines the next priority. If progress is being made but the goal has not been reached, nursing interventions can be continued, discontinued, or modified. If there has been no progress toward the goal, the nurse asks the following questions:

1. Is the goal realistic for this patient and this situation? Does it need to be changed? Does the critical time need to be changed? What factors were involved in progress or lack of progress towards goal?
2. Was the nursing diagnosis accurate? Were data overlooked or are there new data to include? Have new problems emerged that need attention? Is this the patient's priority or is there some other need/problem that seems more important to the patient?
3. Are the nursing actions effective/ineffective? Are there other options to try? Consult with peers, supervisors, and current professional literature.

Revise or modify the care plan as necessary according to answers to these questions. The nursing process is dynamic and cyclic; ongoing evaluation provides valuable information to keep nursing process effective and nursing practice accountable.

The act of planning patient care by using the nursing process is an integral part of modern professional nursing care. The user of this book, be it the nursing student or the experienced nurse, will find it to be an invaluable reference not just to nursing process but to the dynamic, ever-changing arena of individualized nursing care plans.

Bibliography

Carpenito, L. (1984). *Handbook of nursing diagnosis.* Philadelphia: Lippincott.

Carpenito, L. (1983). *Nursing diagnosis: Application to clinical practice.* Philadelphia: Lippincott.

Gordon, M. (1982). *Nursing diagnosis: Process and application.* New York: McGraw-Hill.

The Child with Acquired Immune Deficiency Syndrome

Definition/Discussion

Acquired immune deficiency syndrome (AIDS) is an impairment of the body's immune system. The causative agent is human immunodeficiency virus (HIV), also referred to as human T-lymphotropic virus type III (HTLV-III), lymphadenopathy-associated virus (LAV), or AIDS-related virus. The process by which the virus compromises the immune system is unclear. The result of infection with the virus, however, is a significantly increased susceptibility to infections from a group of opportunistic organisms including bacterias (e.g., *M. avium* or *intracellulare, M. kansasii*), funguses (e.g., candidiasis, cryptococcosis), protozoas and helminthics (e.g., cryptosporidiosis, *P. carinii*, strongyloidosis, toxoplasmosis), and viruses (e.g., cytomegalovirus [CMV], herpes simplex, papovirus). Infection from one of these organisms indicates an underlying cellular immunodeficiency. If no other cause of immunodeficiency can be identified (e.g., immunodeficiencies that are congenital or acquired through medications, malignancy of the lymphoreticular system, or starvation) a diagnosis of AIDS is made.

AIDS is a newly discovered disease: the first case was diagnosed in the late 1970s. Although still relatively uncommon in the general population, the incidence of AIDS has increased dramatically over the past decade. The number of pediatric AIDS cases continues to increase.

HIV has been isolated from the blood, brain tissue, saliva, tears, semen, and breast milk of infected individuals. The majority of children who have become infected with HIV are the infants of mothers who have AIDS or who are in a high-risk group (e.g., IV drug abuser, multiple sexual partners, sexual partner of AIDS-infected male); it is thought that transmission occurs via blood and secretions during the birth process, but may be transmitted via breast milk. A much smaller percentage of children with AIDS have received blood or coagulation factors from infected donors, or are from countries where AIDS is reaching epidemic proportions.

The incidence of AIDS in health care providers who are *not* also members of high-risk groups is exceptionally low. Transmission of HIV to otherwise minimal-risk health care providers has occurred only through accidental injection with HIV-infected blood products (precautions for health care providers caring for the AIDS patient can be found in table 1).

Nursing Assessment

☐ PERTINENT HISTORY

Failure to thrive; chronic diarrhea; persistent respiratory infections; fever; malaise; night sweats; fatigue; muscle and joint weakness; history of blood-product transfusions; pre- or postnatal exposure to HIV-infected parent; growth history (e.g., plot weight, height, and head circumference on growth grid), food likes/dislikes, feeding styles, parents' concerns for nutritional status

☐ PHYSICAL FINDINGS

Lymphadenopathy, hepatosplenomegaly, bacterial sepsis, herpetic lesions, anemia, candidiasis (thrush), encephalopathy, lymphoid interstitial pneumonia; lymphopenia (specifically with a decrease in T-helper lymphocytes), positive HIV antibody, positive HIV culture, normal or increased immunoglobulin levels, laboratory and physical findings consistent with infection with specific opportunistic infections, neurologic status, baseline respiratory function (e.g., relevant history, respiratory rate, respiratory effort, skin color, presence or absence of cough, sputum production, arterial blood gases, pulmonary function tests, presence of dyspnea with activity), quality and quantity of stool, abdominal pain and distension, bowel tones, mucous membranes, urine specific gravity, serum electrolytes, skin condition (e.g., presence or absence of lesions, areas of breakdown, dryness, allergies)

☐ PSYCHOSOCIAL CONCERNS/ DEVELOPMENTAL FACTORS

Anxiety about diagnosis, etiology, and prognosis; response of family, friends, community to diagnosis;

effect of diagnosis and opportunistic infection on ability to master developmental tasks; habits (e.g., play, sleep, what comforts child, favored objects); school activities; ability to utilize available resources; support systems; coping strategies used in the past; perception of child's needs

☐ PATIENT AND FAMILY KNOWLEDGE

Disease process, transmission, associated risk factors, treatment, precautions, screening tests; awareness of informational and support resources; level of knowledge, readiness and willingness to learn

Nursing Care _____

☐ LONG-TERM GOAL

The child/family will function in as optimal a state of biopsychosocial integrity as possible; the child/family will maintain their roles in the home/community to as great a degree as possible.

NURSING DIAGNOSIS #1

Potential for infection related to immunosuppression

Rationale: Because AIDS interferes with cell-mediated immunity, which is responsible for the production of T-cells, children with AIDS are highly susceptible to infection from a variety of opportunistic organisms. Infection by these organisms is difficult to control and is responsible for the high mortality associated with AIDS.

☐ GOAL

The child will remain free from infection.

☐ IMPLEMENTATION

- Identify prenatal patients who are members of high-risk groups and prepare for the possibility of cesarean delivery.
- Counsel women of childbearing age who have AIDS, or who have delivered a child who has developed AIDS, regarding the risk of transmitting AIDS to subsequent children; provide information on birth control; discourage breast-feeding.
- Maintain the child who is infected with HIV in protective isolation; implement additional isolation protocols as dictated by hospital protocol and warranted by the opportunistic organism(s).
- Wash hands before and after care of the child; remove rings/watches while providing direct care.
- Minimize exposure of the child to infection; review isolation and handwashing techniques with family and other visitors.
- Administer antimicrobial therapy, carefully; monitor for side effects/toxicity; administer IV medica-

tions in adequate amount of fluids and over prescribed amount of time.
- Monitor vital signs, changes in physiologic status, and laboratory tests for signs of infection; collect specimens accurately and in a timely manner per hospital protocols.
- Minimize the psychologic effects of isolation by spending additional time talking and playing with the child; avoid use of gown, gloves, and mask if contact with child will not involve contact with body fluids; arrange visits by hospital volunteers, particularly if parents/visitors are absent.
- Provide toys that can be easily decontaminated.

☐ EVALUATION CRITERIA/DESIRED OUTCOMES

The child
- Is protected from nosocomial infections
- Has infection detected early and treatment initiated

NURSING DIAGNOSIS #2

a. **Ineffective airway clearance** related to viscous secretions, ineffective cough, fatigue
b. **Ineffective breathing pattern** related to severe, nonrelieved cough, hepatosplenomegaly
c. **Impaired gas exchange** related to loss of functioning lung tissue

Rationale: Pulmonary disease is the leading cause of morbidity and mortality in the patient with AIDS. Pulmonary infection may lead to damage of actual lung tissue.

☐ GOAL

The child will maintain/regain pulmonary function.

☐ IMPLEMENTATION

- Assess respiratory status every 2 hours, or more frequently if indicated, for signs of respiratory compromise (e.g., tachypnea, tachycardia, dyspnea, apprehension, irritability, confusion, or poor feeding).
- Explain rationale for interventions.
- Assist older child to deep breathe and cough effectively (e.g., splint abdominal muscles, use incentive spirometer); stimulate younger child to cough (e.g., gentle airway suctioning, external laryngeal pressure); observe child closely during coughing episodes and breathing exercises.
- Organize care so that child is allowed adequate rest/sleep periods.
- Monitor use and effectiveness of measures de-

signed to enhance oxygenation (e.g., oxygen, mechanical ventilation, humidification, suctioning).
- Administer medications as prescribed; note effectiveness; report side effects, toxicity.
- Observe agency protocol for tracheal suctioning and care of tracheostomy site if child has a tracheostomy; include hyperoxygenation before and after suctioning; observe for signs of hypoxemia; refer to *The Child with a Tracheostomy*, page 280.
- Wear mask and gloves whenever providing respiratory care.
- Institute postural drainage and percussion as ordered; evaluate breath sounds prior to and following therapy; avoid positions that interfere with adequate respiratory function.
- Understand rationale and intended outcome of chest tubes (e.g., removal of air/fluid); follow hospital protocol related to chest-tube management; maintain patency of chest tubes by gently milking or tapping the tubes; avoid "stripping" chest tubes, which creates dangerously high negative pressures; refer to Nursing Diagnosis #3 in *The Child Undergoing Cardiac Surgery*, page 43.

☐ EVALUATION CRITERIA/DESIRED OUTCOMES

The child
- Demonstrates improved respiratory function
- Has improved blood gas values
- Expectorates secretions
- Experiences decreased dyspnea on exertion or with feedings

NURSING DIAGNOSIS #3
a. **Alteration in nutrition: less than body requirements** related to catabolic state, anorexia, difficulty swallowing, pain, diarrhea
b. **Alteration in oral mucous membranes** related to immunosuppression, opportunistic infection

Rationale: The infectious process increases metabolic demands while rapid passage of nutrients through the gastrointestinal tract impairs absorption. Children with AIDS frequently develop mouth and esophageal lesions caused by herpes or candidiasis infection. These lesions are painful and interfere with chewing and swallowing. Inadequate nutrition further compromises the child's immune status.

☐ GOAL

The child will gain weight; will ingest a diet adequate to meet metabolic demands and facilitate growth.

☐ IMPLEMENTATION

- Document daily weights, enteral/parenteral intake, episodes and amounts of vomiting/diarrhea.
- Utilize creative and developmentally appropriate approaches to enhancing nutritional intake (e.g., offer attractive, colorful foods in small, frequent servings; encourage family and friends to bring in favorite foods; allow child to select foods; reward intake with stickers, stars, special privileges); allow child to utilize already mastered feeding skills (e.g., sit toddler in highchair if able and encourage self-feeding); experiment with food textures and temperatures to find foods most palatable to child.
- Administer supplemental vitamins and minerals as prescribed.
- Brush teeth with soft toothbrush or sponge; provide oral care every 2-4 hours; rinse mouth with water after feedings.
- Apply Nystatin to oral mucosa with soft sponge applicator if child has candidiasis (thrush); offer Nystatin Popsicles to older child.
- Coordinate nutritional approaches with nutritionist; request that special foods be available or stocked on unit around the clock.
- Consult with physician about starting tube feedings or total parenteral nutrition if child is unable to maintain adequate oral intake; refer to *The Child Requiring Tube Feedings*, page 288, or *The Child Receiving Total Parenteral Nutrition*, page 276.
- Monitor laboratory tests indicative of nutritional status (e.g., hemoglobin, red blood cell indices, total protein).

☐ EVALUATION CRITERIA/DESIRED OUTCOMES

The child
- Increases intake
- Gains/maintains weight

NURSING DIAGNOSIS #4
a. **Alteration in bowel elimination: diarrhea** related to bowel infection, prescribed medication, tube feeding intolerance
b. **Fluid volume deficit** related to diarrhea

Rationale: Protozoan and bacterial infections of the bowel will likely present as diarrhea. Diarrhea may also result from antimicrobial drugs/high osmolarity of tube feedings. Frequent episodes of diarrhea are likely to result in inadequate nutritional status, fluid/electrolyte and acid-base imbalances.

☐ GOAL

The child will be free from diarrhea; will maintain fluid, electrolyte, and acid-base balance.

IMPLEMENTATION

- Monitor general condition, vital signs, skin turgor, mucous membranes every shift and as necessary.
- Document weight changes.
- Check stools for reducing substances (Clinitest) and for occult blood (guaiac) every shift.
- Consult with physician about replacing stool losses with IV fluids.
- Change soiled diapers with each stool; clean and dry perianal area; wear gloves and practice scrupulous handwashing when in contact with stool.
- Avoid use of antidiarrheal medications; refer to *The Child with Diarrhea/Gastroenteritis*, page 112.
- Consult with physician about changes if diarrhea is thought to be related to medication or tube feedings.

EVALUATION CRITERIA/DESIRED OUTCOMES

The child
- Has reduced stool output
- Has intact perianal skin
- Maintains normal serum electrolyte values
- Improves skin turgor and condition of skin, hair, nails, and mucous membranes

---

NURSING DIAGNOSIS #5

Impairment of skin integrity related to immunosuppression, opportunistic infection

Rationale: The effect of AIDS on the immune system increases the risk of skin lesions caused by herpes or candidiasis. The overall debilitation associated with AIDS also predisposes the child to skin breakdown.

GOAL

The child will maintain skin integrity.

IMPLEMENTATION

- Clean skin lesions with warm water or saline; rinse and dry gently; apply antimicrobial ointment if prescribed; cover with nonadherant pad and dressing (e.g., Kerlix, Kling) if appropriate; avoid applying tape directly to skin if possible.
- Cleanse perianal area with warm, soapy water (not diaper wipes) after each bowel movement or diaper change; expose perianal area to air when child is lying quietly if excoriated; protect from injury if a heat lamp is used to dry the skin and enhance circulation.
- Apply antimicrobial ointment or a water-occlusive ointment to clean, dry perianal area after each stool.
- Handle child gently when positioning; avoid pulling child against sheets to avoid shearing injuries to skin.
- Reposition at least every 2 hours if child is unable to move independently; utilize egg-crate or alternating-pressure mattress when indicated.
- Massage bony prominences frequently (e.g., with each reposition) to stimulate circulation and enhance comfort.

EVALUATION CRITERIA/DESIRED OUTCOMES

The child
- Is free from skin breakdown

NURSING DIAGNOSIS #6
a. **Grieving** related to anticipated loss of child
b. **Ineffective individual coping** related to perceptions of/reactions to diagnosis
c. **Ineffective family coping** related to perceptions of/reactions to diagnosis

Rationale: The seriousness of an AIDS diagnosis and the associated mortality rate challenges the coping resources of even the strongest individuals and families. The parents of the child with AIDS often experience guilt related to transmission of the disease. Because of the public hysteria associated with AIDS, families with a child diagnosed with AIDS may lose the support of relatives and friends at a time when they need it most.

GOAL

Family members will express feelings, concerns, and fears; will deal effectively with the guilt related to the diagnosis; will develop new or will strengthen existing effective coping strategies; will utilize available resources.

IMPLEMENTATION

- Provide uninterrupted time for family members to talk about their feelings, concerns; encourage to identify their own needs.
- Assist family members to provide care for the child; identify aspects of the parenting role (e.g., feeding, bathing, oral hygiene, play, discipline) that were performed prior to diagnosis and can continue to be performed throughout the course of the illness.
- Promote decision making (e.g., include family members in conferences, encourage them to be advocates for the child).
- Assist the family to identify available support systems; acquaint family members with additional resources; obtain permission from family to contact

other families who are coping adequately with the diagnosis and arrange contact between families.

- Assist to make decisions concerning home care of the child; arrange for an in-hospital visit from the home-health nurse who will be following the child at home.
- Recognize that each family member will cope differently and at own pace; respect differences in coping strategies; assist all family members in dealing with the differences.
- Facilitate/participate in care conferences at admission, throughout the child's hospital stay, and prior to discharge; recognize that staff members may also have difficulty coping, especially if the HIV transmission was likely to be from parent to child; arrange consultation for staff members by appropriate personnel.
- Initiate referrals to mental health resources as necessary.

☐ EVALUATION CRITERIA/DESIRED OUTCOMES

The child/family
- Expresses feelings, concerns, fears
- Maintains social interaction with other family members, friends, and community members
- Identifies resources available for support

NURSING DIAGNOSIS #7
a. **Altered growth and development** related to neurologic changes associated with AIDS, separation from familiar environment, isolation from peer group
b. **Potential for injury** related to neurologic changes associated with AIDS

Rationale: Children with AIDS often experience a progressive encephalopathy that results in neurologic symptoms, loss of developmental gains, or cognitive deficits. The isolation involved in the care of the child inhibits the performance of developmentally appropriate activities while increasing the anxiety and stress associated with separation from the home environment.

☐ GOAL

The child will participate in age-appropriate developmental activities; will avoid injury due to changes in neurologic status.

☐ IMPLEMENTATION

- Institute safety precautions to avoid injury related to ataxia, weakness, and seizures; pad side rails if indicated; have basic resuscitation equipment at bedside, raise side rails when child is unattended, ensure that toys are developmentally safe.

- Arrange for physical therapist to work with child in order to maintain motor skills.
- Provide with opportunities to engage in developmentally appropriate activities consistent with physical status; incorporate developmentally appropriate approaches into nursing care.
- Arrange for the school-age child to have normal educational experiences through hospital-based teachers or teachers from the local school system.
- Develop a schedule for daily activities so that staff approaches are consistent and child maintains some control over own environment.

☐ EVALUATION CRITERIA/DESIRED OUTCOMES

The child
- Attains optimum developmental potential
- Is free from injury

NURSING DIAGNOSIS #8
Alteration in parenting related to unstable family environment, substance abuse

Rationale: Approximately three-fourths of the children with AIDS are infants born to mothers who have or are at high risk for AIDS. Many of these mothers have a history of IV drug use or multiple sexual partners.

☐ GOAL

The child will be free from injury or neglect by parents; will establish a trusting relationship with parents; the parents will provide a safe, nurturing environment for their child.

☐ IMPLEMENTATION

- Monitor parents' interactions with the child.
- Provide a nonthreatening environment so that parents may verbalize their feelings about parenting and their expectations of the parenting experience.
- Role model for the parent while interacting with the child; point out aspects of the child's behavior that are consistent with developmental norms; provide appropriate stimulation; encourage parents to participate in the child's care; provide positive reinforcement.
- Arrange for referral of parents to appropriate professionals as indicated; initiate contact with the health care professional who will be providing home care follow-up.
- Arrange for the child to have consistent visits by volunteers; attempt to provide consistent staffing as much as possible.

EVALUATION CRITERIA/DESIRED OUTCOMES

The child
- Attains appropriate developmental milestones
- Demonstrates evidence of developing a trusting relationship
- Is free from injury or neglect

The parents
- Participate in child's care
- Demonstrate appropriate parenting activities

NURSING DIAGNOSIS #9

Knowledge deficit regarding implications of diagnosis, care of the child in the home, indications for seeking medical attention

Rationale: To decrease the risks of recurrent infection and possible HIV transmission, the family needs guidelines for care of the child at home and reminders of when to contact the physician.

GOAL

The child will receive optimum care at home.

IMPLEMENTATION

- Initiate contact with the appropriate home care agency; begin discharge planning early.
- Emphasize to family members that HIV transmission occurs through intimate contact with body fluids and that nonintimate contact is thought to be safe.
- Instruct family members how to
  - wash hands correctly
  - wear gloves when in contact with body excretions or blood
  - avoid sharing personal care objects such as toothbrushes, pacifiers, razors
  - wash eating utensils in hot, soapy water or dishwasher
  - avoid sharing eating utensils
  - dispose of soiled articles and diapers in tightly secured plastic bags
  - launder clothing and linen separately in hot, soapy water
  - clean soiled surfaces with a solution of 1 part bleach to 9 parts water
  - prepare solution daily
  - discard contaminated cleaning water into the toilet.
- Caution family members to restrict visitors to those who are healthy.
- Instruct family members about signs of infections; stress the need to contact the physician if these signs occur.
- Provide a written list of prescribed medications with times, dosages, and possible side effects; explain measures to minimize toxic effects.
- Evaluate need for education of others who will be in contact with child (e.g., babysitters, school teachers, neighbors); assist parents in providing information as needed.
- Provide parents with access to supplies as necessary; provide them with information on available support/financial resources (e.g., local public health department, toll-free AIDS information line [1-800-342-2437], National Gay Task Force crisis-line [1-800-221-9044]).

EVALUATION CRITERIA/DESIRED OUTCOMES

The child/family
- Lists signs of infection, guidelines for providing care at home, and indications for contacting physician
- Discusses plan for home care
- Demonstrates safe care of child

Table 1
Precautions for Health Personnel Caring for the AIDS Patient

- Maintain good handwashing techniques.
- Arrange nursing care of the AIDS-infected child so that pregnant health-care providers do not provide direct care.
- Wear gown and gloves whenever contact with the child's body fluids, secretions, or excretions is anticipated.
- Wear mask if contact with respiratory secretions is anticipated.
- Communicate that child has AIDS or is HIV-positive to other health-care providers via notes (e.g., Kardex, chart, outside room) using approved designation, but avoid engendering anxiety among families of other patients on the unit.
- Maintain scrupulous attention to disposal of needles and other sharp instruments; place contaminated needles and other "sharps" into designated containers without recapping.
- Label specimens and laboratory slips with "biohazard" or other approved designation to prevent injury to laboratory personnel.
- Avoid contamination when drawing blood or collecting other specimens; dispose of diapers and linen as dictated by hospital protocols.
- Supervise patient environment during emergency situations so that unwary personnel responding to the crisis are not inadvertently contaminated.
- Wash contaminated surfaces with a solution of 1 part bleach to 9 parts water; prepare new solution daily.

The Child with Acute Renal Failure

Definition/Discussion

Acute renal failure (ARF) is a sudden loss of the kidney's ability to excrete the waste products of cell metabolism. It is frequently associated with another disease process. Presenting symptoms in the child include sudden oliguria and a loss of internal homeostasis, resulting in a rise in nitrogenous waste products and a hypervolemic state.

ARF may result from acute glomerulonephritis, diseases affecting the vascular system, obstructions, allergic conditions, hypovolemia, toxic drug or chemical exposure, and trauma. Prognosis is guarded but ARF is reversible if the disease process that originally triggered it is recognized early and treatment is initiated immediately. Complete recovery from all urinary and renal abnormalities as well as functional alterations may not be apparent for at least 6 months.

Nursing Assessment

☐ PERTINENT HISTORY

Kidney or urinary tract infections; major abdominal or vascular surgery; critical illness; family history of renal disease; current medications; recent flu episode; sepsis; recent, unexplained weight gain; hypertension; hypovolemia; respiratory, cardiac, or liver disease; usual pattern and amount of voiding

☐ PHYSICAL FINDINGS

Hematuria, oliguria, or anuria; bruising, petechiae; edema, swollen eyelids, pallor, pruritus, dry skin; dyspnea, increased rate and depth of respirations; hyper/hypotension; lethargy, drowsiness, headache, muscle twitching, restless leg syndrome, convulsions; nausea, anorexia, taste of ammonia in mouth or urine odor on breath, stomatitis, diarrhea; laboratory studies: elevated sediment, osmolarity, and creatinine on urinalysis; elevated serum ammonia, albumin, creatinine, bilirubin, and uric acid; elevated BUN; electrolyte disturbances and resultant ECG changes; anemia, prolonged coagulation studies

☐ PSYCHOSOCIAL CONCERNS/ DEVELOPMENTAL FACTORS

Anxiety, fear of death or the unknown precipitated by the critical-care environment; associated changes in physical appearance precipitating body-image disturbance; habits (e.g., what comforts child, bedtime routine, favored objects)

☐ PATIENT AND FAMILY KNOWLEDGE

Possible course of episode prognosis, level of knowledge, readiness and willingness to learn

Nursing Care

☐ LONG-TERM GOAL

The child will regain normal kidney function and resume usual activities and roles.

NURSING DIAGNOSIS #1
a. **Alteration in fluid volume: excess** related to decreased urine output
b. **Alteration in cardiac output: decreased** related to fluid volume excess, disturbances in renin-angiotensin system, hyperkalemia
c. **Potential for noncompliance** related to thirst, need for fluid restriction

Rationale: Damaged renal tissue is not able to maintain homeostasis. Fluid, sodium, potassium, magnesium, and phosphates are retained and an abnormal amount of calcium is excreted. Disturbances in the renin-angiotensin system result in hypertension, which may increase cardiac afterload and contribute to the development of heart failure with resultant decreased cardiac output and the possibility of pulmonary edema. Cardiac dysrhythmias secondary to electrolyte imbalances can be life threatening. In addition, increased levels of metabolic waste products present in renal failure are toxic to the pericardial sac and may produce pericarditis with possible tamponade. Once fluids are limited, the child will have complaints of thirst and may search for liquids in the environment (toilet, sink).

7

GOAL

The child will maintain a fluid intake adjusted to body need during the acute phase of illness; will maintain electrolyte balance and normal blood pressure; will be relieved of chest pain or discomfort; will be free from cardiac failure/tamponade.

IMPLEMENTATION

- Record intake and output accurately every hour initially, then every 4 hours; note and record color and clarity of urine.
- Plan fluid allotment around mealtime, snack, medications, and bedtime; daily intake should equal ml-for-ml replacement for urinary output plus 400 ml/m² (average daily insensible loss through skin and lungs).
- Weigh child daily, at same time, on same scale, in the same clothes (1 kg = 1,000 cc fluid); use bed scale if necessary.
- Administer diuretics, carefully monitoring toxic effects and urinary output after administration.
- Encourage intake of diet low in sodium; restrict oral intake of fluids within imposed limits; subtract total IV fluids from 24-hour total to adjust oral fluid limit.
- Check tray for hidden fluids (e.g., fruit in its own juice) and restricted foods; keep empty cups out of child's room.
- Substitute frozen Popsicles or juice over crushed ice for fluids.
- Explain restrictions in terms that the child can understand.
- Use game playing to see how long the child can "wait" for a drink; give positive reinforcement (e.g., praise, medal, toy) at end of time.
- Monitor vital signs, neurologic status (level of consciousness, headache, visual or pupillary changes, restlessness, seizures) every hour initially, then every 4 hours or as directed; report significant changes.
- Monitor cardiac rhythm continuously; record a rhythm strip every 4 hours or more frequently if irregular pattern develops; measure central venous and pulmonary artery pressures, and cardiac output every 1-2 hours; report changes to physician.
- Regulate IVs carefully; maintain fluid restrictions; check with the pharmacist to determine if medications may be mixed in less than usual amounts of fluid.
- Administer antihypertensive medications; consult physician if diastolic blood pressure is less than the parameters ordered; hold antihypertensive medications 2 hours prior to dialysis therapy; monitor effects.
- Monitor serum electrolyte levels, ammonia, creatinine, BUN; report abnormal values.
- Assess for presence of chest pain (cardiac or pleuritic), dyspnea, paradoxical pulse (weaker with inspiration), pericardial friction rub, narrowing pulse pressure, distended neck veins, peripheral edema, rales, cardiac dysrhythmias, and fever.
- Medicate for pain as needed; monitor effects; consult with physician for changed order if relief not obtained.
- Auscultate breath and heart sounds at least every 2-4 hours.
- Assess peripheral pulses, check for periorbital and peripheral edema or distended neck veins every 4 hours; note skin turgor at least every 4 hours; ask parents if child looks different than usual.
- Promote rest by keeping environment as quiet as possible and by organizing care to allow child uninterrupted periods of rest.
- Position for comfort with head of bed elevated 30°-40°; administer oxygen as ordered.
- If tamponade presents, assist with emergency pericardiocentesis; provide emotional support to child/family.
- Prepare child for dialysis if necessary; refer to *The Child Requiring Peritoneal Dialysis*, page 219, or *The Child Requiring Hemodialysis*, page 144.

EVALUATION CRITERIA/DESIRED OUTCOMES

The child

- Has normal serum electrolytes
- Is free from periorbital and peripheral edema, respiratory difficulty, increase in body weight
- Maintains/regains urinary output
- Has a balanced intake and output
- Maintains fluid restriction
- Has vital signs within normal limits
- Is free from chest pain or discomfort

NURSING DIAGNOSIS #2

a. **Potential for infection** related to decreased functioning of immune system
b. **Potential for injury (bleeding)** related to anemia and increased coagulation times

Rationale: Renal failure causes decreased inflammatory response and a reduction in antibody production. Wound healing is delayed, precipitating the development of infections, especially pneumonia, septicemia, and urinary tract and wound infections. Renal failure causes decreased production of erythropoietin, resulting in a decrease in the production of red blood cells. Coagulation factor production is also decreased. Prolonged clotting times may result in excessive bleeding from what might normally be considered minimal trauma, especially in the presence of sepsis or disseminated intravascular clotting (progressive stages of shock).

GOAL

The child will be free from infection and bleeding.

IMPLEMENTATION

- Assess closely for any signs of overt or covert bleeding (frank blood, fluid "weeping" around sites of penetration of the skin, weakness, pallor); know that a narrowing pulse pressure combined with increased heart and respiratory rates suggests covert bleeding; note orthostatic changes in blood pressure.
- Monitor for signs of infection (malaise, elevated temperature, abnormal white blood cell count, redness or inflammation, drainage or secretions with positive bacterial cultures); know that sepsis may be present without febrile response.
- Change child's position, encourage use of blow bottles or incentive inspirometer, and have child cough and deep breathe every 2 hours to prevent pulmonary complications; in children unable to expectorate use nasal-tracheal suction every 2 hours or as needed; for children requiring mechanical ventilation suction the endotracheal tube every 2 hours or as needed; encourage family involvement in respiratory hygiene measures with the toddler and preschooler.
- Protect child from chilling and drafts; provide extra covers as needed.
- If indwelling urinary catheter is used, ensure maintenance of a closed drainage system; refer to *The Child with a Urethral Catheter*, page 294; empty collection bag at least every 8 hours and measure carefully; observe urinary drainage for color, odor, and particles; record specific gravity, reporting highly concentrated or very dilute urine.
- Provide care to all wound and puncture sites using strict aseptic technique; assess IV sites every hour for redness, tenderness, and edema; rotate IV sites as needed and change tubing every 48 hours or according to hospital protocol.
- Administer prophylactic antibiotics in a timely manner to ensure maintenance of therapeutic blood levels; monitor for signs of toxicity; note that the frequency of administration of some antibiotics (e.g., Gentamicin, Tobramycin) may be less when the child is anuric/oliguric.
- Monitor hematologic studies; administer blood components as ordered; refer to *The Child Receiving Blood and Blood-Product Transfusions*, page 24.

EVALUATION CRITERIA/DESIRED OUTCOMES

The child
- Is afebrile, has other vital signs within normal limits
- Is free from bleeding
- Has negative urine, sputum, blood, and wound cultures

- Maintains/regains normal hematology studies

NURSING DIAGNOSIS #3
a. **Alteration in nutrition: less than body requirements** related to anorexia, stomatitis, dislike of dietary restrictions
b. **Impairment of skin integrity** related to poor nutritional status, immobility

Rationale: Symptoms of anorexia, metallic taste, nausea, vomiting, stomatitis, gastrointestinal ulcers, diarrhea, and a dislike for restricted diet may result in inadequate nutritional intake leading to breakdown of body protein and negative nitrogen balance, with resultant impaired skin integrity.

GOAL

The child will ingest adequate amounts of prescribed diet; will maintain positive nitrogen balance.

IMPLEMENTATION

- Provide a diet high in carbohydrates, vitamins, and fat, and low in sodium, potassium, and protein (allowed protein should be high in essential amino acids); consult with dietician if child refuses foods provided, and modify diet based on the child's likes, eating patterns, and fluid restrictions; give frequent, small feedings and provide dietary supplements if individual dietary regimen permits.
- Record daily solid intake; monitor serum protein levels.
- If child is unable to tolerate oral intake, administer tube feedings, total parenteral nutrition, intralipids as ordered; refer to *The Child Requiring Tube Feedings*, page 288, and *The Child Receiving Total Parenteral Nutrition*, page 276.
- If antacids are prescribed, ensure they are low in magnesium.
- Change child's position every 2 hours; support and protect bony prominences; provide preventive skin care (e.g., back rub/massage, application of lotion); encourage ambulation as tolerated.

EVALUATION CRITERIA/DESIRED OUTCOMES

The child
- Ingests 90% of prescribed diet
- Maintains body weight
- Has normal muscle tone, serum protein levels
- Maintains skin integrity

NURSING DIAGNOSIS #4

Anxiety related to unexpected serious illness, uncertain prognosis, and separation from family and friends during hospitalization

Rationale: Since ARF can lead to chronic renal failure or death, the older child/family is likely to experience feelings of anxiety about outcome of acute situation. When children are hospitalized, they are separated from their family and friends. This separation, along with the "strangeness" of the hospital environment (e.g., new people, painful procedures), causes an increase in anxiety for children of all ages.

☐ GOAL

The child/family will experience only a moderate amount of anxiety; will understand condition and treatments as necessary and desired as appropriate for age and developmental level.

☐ IMPLEMENTATION

- Plan supportive care and explanations according to child/family anxiety levels; involve the social worker in care.
- Ask the older, verbal child what s/he is feeling and explain that children usually have a variety of feelings, often similar to those just expressed; provide adequate time to permit child free expression.
- Assess nonverbal behaviors of the infant/toddler; ask family members to assist in defining behaviors that indicate child is anxious.
- Communicate progress to child/family; interpret lab results, vital signs, urinary output, etc., as requested.
- Encourage family members to bring in familiar objects from home (e.g., toys, games, photographs, radio) to keep in child's room.
- Answer all questions as honestly as possible including fears and questions about death.
- Explain the purpose and sequence of all procedures and treatments; allow the child to participate in decision making as much as possible.
- Encourage family members to participate in as much care as possible (e.g., feeding, bathing, playing).
- Allow control over daily schedule as possible.
- Consult child development specialist to assist with diversional activities.

☐ EVALUATION CRITERIA/DESIRED OUTCOMES

The child/family
- Describes specific condition and likely prognosis accurately

- Participates in decision-making process
- Exhibits decreased anxiety through calm facial expression, relaxed posturing, normal respiratory and heart rates
- Undertakes appropriate activities for age

NURSING DIAGNOSIS #5

Knowledge deficit regarding prescribed convalescent regimen

Rationale: The child/family needs to understand the importance of continued vigilance to preserve existing renal function and to prevent recurrence or progression to chronic renal insufficiency.

☐ GOAL

The child/family will understand and comply with convalescent regimen.

☐ IMPLEMENTATION

- Assess specific learning needs of child/family; modify teaching plan accordingly.
- Teach about normal kidney function and discuss alterations that the child experienced.
- Provide child/family with written guidelines for prescribed medications, diet and fluid restrictions; review these several times prior to discharge; provide opportunities for questions.
- Review toxic effects of medications; instruct family member to inform physician if toxicity is evident.
- Explain the importance of rest during the recovery phase; assist the child in planning for exercise as tolerated.
- Review signs and symptoms of edema.
- Review signs of infection; instruct child/family to report their occurrence to physician.
- Tell child/family that full recovery may take up to a year; emphasize importance of obtaining follow-up care as scheduled.
- Provide phone numbers of contact persons (e.g., nephrologist, renal clinical nurse specialist, social worker) and instruct to call if problems/questions arise.

☐ EVALUATION CRITERIA/DESIRED OUTCOMES

The child/family
- Describes acute renal failure and prescribed treatment during convalescent phase
- Lists toxic effects of medications, signs and symptoms of edema and infection, and indications for contacting physician
- Expresses awareness of time required for healing and measures designed to facilitate full recovery.

The Child Experiencing Anxiety

Definition/Discussion

Anxiety is the uncomfortable feeling of tension or dread that is unconnected to a specific stimulus; it can be vague or intense. It occurs as a reaction to some unconscious threat to biologic integrity/self-concept. Anxiety can be assessed according to level.

- *Mild:* increased alertness and motivation; increased ability to cope with daily problems
- *Moderate:* decreased perception of the environment with selective inattention; decreased ability to think clearly
- *Severe:* drastically reduced perceptual field; able to focus on only one detail at a time
- *Panic:* inability to integrate environment with the self; cannot function; physical activity is disorganized; the child may be "frozen"

Anxiety can be used as a motivating rather than a destructive force if it is recognized and successful coping mechanisms developed.

Nursing Assessment

☐ PERTINENT HISTORY

Recent environmental/family/school/life-style changes, family/employment stability, losses, absence of supportive relationships, confusion of values/beliefs, previously experienced anxiety and coping methods, financial/health status, accident proneness, child abuse/neglect, chronic fatigue, change in appetite, grinding of teeth during sleep, pain

☐ PHYSICAL FINDINGS

Increased vital signs, muscle tension, sweating, headaches, dizziness, tremors, sweaty palms, flushing, fatigue, GI discomfort/dysfunction, hyperventilation, somnolence or insomnia, nightmares, crying, irritability, dry mouth, capillary dilation, inability to concentrate/understand explanations, shortened attention span for age, bed wetting, frequent urination, headache, stuttering

☐ PSYCHOSOCIAL CONCERNS/ DEVELOPMENTAL FACTORS

Developmental level, age-appropriate ability to express self, degree of perceived disruption, feelings/attitudes associated with the disruption, patterns of dependency, coping patterns of family, socialization pattern (e.g., values, belief systems, culture), habits/routines (e.g., play times, favorite games, sleep/naps, preferred foods), deterioration in school performance, emotional instability/tension, impulsive/regressive/neurotic/psychotic behaviors, sexual acting out, withdrawal from peer/social groups

☐ PATIENT AND FAMILY KNOWLEDGE

Identifiable cause(s), realization that both positive and negative stressors lead to anxiety, involvement of community agencies, level of knowledge, readiness and willingness to learn

Nursing Care

☐ LONG-TERM GOAL

The child will cope effectively with anxiety and use it as a motivation for change as appropriate.

NURSING DIAGNOSIS #1

Ineffective individual coping related to perception of situation

Rationale: Anxiety of more than a mild level will impair the individual's ability to cope.

☐ GOAL

The child will cope with the anxiety and reduce it at least one level.

☐ IMPLEMENTATION

- Use interventions appropriate to level of anxiety
  mild: does not require any intervention
  moderate
  - determine cause if possible
  - do not allow your own personal anxieties to be perceived by the child
  - spend 5-10 minutes with the child at least 3 times daily; show interest and support

- use age-appropriate techniques to discuss situation (e.g., drawing, telling a story, or situation completion ["There once was a little boy/girl who was upset over. . ."], throw bean bags at targets, play tag); refer to *The Child Requiring Play Therapy*, page 226
- allow child to cry
- do not make demands
- do not argue with/confront the child regarding unrealistic perceptions
- focus on the immediate problem; stay in the "here and now"
- explain all treatments/procedures to child in developmentally appropriate language
- do not give more information than child can handle
- be clear and concise in communication/explanations; repeat if needed
- attend to physical comforts and needs
- teach relaxation exercises; refer to Table 2, *Stress Reduction Activities*, page 13

severe
- use previously stated interventions as applicable
- stay with child until anxiety is lessened
- provide a calm, quiet environment
- have child take slow deep breaths if hyperventilating; ask to focus on how body feels on expiration; breathe with child to provide support
- use brief, simple communications
- structure activities into concrete tasks that do not require concentration
- attend to somatic complaints
- administer medication if ordered; evaluate effectiveness

panic
- use previously stated interventions as appropriate
- do not leave child alone
- demonstrate competence; remain calm; use firm, professional manner
- use a small room or separate area to provide privacy and security
- use physical touch judiciously; some children are comforted by touch and some are threatened by it
- reassure child that control will be maintained
- direct child's energy into repetitive motor activities
- observe closely

☐ EVALUATION CRITERIA/ DESIRED OUTCOMES

The child
- States anxiety is decreased to a tolerable level
- Demonstrates behaviors indicating a decrease in anxiety
- Channels energy into goal-directed activity

NURSING DIAGNOSIS #2
Sleep pattern disturbance related to anxiety

Rationale: Physiologic disturbances caused by anxiety may be reflected in a disturbance in sleep patterns.

☐ GOAL

The child will achieve a sleep/rest pattern appropriate to age/developmental needs.

☐ IMPLEMENTATION

- Determine type of sleep disturbance child is experiencing.
- Ask what the child/parents perceive as the reasons for the disturbed sleep pattern.
- Provide measures appropriate to reduce insomnia
  - maintain a quiet, secure environment
  - use relaxation techniques (e.g. rocking to sleep, rubbing back, singing lullabies, night light)
  - decrease the number of distractions (e.g., temperature taking during night)
  - structure bedtime routine to match home routine (e.g., consistent time, bath, reading, warm drink, music, security blanket, amount of covers, type of bed clothing)
- Provide daytime stimulation; schedule time for physical activities; discourage napping and dozing (as age appropriate).

☐ EVALUATION CRITERIA/DESIRED OUTCOMES

The child
- Falls asleep within 20 minutes
- Appears rested, has energy for daytime activities

NURSING DIAGNOSIS #3
Knowledge deficit regarding recognition and effective management of anxiety

Rationale: Children/parents can cope effectively with anxiety if they learn to recognize it. New coping strategies can replace old ineffective coping skills.

☐ GOAL

The child/parents will identify sources of anxiety; will employ effective measures to manage anxiety.

☐ IMPLEMENTATION

- Be aware of the impact of anxiety on ability to learn

- mild: learning can occur at this level
- moderate: learning can occur but it must be directed
- severe: inability to learn at this level
- panic: unable to learn
  - Continue planned interactions with child.
  - Teach parents to recognize that a change in school performance may indicate anxiety.
  - Help identify those tensions and environmental factors that create a feeling of anxiety; attempt to identify precipitating factors/situations.
  - Give careful, age-appropriate explanations; encourage questions and verbalization of any concerns that child may have.
  - Stress the importance of patience since the child may not respond as before.
  - Involve family in prevention/management of anxiety as much as possible; include in decisions about care.

- Teach the importance of regular physical activity.
- Provide positive reinforcement to parents who maintain an environment that allows an understanding of/control over the anxiety.
- Discuss alternatives to, advantages, and disadvantages of reducing stressors; explore ways to alter stressors.
- Provide information regarding available community support services.

☐ EVALUATION CRITERIA/DESIRED OUTCOMES

The child/parents
- List environmental factors that elicit anxiety
- Discuss ways of keeping anxiety at a mild or moderate level
- State willingness to learn new coping strategies
- Verbalize ways to cope with severe anxiety if it occurs

Table 2
Stress-Reduction Activities

Stress is a generalized, nonspecific response of the body to any demand, change, or perceived threat and is unavoidable. Stressors are the circumstances or events that elicit this response and may be real or anticipated, positive or negative. Distress is damaging or unpleasant stress. Stress-reduction techniques are usually most effective for children over 6.

Techniques	Nursing Implications
Develop effective coping mechanisms.	Role play various different ways of dealing with stressors. Discuss which ones would be the easiest/most useful for child/parent.
Begin daily exercise program.	Suggest methods to reduce stress through exercise (e.g., walking, running, dancing, swimming, gardening, participating in sports, body movement exercises, yoga). Assist in developing a plan of regular activity. Evaluate extracurricular school activities that would assist the child deal with stressors. Refer to school/community gyms, health clubs, and YMCAs. Advise consultation with personal physician for contraindications to exercise program.
Develop alternative ways to relax.	Identify activities the child enjoys (e.g., drawing, pottery, carpentry, writing, music, photography, reading); assess for relaxing activities (e.g., watching the sunset, taking a bubble bath). Refer to recreation departments, education programs, community colleges.
Practice relaxation techniques.	Guide through a relaxation exercise to experience its usefulness. Begin relaxation with deep breathing. Use guided imagery to induce relaxation (e.g., "Take another deep breath and let all the tension release. With each breath you become more relaxed. Now imagine yourself in a peaceful, quiet setting [garden, beach, etc.].."). Refer to cassettes/books/classes on learning and practicing relaxation techniques.
Practice diaphragmatic breathing; periodic deep breathing.	Practice diaphragmatic breathing with child • sit or recline in a comfortable position with legs uncrossed • place one hand on chest and other hand on diaphragm, approximately 2 inches below bottom center of breastbone • inhale so diaphragm expands and hand covering diaphragm moves out while other hand remains almost still • as you exhale, diaphragm relaxes and hand covering it moves inward

Make positive affirmations.	Teach to • write out the statements and place them in a visible area (e.g., mirror, steering wheel, refrigerator, desk) • repeat the statements several times daily. • be specific, positive, and brief (e.g., ''I am relaxed,'' not ''I am not tense.'') • use the present tense ''I am,'' not ''I will'' (e.g., ''I am learning to express my feelings.'' ''I am expressing anger in a positive way.'' ''I am loveable.'')
Balance school and recreation.	Teach importance of • regular study schedule so as not to overwhelm self with all the work at one time and to be able to see progress • learning to take relaxation breaks
Improve self care.	Discuss personal habits that contribute to distress • poor nutrition • neglecting early warning signs of tension • nonassertiveness • drinking, smoking, drug use • sexual activity (promiscuity due to peer pressure, lack of birth control) Demonstrate positive ways to express/become more aware of feelings. Discuss importance of setting priorities, taking one thing at a time.

The Child Undergoing an Appendectomy

Definition/Discussion

Appendectomy is the removal of the appendix that is inflamed following infection or obstruction of the appendiceal lumen. Peritonitis results if the appendix ruptures.

Nursing Assessment

☐ **PERTINENT HISTORY**

Fever, abdominal pain/cramping, vomiting, anorexia, diarrhea or constipation, exposure to infection (e.g., drinking contaminated water, eating contaminated food), unsuccessful home treatment

☐ **PHYSICAL FINDINGS**

Rebound tenderness in right lower quadrant (McBurney's point), decreased or absent bowel sounds, rigid position or abdominal guarding, dehydration, changes in vital signs, elevated white blood cell count, abdominal x-ray

☐ **PSYCHOSOCIAL CONCERNS/ DEVELOPMENTAL FACTORS**

Age, daily routine, meaning of disease and hospitalization to child/family, previous hospitalization experiences, habits (e.g., what comforts child, bedtime routine, favored objects)

☐ **PATIENT AND FAMILY KNOWLEDGE**

Understanding of disease and need for immediate attention, past experiences with persons who had appendicitis; level of knowledge, readiness and willingness to learn

Nursing Care

☐ **LONG-TERM GOAL**

The child will recover from appendectomy free from preventable complications; the child will return to normal daily activities after a short convalescence.

NURSING DIAGNOSIS #1

Fluid volume deficit related to pre-op dehydration, post-op NPO status, nasogastric (NG) decompression

Rationale: Vomiting, diarrhea, and inadequate oral intake preoperatively deplete total body water; peritonitis will cause a shift of water out of the extracellular space into the abdominal "third space"; NG suction removes gastric contents that contain water, hydrochloric acid, and potassium.

☐ **GOAL**

The child will maintain adequate hydration status; will maintain/regain vital signs within normal limits for age; will have adequate urine output, normal skin turgor, moist mucous membranes; will regain preillness weight.

☐ **IMPLEMENTATION**

- Weigh preoperatively and every day postoperatively at the same time, on same scale, in the same clothing, and record.
- Calculate maintenance fluid requirement for weight; add additional fluids to compensate for losses and fever; calculate expected urine output for weight.
- Maintain accurate intake and output; weigh diapers of younger child and subtract dry weight from wet weight (1 gram = 1 cc); estimate wound drainage and include as part of output.
- Check urine specific gravity every 8 hours.
- Measure NG output every 4-8 hours and replace with ordered IV solution over 4-8 hours.
- Maintain patent IV line; check for infiltration or dislodgment; check rates of maintenance and replacement solutions every 1-2 hours.
- Dilute antibiotics in appropriate amount of fluid to decrease risk of phlebitis.
- Maintain patent NG tube; irrigate with 5-10 cc normal saline every 2-4 hours and note how much irrigant can be withdrawn (subtract amount of re-

maining irrigant from total NG output before calculating replacement).

- Monitor for signs of dehydration every 4 hours (e.g., poor skin turgor, dry mucous membranes, elevated heart rate, decreased blood pressure).
- Give oral fluids when normal bowel sounds return; offer small amounts of preferred liquids initially and increase slowly.
- Monitor serum electrolytes.

☐ **EVALUATION CRITERIA/DESIRED OUTCOMES**

The child

- Has intake and output adequate for age and weight
- Maintains moist mucous membranes, good skin turgor
- Has heart rate and blood pressure within normal limits for age
- Has urine specific gravity of 1.003-1.020
- Regains preillness weight

NURSING DIAGNOSIS #2

Ineffective breathing pattern related to abdominal pain

Rationale: Abdominal pain secondary to the incision and possible peritonitis inhibits full expansion of the thoracic cage and discourages effective coughing.

☐ **GOAL**

The child will have clear breath sounds, pink color with no cyanosis; will cough up secretions.

☐ **IMPLEMENTATION**

- Monitor vital signs every 4 hours, more frequently if unstable or if febrile.
- Medicate for pain 30 minutes prior to deep breathing, coughing, and ambulation.
- Encourage to deep breathe; assist to splint incision with pillow or hand; encourage deep breathing by blowing bubbles, blowing a Ping-Pong ball tied to a string, using an incentive spirometer; reward attempts at deep breathing and coughing with stickers or stars on a chart.
- Assist to ambulate; set short distance goals initially and gradually increase distance; incorporate an interesting destination into ambulation (e.g., playroom, sunporch, nurses' station).
- Auscultate breath sounds before and after pulmonary interventions.
- Explain to older child the rationale for deep breathing and coughing; allow to participate in planning for pulmonary exercises.

☐ **EVALUATION CRITERIA/DESIRED OUTCOMES**

The child

- Has clear breath sounds
- Is afebrile

NURSING DIAGNOSIS #3

Alteration in comfort: pain related to incision, presence of NG tube, peritonitis

Rationale: The pain from the abdominal incision, irritation of the NG tube, and peritonitis (if present) will interfere with pulmonary exercises, ambulation, and adequate rest/sleep.

☐ **GOAL**

The child will verbalize relief from pain; will cough and deep breathe adequately; will walk an increased distance each ambulation; will rest/sleep adequately.

☐ **IMPLEMENTATION**

- Assess pain every 2-4 hours and as necessary; observe posture, breathing patterns, movement; check heart rate and blood pressure (refer to *The Child Experiencing Pain*, page 216); ask parents' perception of child's comfort level.
- Medicate child initially with IV or IM narcotic analgesics as ordered; administer IV narcotics slowly (over 5 minutes) and observe for changes in respiratory pattern; when oral intake is established, begin oral analgesics, assess effectiveness; reassure parent/child that addiction to narcotics is not a concern.
- Administer antibiotics as ordered to resolve peritonitis; monitor for side effects.
- Assist child to assume a position of comfort; utilize nonmedicinal approaches to comfort (e.g., backrubs, distraction with toys and games, imagery, soothing music, relaxation breathing).
- Allow child to assist with dressing changes (e.g., removing old dressing, holding tape); encourage child to apply dressing to doll or stuffed animal.
- Assess NG intubation site and keep anterior nares clean; apply lubricant.
- Plan activities so that child has uninterrupted rest/sleep patterns.

☐ **EVALUATION CRITERIA/DESIRED OUTCOMES**

The child

- Ambulates free from complaints of pain
- Coughs and deep breathes adequately
- Rests and sleeps comfortably

NURSING DIAGNOSIS #4

Alteration in nutrition: less than body requirements related to NPO status, pre-op anorexia and vomiting

Rationale: The child whose pre-op nutritional status is good will have adequate nutritional stores for approximately 1 week postoperatively. Wound healing and strength will be compromised if nutritional stores are depleted.

☐ GOAL

The child will experience quick incision healing free from secondary infection; will increase strength and ambulate without fatigue; will regain preillness weight.

☐ IMPLEMENTATION

- Monitor daily weight.
- Check urine daily for presence of ketones.
- Assess strength (e.g., ability to ambulate, hand grasp, effectiveness of coughing) every 8 hours.
- Ascertain child's favorite foods and develop diet plan that includes foods containing protein and vitamin C as soon as oral intake is allowed; know typical eating pattern for age.
- Offer small, frequent meals; utilize novel ways of serving meals (e.g., colorful plates and napkins, having a party, encouraging family members to have meals with child).
- Request a nutrition consultation and anticipate initiation of total parenteral nutrition if NPO status continues for longer than 1 week.

☐ EVALUATION CRITERIA/DESIRED OUTCOMES

The child
- Shows adequate wound healing
- Is free from ketonuria
- Returns to/maintains preillness weight
- Ambulates with progressive energy

NURSING DIAGNOSIS #5

Fear related to abruptness of hospitalization, pain, separation from parents, unfamiliar environment

Rationale: The child's response to hospitalization and illness will depend upon developmental level and prior experiences with the health care system. Fear can create both psychologic and physiologic (stress response) barriers to healing, as well as interfering with the child's ability to develop efficient coping skills.

☐ GOAL

The child will identify feelings of fear; will employ effective coping skills; will participate in care and cooperate with necessary interventions.

☐ IMPLEMENTATION

- Recognize signs of fear (e.g., increased heart/respiratory rate, increased blood pressure, muscle tightness, pallor).
- Explain that experiencing fear is normal in the situation and offer support.
- Demonstrate what will happen to the child using a doll or stuffed animal; recognize that this approach is appropriate for the preschooler and older child, but will heighten the anxiety of the younger child.
- Encourage to communicate fears using stories, drawings, or any other medium with which the child is comfortable.
- Inform child that although pain is expected, you will help the child handle/minimize it.
- Assist parents to deal with their own fear of the situation so that their own anxiety does not heighten the child's.
- Incorporate home routines into hospital routines as often as possible.
- Assure the child that each day s/he will feel better than the previous day.

☐ EVALUATION CRITERIA/DESIRED OUTCOMES

The child
- Expresses feelings
- Participates in/cooperates with care

NURSING DIAGNOSIS #6

Knowledge deficit regarding care of child after discharge

Rationale: The child will be discharged as soon as wound healing is established, adequate solid intake is tolerated, and a course of antibiotics is completed. The child will require some time, however, to convalesce before returning to normal daily activity.

☐ GOAL

The child's incision will heal with minimal scarring, free from secondary infection; the child will return to normal daily activity and level of development.

☐ IMPLEMENTATION

- Teach parents home care of incision; provide with supplies or source of supplies; teach handwashing and disposal of contaminated dressing.

- Reinforce need for diet high in protein and vitamin C.
- Instruct regarding administration of prescribed antibiotics and pain medications.
- Teach signs of infection (e.g., fever, redness and warmth at incision, change in normal behavior).
- Reassure parents that a temporary loss of mastery of recently acquired developmental skills is a normal response to hospitalization.
- Provide parents with phone numbers of persons to contact if they have questions or concerns; instruct regarding return appointment.

☐ EVALUATION CRITERIA/DESIRED OUTCOMES

The child/parents
- State comfort with caring for incision, perform return demonstration showing correct techniques
- State correct dose/time for medication administration

The child
- Shows normal wound healing
- Returns to normal activities

The Child with Asthma/Bronchiolitis

Definition/Discussion

Asthma is an intermittent, reversible, obstructive disorder of the respiratory tract caused by bronchial smooth muscle constriction, mucosal edema, and excess mucus production. It is characterized by wheezing, dyspnea, and coughing. Bronchiolitis is a viral illness characterized by inflammatory obstruction of the small airways. Asthmatic episodes fall on a continuum of infrequent, mild episodes to severe, life-threatening crises. Asthma affects all age groups but onset is rare in the first year of life, whereas bronchiolitis is found in children under 2 years of age, most commonly between 2-12 months. Some researchers feel that bronchiolitis may trigger the development of asthma.

Nursing Assessment

☐ PERTINENT HISTORY

Precipitating events (e.g., upper respiratory infection, allergens, stress), duration of wheezing, medications used and time last taken, prior experiences with asthmatic episodes, family/child history of allergies

☐ PHYSICAL FINDINGS

Respiratory rate and effort, use of accessory muscles, shape of chest (may be barrel shaped), breath sounds (rales, rhonchi, wheezing), degree of restlessness/anxiety, heart rate, blood pressure, signs of respiratory failure (e.g., diaphoresis, fatigue, decreased responsiveness, cyanosis), arterial blood gases (ABGs), theophylline level (if home regimen includes theophylline), chest x-ray, white blood cell count (especially eosinophil)

☐ PSYCHOSOCIAL CONCERNS/ DEVELOPMENTAL FACTORS

Age, degree to which asthma has interfered with normal life-style of child/family, degree of incorporation of therapeutic regimen into life-style, child/family coping mechanisms, usual comfort measures, habits (e.g., bedtime routine, favored objects), previous experience with hospitalization, other family/friends with asthma, past experiences with asthma

☐ PATIENT AND FAMILY KNOWLEDGE

Precipitants of asthmatic episodes, understanding of prescribed medications (names, actions, dosage, route, frequency, side effects, signs of toxicity), non-medicinal interventions (e.g., exercise, avoidance of irritants/allergens), support services, level of knowledge, readiness and willingness to learn

Nursing Care

☐ LONG-TERM GOAL

The child will recover free from preventable complications; the child will attain optimal health and maintain a normal life-style through control of asthmatic episodes; the child in a severe asthmatic crisis will regain adequate respiratory function.

NURSING DIAGNOSIS #1
a. **Ineffective airway clearance** related to bronchospasm, mucosal edema, accumulation of mucus
b. **Impaired gas exchange** related to mucus obstruction of alveolar function

Rationale: Inflammation of the airways interferes with normal airflow and thus gas exchange. Mucus plugs can cause atelectasis and alveolar collapse. When bronchioles are partially obstructed, they trap air distal to the plug causing hyperinflation. Shunting of blood/hypoxemia will occur because the alveoli are poorly ventilated but well perfused. Pulse and blood pressure may increase to compensate. In asthma, irritants/allergens/stressors create a change in the airway environment, triggering an increase in cholinergic and decrease in beta-adrenergic activity. This autonomic nervous system response leads to bronchial constriction, mucosal wall edema, and increased mucus production, thus preventing normal flow of air into and out of the alveoli. Wheezing occurs as air flows through constricted airways. Accessory muscles constrict to assist respiratory effort.

□ GOAL

The child will inspire and exhale air without wheezing or using accessory muscles; will maintain/regain normal respiratory rate, color, cardiac function.

□ IMPLEMENTATION

Acute Attack

- Monitor respiratory rate, heart rate, blood pressure every 15-30 minutes.
- Auscultate breath sounds and observe color every 15-30 minutes; observe respiratory effort and document.
- Assist to assume whatever position is most comfortable (e.g., high-Fowler's, in a chair or infant seat, on side of bed, leaning on a pillow on an overbed table).
- Administer medications as ordered; monitor for response and side effects.
- Maintain patent IV line for administration of bronchodilators; refer to *The Child with an Intravenous Catheter*, page 174.
- Administer oxygen at ordered flow (if child has chronic CO_2 retention, do not exceed 2 liters/minute); utilize nasal prongs for oxygen administration (mask will contribute to a sense of suffocation) or use oxygen hood/mist tent for infant.
- Obtain ABGs and other bloodwork as ordered.
- Utilize cardiac monitor to observe for dysrhythmias.
- Maintain a calm atmosphere to decrease child's anxiety.
- Have emergency equipment available (e.g., appropriate sized ventilation bag, endotracheal tubes, laryngoscope, emergency medications).
- Know that infants are obligatory nose breathers, bulb suction nares as needed.

As acute attack resolves

- Monitor respiratory rate and effort, auscultate breath sounds every hour.
- Allow to assume position of comfort; child may be more comfortable sitting in parent's lap, an infant upright in infant seat.
- Administer oxygen as ordered and observe effectiveness.
- Document amount and appearance of expectorated sputum; keep ample supply of tissues and disposal bag at bedside.
- Administer nebulized bronchodilators as ordered (rarely used in bronchiolitis); assist child with all treatments (may be more cooperative taking nebulizer treatment while sitting on parent's or nurse's lap, playing with toys, or giving treatment to doll or stuffed animal); evaluate heart rate and blood pressure before and after administration.
- Begin instruction on breathing exercises; have the child practice abdominal or diaphragmatic breathing (instruct to push out abdominal muscles on inspiration, to pull in abdominal muscles on exhalation; exhale against pursed lips, 2-3 times longer than inhalation); use games to teach breathing (e.g., blowing a Ping-Pong ball across a table, blowing bubbles).
- Initiate chest physical therapy when severe obstruction resolves and cough becomes looser and moist.
- Assist with spirometric pulmonary function tests.

□ EVALUATION CRITERIA/DESIRED OUTCOMES

The child

- Maintains patent airway
- Has normal respiratory rate and effort, normal ABGs, no use of accessory muscles, pink color
- Has clear breath sounds with free movement of air

NURSING DIAGNOSIS #2

Anxiety related to feeling of suffocation, unfamiliar hospital environment

Rationale: The child with severe dyspnea experiences feeling of suffocation; once the dyspnea is relieved, the anxiety will diminish. The unfamiliar hospital setting and routines may also produce anxiety.

□ GOAL

The child will experience a decreased feeling of anxiety; will cooperate with interventions designed to alleviate dyspnea.

□ IMPLEMENTION

- Teach how to control anxiety/panic with first signs of asthmatic attack (e.g., to visually imagine staying calm and under control; to begin slow, deep breathing exercises).
- Avoid covering face with mask or placing in mist tent if this exacerbates distress.
- Loosen restrictive clothing.
- Avoid use of sedatives.
- Stay with child; speak in calm, soothing tone of voice; explain that the bronchi are temporarily in spasm but will soon begin to relax.
- Allow parents to remain with child; enable parents to assist by explaining all procedures.
- Encourage child/parents to express feeling about severe episode when it has been resolved; provide child with opportunity to work through experience using drawings, dolls, hospital equipment; refer to *The Child Requiring Play Therapy*, page 226.
- Orient to place, time, and physical status; provide with concrete ways of establishing time of day, when parents will be returning (e.g., use clock, calendar, "after Sesame Street is over").

- Facilitate development of trust by being truthful, acknowledging pain/discomfort of procedures, and providing assurance that someone will come whenever needed; reassure that nurse will be observing closely at night so that child is not afraid to sleep.

☐ EVALUATION CRITERIA/DESIRED OUTCOMES

The child
- Appears relaxed
- Has adequate rest/sleep pattern
- Expresses feelings/concerns
- Cooperates with procedures

NURSING DIAGNOSIS #3

Fluid volume deficit related to dyspnea, tachypnea, decreased oral intake

Rationale: Insensible water loss from tachypnea and diaphoresis will deplete total body water. Increased oral liquids will help to loosen and liquify secretions.

☐ GOAL

The child will ingest adequate fluid for age/weight; will have urine output adequate for weight with a specific gravity of 1.003-1.020; will have moist mucous membranes, good skin turgor; will maintain/regain preillness weight.

☐ IMPLEMENTATION

- Calculate maintenance fluid requirement for weight; plan additional fluid replacement to compensate for insensible and diaphoretic losses.
- Maintain IV at ordered rate; decrease as oral intake increases; protect IV from infiltration or dislodgment; explain purpose to an older child; restrain affected extremity of younger child.
- Dilute medications in adequate amount of fluids.
- Ascertain preferred fluids; offer frequently in order to meet daily fluid requirement; utilize novel approaches to drinking (e.g., playing tea party, Popsicles, frozen juices [unless they cause coughing], funny straws); avoid milk if it tends to thicken secretions.
- Monitor intake and output, mucous membranes, skin turgor daily; measure specific gravity of each voided specimen.
- Weigh daily at the same time, on the same scale, with the same clothing; record.
- Monitor serum electrolytes.

☐ EVALUATION CRITERIA/DESIRED OUTCOMES

The child
- Has adequate intake and output for age/weight
- Maintains moist mucous membranes, good skin turgor
- Maintains weight
- Has serum electrolytes within normal limits

NURSING DIAGNOSIS #4

Noncompliance related to lack of knowledge, negative side effects of prescribed treatment, lack of trust in health care providers

Rationale: A variety of factors may interfere with adequate control of asthmatic episodes. Many are related to poor appreciation of the need to adhere closely to the treatment plan, or other life-style factors that make compliance difficult.

☐ GOAL

The child/parents will identify factors that interfere with compliance, will develop feasible alternatives to the treatment plan, and improve control of asthmatic episodes.

☐ IMPLEMENTATION

- Explore child's/parents' knowledge and feelings about asthma, the treatment plan; assist to identify misconceptions.
- Assist to identify barriers that prevent adherence to the treatment regimen
- Explore impact that asthma and the treatment plan have on the family system; assist to develop ways of lessening impact.
- Assist to identify possible concerns about working with the health care system.
- Identify reasons for any missed appointments (e.g., transportation difficulties, child care, forgetfulness); assist to identify resources; mail appointment-reminder cards to alleviate the problem of forgotten appointments.
- Schedule an interpreter for appointments if the child/family is non-English speaking or hearing impaired.
- Introduce child/parents to others who are coping successfully with asthma.

☐ EVALUATION CRITERIA/DESIRED OUTCOMES

The child/parents
- Identify specific factors that interfere with compliance to the treatment plan
- Demonstrate improved adherence to treatment plan

The child
- Has fewer asthmatic episodes

NURSING DIAGNOSIS #5

Ineffective family/individual coping related to asthma, risk of life-threatening complications

Rationale: Chronic illness such as asthma disrupts the normal life-style of the entire family as well as the ill child. Financial expenditures related to treatment or time lost from work may upset the family's financial stability. Healthy family members may feel that too much attention is being paid to the ill family member.

☐ **GOAL**

Family members will verbalize the impact the chronic illness is having on their lives and the life of their child; will have emotional needs met; will identify community information and support resources and utilize them appropriately.

☐ **IMPLEMENTATION**

- Provide opportunities for recognition and acceptance of negative feelings family members may have about the ill child; listen to family discuss problems and support them in working out their own best solutions; refer for counseling as needed.
- Arrange for the family to meet others whose lives have been impacted by asthma.
- Explore with family opportunities for age-appropriate activities (e.g., summer camp for the child with asthma).
- Identify available community information and supportive resources.

☐ **EVALUATION CRITERIA/DESIRED OUTCOMES**

The family
- Shows improved communication among members
- Uses resources appropriately
- States they are receiving adequate family support
- Maintains normal life-style for child
- Functions well with necessary alterations

NURSING DIAGNOSIS #6

Knowledge deficit regarding asthma treatment regimen, exercise, avoidance of irritants/allergens

Rationale: Knowledge of factors that precipitate asthmatic episodes and the rationale for interventions will enable child/family to have greater control over asthmatic episodes, utilize health care assistance more appropriately, and maintain a more functional life-style.

☐ **GOAL**

The child/parents will identify names, dosages, expected effects, toxic effects, and frequency of use of prescribed medications; will describe available resources and indications for seeking health care assistance; will practice an appropriate exercise regimen including breathing exercises; will list irritants/allergens that precipitate asthmatic episodes, and prevention measures.

☐ **IMPLEMENTATION**

- Teach about use of prescribed medications (names, actions, side effects, dosage, schedules); identify signs of toxicity and encourage to contact health care providers if signs occur (side effects and toxic effects can often be eliminated by a change in dose or medication).
- Teach regarding PRN use of medications (e.g., using cromolyn sodium prior to exercise); caution regarding use of over-the-counter inhalers, decongestants, cough suppressants.
- Reinforce breathing exercises and benefits of doing regular physical exercise; caution to stop before fatigue; encourage lung-developing exercises and games (e.g., jogging, soccer, swimming); for children with musical ability, playing a wind instrument can develop lungs and be relaxing.
- Instruct how to minimize contact with irritants/allergens in home, school, work-place (e.g., use of nonallergenic pillows, plastic mattress covers, avoidance of smoking areas, use of face mask when pollutant level is high).
- Teach to avoid contact with others who have upper respiratory infections.
- Teach about immunotherapy if ordered.
- Provide with available information/support resources in the community.
- Instruct regarding use and cleaning of equipment used to administer medications; provide with 24-hour number to contact if equipment breaks.
- Allow sufficient time for questions and concerns.

☐ **EVALUATION CRITERIA/DESIRED OUTCOMES**

The child/parents
- Seek appropriate health care assistance
- Identify situations or agents that precipitate an asthmatic attack and conscientiously try to avoid these
- Recognize signs of an impending attack (e.g., cough, wheezing, fever, nausea and vomiting, increased anxiety or tension) and list steps to take to minimize distress (e.g., position, rest, medications, fluids, visualization)
- State the importance of both rest and exercise; plan activities around a sensible schedule
- List the individual medications and treatments required, possible side effects, purposes, amount, and indications for administration

- State measures to prevent exposure to infection; identify when to seek medical assistance

The child
- Has decreased number and severity of asthmatic episodes

NURSING DIAGNOSIS #7

Knowledge deficit regarding bronchiolitis treatment regimen

Rationale: The child will be discharged as respiratory status starts to return to normal and close observation/oxygen therapy is no longer required. The child will need to convalesce before returning to usual activities.

☐ **GOAL**

The child will return to normal activity; will avoid future respiratory infections.

☐ **IMPLEMENTATION**
- Assist parents to develop a plan for home care that includes rest/sleep periods, a well-balanced diet, appropriate activities.
- Reinforce need to protect child from contagious illnesses until respiratory status has returned to normal.
- Instruct parents regarding signs of recurrent illness (e.g., fever, shortness of breath, coughing, poor color, poor feeding, change in normal behavior).
- Reassure parents that a temporary loss of mastery of recently acquired developmental skills is a normal reaction to hospitalization.
- Provide parents with phone numbers and names of contact persons if they have questions, instruct concerning follow-up appointment.

☐ **EVALUATION CRITERIA/DESIRED OUTCOMES**

The child
- Returns to normal daily activities
- Is free from recurrence of respiratory illness

The Child Receiving Blood and Blood-Product Transfusions

Definition/Discussion

Homologous (another individual's) donated blood or *autologous* (self-donated and stored) blood or blood components are infused in order to enhance the achievement of hemodynamic equilibrium in the recipient. The varieties of blood-component products are detailed in Table 3.

Nursing Assessment

☐ PERTINENT HISTORY

Recent trauma, hemorrhage; impaired coagulation of blood, clotting disorders; chemotherapy, decreased platelet counts, thrombocytopenia; aplastic anemia, bone-marrow suppression, severe anemia; granulocytopenia, immunosuppression; hypoalbuminemia, agammaglobulinemia; severe burns, fluid shifts/imbalances

☐ PHYSICAL FINDINGS

Signs/symptoms related to pertinent history; lab studies: blood type, Rh factor, blood grouping in relationship to compatibility of available donor blood/components, hemoglobin, hematocrit, electrolytes

☐ PSYCHOSOCIAL CONCERNS/ DEVELOPMENTAL FACTORS

Emergency situation versus result of long-term therapy; age, developmental stage; moral, ethical, and religious principles affecting transfusion therapy (e.g., Jehovah's Witnesses); fears of contracting disease (e.g., AIDS, hepatitis)

☐ PATIENT AND FAMILY KNOWLEDGE

Potential benefits and risks of transfusion therapy; availability of family/support groups to donate blood or to initiate blood-donor drives when large quantities are required; level of knowledge, readiness and willingness to learn

Nursing Care

☐ LONG-TERM GOAL

The child will safely receive blood transfusion therapy free from the development of related major complications; the child will regain or maintain hemodynamic equilibrium.

NURSING DIAGNOSIS #1
a. **Anxiety** related to perceptions of receiving transfusion
b. **Knowledge deficit** regarding transfusion procedure

Rationale: Whether or not this is the first time the child has received blood/blood products, the child/family is likely to express some concerns about the procedure. With the current public awareness of the risk of contracting AIDS, it may be expected that the child/family will require explanations and reassurance to allay anxiety. Transfusions are legal matters requiring consent for treatment or documented refusal to receive blood or blood-component therapy. Sufficient information prior to administration is required for informed consent.

☐ GOAL

The child/family will have decreased anxiety regarding transfusion; will understand transfusion procedure.

☐ IMPLEMENTATION

• Reinforce physician explanations about proposed transfusion; allow time for child/parents to express concerns and ask questions.
• Offer brief explanation of precautionary measures employed by blood bank to ensure safety of blood products.

- Acknowledge concerns; reassure that others have expressed similar feelings.
- Explain usual protocol for administering blood products (e.g., taking vital signs [including temperature] before, during, and after administration; having 2 nurses validate that the correct product is being administered) so that child/parents will not become concerned when these measures are enacted.

☐ EVALUATION CRITERIA/DESIRED OUTCOMES

The child/parents
- Describe procedure for administering transfusion
- List precautions taken to prevent errors
- Express decreased level of anxiety regarding transfusion

NURSING DIAGNOSIS #2
a. **Potential for injury** related to administration of incompatible blood/blood component
b. **Impaired gas exchange** related to hemolytic/allergic reaction or pulmonary congestion following circulatory overload
c. **Alteration in fluid volume: excess** related to infusion of blood products

Rationale: Serious complications of transfusion include hemolytic reactions and circulatory overload. Allergic reactions are usually more benign (see Nursing Diagnosis #5) although bronchoconstriction and inflammation of the respiratory passages may occur.

Hemolytic reactions are usually caused by donor-recipient ABO and Rh incompatibilities (i.e., child receiving the wrong blood), faulty transfusion procedures, or improper storage of donor blood. When the hemolytic reaction occurs, there is an antibody-antigen response that causes blood cells to agglutinate, resulting in obstruction of blood flow to vital organs including the lungs.

Some children, especially infants and those with chronic cardiac, respiratory, or renal diseases, are susceptible to circulatory overload. Administration of blood/blood components increases the circulating blood volume. If the child is unable to compensate for this additional fluid, pulmonary congestion (pooling of blood in the alveoli) may develop, altering the ventilation/perfusion ratio and impairing gaseous exchange. These children may be candidates for receiving packed cells rather than whole blood or plasma, which, because of its hyperosmolarity, tends also to increase circulating blood volume.

☐ GOAL

The child will not experience complications of blood/blood product administration; will maintain ventilation/perfusion ratio with resultant oxygenation of all body tissues.

☐ IMPLEMENTATION

- Refer to hospital policy.
- Prevent transfusion reactions
  - identify child and verify blood (e.g., type, Rh factor, donor number, expiration date) with another nurse or physician
  - prime infusion line with normal saline (dextrose solutions tend to cause hemolysis)
  - administer prescribed antihistamine when child has known history of transfusion reactions
  - monitor prescribed flow rate of infusion; use an infusion pump to regulate flow; administer slowly during first 15 minutes of infusion for all children; continue slow rate for children at risk for fluid overload
- Identify possible transfusion reactions promptly
  - monitor vital signs before, during (every 15 minutes for 2 hours, then every 30 minutes) and after transfusion; compare readings to baseline; watch for increased, shallow, labored respirations; laryngeal stridor, wheezing; tachycardia, decreased blood pressure
  - remain with child during first 15-30 minutes of transfusion
  - note and report changes in skin color (e.g., pallor, duskiness) and mentation (e.g., restlessness, confusion, agitation) when taking vital signs; note facial flushing, bounding pulse, complaints of headache and flank/chest pain
  - auscultate lungs for presence of rales, rhonchi, or muffled/distant breath sounds prior to initiating transfusion and when changes in vital signs/skin color/mentation occur
  - inform child/parents of key symptoms of adverse reactions before leaving child and show how to notify nurse should these occur
- Initiate immediate measures to correct transfusion reactions
  - stop transfusion and infuse normal saline
  - remain with child while someone else contacts physician
  - position for comfort and to decrease respiratory distress (e.g., Fowler's position)
  - administer oxygen at ordered flow rate and monitor effectiveness
  - administer prescribed medications; monitor for expected and untoward effects; notify physician of child responses
  - prepare for possible endotracheal intubation/mechanical ventilation
  - continue to monitor vital signs; report significant changes
  - record intake and output; obtain first voided specimen for urinalysis

– obtain blood sample and forward specimen and remaining blood product with attached tubing to laboratory.

☐ EVALUATION CRITERIA/DESIRED OUTCOMES

The child
- Maintains vital signs within normal limits
- Displays normal skin color
- Remains alert and free from change in mental status compared with pretransfusion level of consciousness

---

NURSING DIAGNOSIS #3

Potential for infection related to contaminated blood

Rationale: Pyrogenic (i.e., febrile) reactions can occur if the blood is or becomes contaminated with bacteria during the processing or administration phases. As with any IV, the area around the catheter insertion site must be protected as the break in the skin provides an entry for pathogens. The blood bank refrigerators maintain a constant temperature to discourage growth of bacteria.

☐ GOAL

The child will remain free from infection as a complication of transfusion.

☐ IMPLEMENTATION

- Avoid obtaining blood/blood components from blood bank until ready to administer transfusion.
- Inspect catheter insertion site for signs of inflammation (e.g., swelling, redness, warmth, tenderness) or infection (e.g., pain, drainage) prior to initiating transfusion; refer to *The Child with an Intravenous Catheter*, page 174.
- Assess for signs and symptoms of pyrogenic reactions (e.g., fever, chills, nausea and vomiting, headache, severe hypotension, pain in abdomen/extremities) every 15-30 minutes; discontinue transfusion, maintain IV line with normal saline, and notify physician if these signs and symptoms occur.
- Administer prescribed medications; monitor for desired and untoward effects; report response to physician.
- Follow hospital protocol/guidelines described in Nursing Diagnosis #2 after the transfusion is discontinued.

☐ EVALUATION CRITERIA/DESIRED OUTCOMES

The child
- Remains afebrile
- Has stable vital signs

- Is free from signs of inflammation/infection

NURSING DIAGNOSIS #4

Alteration in cardiac output: decreased related to hyperkalemia

Rationale: Changes in the composition of the donated blood begin within 24 hours of collection. As the expiration date approaches, serum potassium levels increase as lysis of blood cells occurs. Potassium, the major intracellular ion, is released into the extracellular fluid and may reach levels of 30-40 mEq/liter (as compared with normal values of 3.5-5.5 mEq/liter).

For most children, excreting the increased potassium is not a problem. However, children with known renal dysfunction may be unable to excrete the excess potassium and are at risk for developing fatal cardiac dysrhythmias. Children requiring massive transfusions after severe trauma may also display elevated serum potassium levels.

Hyperkalemia causes flaccidity of the heart muscle, resulting in dilation of the heart. As the injured heart contracts, dysrhythmias (e.g., bradycardia initially, followed by ventricular tachycardia/fibrillation) result. Stroke volume and cardiac output are low as the decreased tonicity of the heart muscle precludes complete emptying of the chambers. Unless the hyperkalemia is corrected, cardiac arrest may occur.

☐ GOAL

The child will maintain circulation to all body tissues.

☐ IMPLEMENTATION

- Review pertinent history and physical findings for history of renal disease/elevated serum potassium level; question administering blood near expiration date to children identified as at increased risk for developing hyperkalemia.
- Assess every 4 hours for signs and symptoms of hyperkalemia (e.g., malaise, muscle weakness/flaccid paralysis, paresthesia, mental confusion/irritability, nausea, diarrhea, irregular pulse); report existing signs and symptoms.
- Use continuous cardiac monitoring; record a rhythm strip at least every 4 hours if heart rate/rhythm are irregular.
- Monitor central venous, pulmonary artery pressures and cardiac output every 2-4 hours as ordered; report significant changes; collaborate regarding adjusting IV flow rate in response to child's readings/urinary output.
- Hold oral/IV potassium preparations; check with physician before administering.
- Administer oral/rectal cation-exchange resins as

ordered to remove excess potassium; monitor serum potassium levels for indication of effectiveness.
- Prepare child for hemodialysis if chemical measures are unsuccessful in lowering serum potassium levels.

☐ EVALUATION CRITERIA/DESIRED OUTCOMES

The child
- Has regular pulse and cardiac monitor pattern
- Maintains normal serum potassium level
- Remains free from symptoms of hyperkalemia

NURSING DIAGNOSIS #5

Hypothermia related to infusion of cool blood

Rationale: Blood is stored at a constant cool temperature and should be used within 45 minutes of arrival from the blood bank. Young children with relatively small circulating blood volumes may readily become hypothermic if chilled blood or large amounts of cool blood are infused.

☐ GOAL

The child will maintain normal body temperature.

☐ IMPLEMENTATION

- Allow blood to warm to room temperature, but do not wait more than 45 minutes; warm blood with an electric warming coil if appropriate.
- Monitor for signs of hypothermia (e.g., chills, low temperature, irregular heart rate) every 15-30 minutes; if child shows signs of hypothermia, stop infusion and maintain patency of line with normal saline; notify physician.
- Initiate warming measures (e.g., additional blankets, heat lamp).
- Continue to take temperature every 30 minutes to 1 hour until normal.

☐ EVALUATION CRITERIA/DESIRED OUTCOMES

The child
- Maintains temperature at pretransfusion level

NURSING DIAGNOSIS #6

Alteration in comfort (pruritus) related to allergic reaction

Rationale: Urticaria (i.e., hives) is a common allergic reaction to blood tranfusion and is usually not an indication for discontinuation. The child may, however, be uncomfortable, complaining of skin irritation/itching.

☐ GOAL

The child will be free from discomfort associated with allergic transfusion reaction.

☐ IMPLEMENTATION

- Review pertinent history; if previous allergic reaction reported, collaborate with physician regarding administration of prophylactic antihistamine.
- Administer transfusion slowly (reactions are less likely to occur or be as severe when donated blood is diluted by child's own).
- Administer prescribed medications PRN; monitor for desired relief; contact physician for additional orders if symptoms are exacerbated or do not subside.
- Keep room temperature cool but avoid chilling child; keep skin dry.

☐ EVALUATION CRITERIA/DESIRED OUTCOMES

The child
- Has clear skin
- States relief from discomfort associated with allergic transfusion reaction

Table 3
Blood and Blood Components

Blood/Blood Component	Indications	Administration Information
Whole blood • Cellular and plasma constituents plus anticoagulant • Type and crossmatch ABO *identical*	Acute massive hemorrhage with hypovolemia	1 unit = 500 cc IV piggybacked with NS, infuse first 50 cc or 1/5 volume (whichever is smaller) slowly over 30 min to test for reaction; stay with child; if no reaction, increase rate to get amount in ordered time (e.g., infants/children cc/hr is based on weight; adolescents infuse not less than 1 hr and not more than 4 hr) *Expiration*: 35 days after collection *Storage*: 1°-6°C
Red blood cells • Packed red blood cells (PRBC) • Type and crossmatch ABO *identical*	Debilitated; congestive heart failure; chronic anemia; replace blood loss from surgery; treat chemotherapy-induced erythrocytopenia; generally (assuming a packed cell hematocrit of 70%-75%) % increase in hematocrit = cc/kg of packed cells transfused	1 unit = 250-300 cc IV piggybacked with NS *Expiration*: 35 days after collection *Storage*: 1°-6°C
Saline washed red cells • Red cells washed with saline to remove leukocytes, cellular debris, plasma • Type and crossmatch ABO *compatible*	IgA deficiencies; history of multiple severe urticarial/febrile reactions to blood; renal patients; hyperkalemia; bone-marrow transplant patients; paroxysmal nocturnal hemoglobinuria	1 unit = 270 cc IV piggybacked with NS *Expiration*: 24 hr after washing *Storage*: 1°-6°C
Irradiated red blood • RBCs exposed to 1,500 rad to eliminate viable lymphocytes • Type and crossmatch ABO *compatible*	Bone-marrow transplant patients; neonates; AIDS patients	Same as whole blood
Granulocytes • WBCs extracted from unit of whole blood • Type and crossmatch ABO *compatible*	Septic patients with low WBC not responding to antibiotics; oncology patients with severe bone-marrow depression and progressive infection	1 unit = 300 cc Use within 24 hr of collection IV piggybacked with NS; infuse slowly over 2-4 hr, observe closely for signs of reaction (e.g., chills, fever); if reaction occurs, infusion is usually slowed, not stopped
Platelets • Platelet component harvested from whole blood • No typing required • May be single or multiple donors	Patients actively bleeding with thrombocytopenia/coagulopathies; nonbleeding patients with platelet count less than 10,000-20,000; platelets may not be as effective if child is febrile, has infection, DIC or active bleeding, splenomegaly; becomes refractory to random donors	1 unit = 50 cc Usually administered in multiple units; administer antihistamine prior to transfusion if history of side effects IV piggybacked with NS *Expiration*: 3-5 days (2 hr after pooling) *Storage*: room temperature

Table 3
Blood and Blood Components

Blood/Blood Component	Indications	Administration Information
Fresh frozen plasma (FFP) • Plasma separated from whole blood and frozen • Contains all plasma-clotting factors • Type and crossmatch ABO compatible	Bleeding patients with coagulation deficiencies; unknown type of hemophilia	1 unit = 180-275 cc IV piggybacked with NS *Expiration*: 1 yr (frozen); 24 hr (thawed) *Storage*: 18°C (frozen); 1°-6°C (thawed)
Cryoprecipitated antihemolytic factor (AHF) (Factor VIII; fibrinogen) • Prepared by thawing FFP and collecting precipitated protein • No typing required (ABO compatibility preferred but not essential)	Treatment of hemophilia A (Factor VIII deficiency); von Willebrand's disease	1 unit = 10 cc *Expiration*: 1 yr (frozen); 2 hr (thawed) *Storage*: −18°C
Factor VIII AHF concentrate (Profilate, Factorate, Koate, Hemofil, Humafac)	Hemophilia A	1 unit = 10 cc *Storage*: 4°C for 2 yr as dry crystals; 3 hr room temperature after reconstitution
Factor IX (Koynex Concentrate, Problex) • Comes from pooled plasma, may be thousands of donors/unit	Hemophilia B; hemophilia A with inhibitor	1 unit = 20-30 cc *Storage*: 4°C for 2 yr; room temperature for variable periods
Human albumin • Made from pooled normal human blood, plasma, or serum • 5% and 25% solution	Expand plasma volume; treat hypoalbuminemia and severe protein loss	Given IV with or without dilution (NS) using a filter

The Child Experiencing a Body-Image Disturbance

Definition/Discussion

Body image is a person's image or concept of his/her own body. It is formed from internal development as well as from environmental experiences including input from others, societal views, cultural practices, and previous experience with persons whose bodies have changed.

Although the term "body image" is rarely used in conjunction with very young children, the child's sense of body is critical to early development. During the toddler phase of development, autonomy is the goal as the child strives for some body control. The child becomes aware of his/her body and its totality. The disappearance/removal of any body part threatens the child's existence (e.g., during toilet training, ritualistic activities may be necessary before the child will flush or allow the toilet to be flushed).

The preschool child begins to see self in relation to the rest of the world. However, thinking is not consistent with adult realities; magical thinking is the rule and the child views the world in relation to those things that are familiar (e.g., compares own body to a balloon—if there is a hole, all the air inside will leak out; a preschooler with a cut finger will not be consoled until a Band-Aid is placed on the cut to keep everything inside from leaking out). Children of this age also take things/words literally (e.g., on hearing "Jake will cut off his nose to spite his face," the child will picture Jake without his nose).

School-age children begin to look at the world in a more rational manner; at the same time, peers begin to play a significant role in the child's life. The child compares self to same-sex peer group (e.g., being the tallest boy or girl in the class may be very exciting or upsetting to the child). There is some evidence suggesting that children become weight conscious during the middle school-age years. Adolescents are very body conscious; the onset of puberty creates a great deal of confusion and body changes are magnified. The adolescent has a need to be the same as peers and deviations are not acceptable.

A body-image disturbance reflects the inability of an individual to perceive/adapt to an alteration in structure, function, or appearance of a part of or the entire body.

Nursing Assessment

☐ **PERTINENT HISTORY**

Surgeries, illness, trauma causing change in body form; rapidity of change; permanent or temporary refusal to participate in care; denial of change(s)

☐ **PHYSICAL FINDINGS**

Loss of body part or its function; neurologic, metabolic, or toxic disorders; anorexia/obesity; progressively deforming disorders; acute dismemberment; disability or handicap; visibility of change; withdrawal, apathy, crying, agitation

☐ **PSYCHOSOCIAL CONCERNS/ DEVELOPMENTAL FACTORS**

Cognitive/social/emotional/developmental level, academic achievement, peer relationships, previous experience with someone with altered physical appearance, cultural practices, coping patterns, personality style, dependency patterns, depression, shame, physical/sexual abuse, habits (e.g., what comforts child, eating/bedtime routines, favored objects)

☐ **PATIENT AND FAMILY KNOWLEDGE**

Possibility of rehabilitation or repair, degree of change in life-style and functional significance, value placed on alteration, perception of what change means, available community agencies, level of knowledge, readiness and willingness to learn

Nursing Care

☐ **LONG-TERM GOAL**

The child will acknowledge and integrate body change(s) into adaptive and realistic management of own life.

NURSING DIAGNOSIS #1

Disturbance in self-concept: body image related to altered body structure or function

Rationale: A real or perceived change in body image results in a need to modify one's self-concept. Certain areas of the body have greater value and meaning to an individual; threats to these areas cause more disruption and require more adjustment.

☐ **GOAL**

The child will acknowledge and begin to accept body change(s).

☐ **IMPLEMENTATION**

- Provide openings to enable child to express feelings by validating your observations and feelings (e.g., "You look down in the dumps. How are things going for you today?" or "You seem upset/sad. Are you?" Show child pictures and have him/her describe how the child in the picture is feeling and why); recognize that acting out behavior may be the child's way of expressing frustration; refer to *The Child Requiring Play Therapy*, page 226).
- Be a good listener and accept what child verbalizes; remember not to take anger or hostility personally (this may be the only way possible for the child to handle these feelings).
- Focus on the child's feelings and deal with the presenting behavior (e.g., do not challenge child's denial that a body change has actually occurred).
- Determine what the body-image change means to the child and what effect the child thinks it will have on life; do not challenge perceptions you think are unrealistic, but continue to provide opportunities for child to share these perceptions and feelings with you.
- Be accepting of child's body changes; if child is repulsed or ashamed of physical changes, s/he will be watching the faces of others for negative signs; assist the family to accept changes also and to avoid reinforcement of the child's negative feelings.
- Provide basic needs for child; dependent behaviors/regression in developmental achievements may be exhibited at this time.
- Assist child to normalize the change; use developmentally appropriate strategies (e.g., develop rituals, provide rational explanations, use make-up/adaptive devices to appear just like everyone else).
- Let the child know that the feelings and concerns that are being experienced are normal and that you are there to listen as well as to help cope with the changes.

☐ **EVALUATION CRITERIA/DESIRED OUTCOMES**

The child

- States that a change in the body has occurred
- Begins verbalization of feelings regarding the change

- Exhibits fewer negative reactions to staff and environment
- Shows occasional interest in self-care

NURSING DIAGNOSIS #2

Grieving related to loss or alteration in body form, function

Rationale: Resolution of a loss through successful management of the grief process will allow the child to progress effectively toward adjustment to changes in body structure and function.

☐ **GOAL**

The child will acknowledge, express, and resolve grief related to change(s) in body form or function.

☐ **IMPLEMENTATION**

- Recognize individual responses to grief; these are determined by ego strengths, perception and meaning of loss, previous experiences, and present support systems; refer to *The Parent Experiencing Grief and Loss*, page 139, for review of the grief process.
- Know that the nurse's personal feelings toward loss must be recognized before the nurse can accept those of others.
- Be empathic and understanding; educate child/family regarding normal grief reactions to permit more realistic expectations.
- Encourage verbalization of feelings toward the loss of the body part or function (e.g., the pleasures provided and the needs it fulfilled in the past) in order to promote acceptance and to lessen denial.
- Allow child to cry.
- Be alert for signs of depression (e.g., isolation or withdrawal, inability to grieve, fatigue, anorexia).
- Do not encourage fantasizing or false hopes regarding reversal of change in body form or function.
- Know that resolution of loss is accomplished a little at a time; be realistic about time required to achieve resolution.

☐ **EVALUATION CRITERIA/DESIRED OUTCOMES**

The child

- Verbalizes/demonstrates, through play, sadness and feelings of loss
- States what the body change means
- Shows evidence of adapting to body change

NURSING DIAGNOSIS #3

Knowledge deficit regarding adaptation to alteration in body image

Rationale: When body changes occur, new coping mechanisms and changes in life-style may be required for successful adjustment.

☐ **GOAL**

The child/family will accept the alteration in body and successfully adapt to required changes in life-style.

☐ **IMPLEMENTATION**

- Give positive reinforcement for efforts to adapt; child/family behavior will indicate when acceptance of body alterations has begun (e.g., may ask questions; will start to look at the incision, dressings, etc.).
- Accept, but do not support, expressions of denial.
- Assist child in choice of prosthesis (if one is to be used) by providing information and arranging for a visit by a member of an ostomy club, or other appropriate group; let child/family determine time of visit as appropriate, but try to arrange it as soon as possible.
- Involve child/family in child-care activities; begin slowly and add new activities one at a time; reinforce any efforts to participate.
- Assist adjustment to awareness of the extent of the loss since there is frequently a lag between initial alteration and realistic perception.
- Tell family how they can help by listening, supporting reality, allowing expressions of anger, denial, and not challenging them, permitting child to cry and giving positive reinforcement for all efforts to cope/adapt; praise the family for participation in efforts to assist.
- Hold a team conference, including family if you wish, and share information on grief and loss (see page 139) and crisis intervention (see page 85) with each other; discuss what parts of these concepts apply at this time; revise the care plan as necessary.
- Refer for continued contact with community support group, home health nurse, and appropriate community agencies.

☐ **EVALUATION CRITERIA/DESIRED OUTCOMES**

The child

- Accepts continued support and positive input from family
- Utilizes community resources such as ostomy club, therapy, to provide ongoing support, reassurance, and assistance in recovery
- Resumes predisturbance activities

The family

- Supports the child and provides positive input

The Child with Burns: Acute Phase

Definition/Discussion

Burns are injuries to tissues caused by thermal (e.g., flame, liquid)/chemical/electrical/radioactive agents. The outcome of burn injury is the denaturation of protein, resulting in cell injury or death.

Nursing Assessment

☐ **PERTINENT HISTORY**

Mechanism of burn injury, past medical history, allergies, medications

☐ **PHYSICAL FINDINGS**

Vital signs, level of consciousness (LOC); depth of burn (i.e., layers involved); area and extent of burn (i.e., percentage of total body surface area involved); presence of factors indicative of smoke inhalation (e.g., stridor, nasal flaring, carbonaceous sputum, blackened tongue, dry cracked lips, singed nasal hairs, erythema of pharynx, cherry-red lips); urinary output; circumferential burns; arterial blood gases; serum electrolytes; fluid status; bowel sounds

☐ **PSYCHOSOCIAL CONCERNS/ DEVELOPMENTAL FACTORS**

Age, developmental level, regression, family interaction pattern, ethnicity, cultural background, financial status, usual coping mechanisms, sleeplessness, pain, perception of body image change, habits (e.g., what comforts child, eating/bedtime routine, favored objects)

☐ **PATIENT AND FAMILY KNOWLEDGE**

Perception of health status, disease condition, hospital routines; level of knowledge, readiness and willingness to learn

Nursing Care

☐ **LONG-TERM GOAL**

The child will recover from the burn without loss of function of any body part; the child will recover maximum potential use of the involved body part(s).

NURSING DIAGNOSIS #1

a. **Impaired gas exchange** related to heat exposure, inhalation injury, edema of laryngeal structures
b. **Ineffective breathing pattern** related to heat exposure, inhalation injury, edema of laryngeal structures
c. **Ineffective airway clearance** related to retained secretions, imposed position

Rationale: Byproducts of combustion cause pneumonitis, resulting in destruction of respiratory cell protein and loss of cilia. Heat exposure results in an increased capillary leak in the respiratory structures causing edema of the respiratory passages. Inability to expectorate retained secretions as a result of a decreased cough reflex may lead to an altered respiratory status.

☐ **GOAL**

The child will maintain a patent airway and adequate oxygenation.

☐ **IMPLEMENTATION**

- Maintain patent airway with high-flow oxygen (100%) unless contraindicated.
- Monitor respiratory rate and characteristics of respiration every hour and as necessary.
- Monitor for LOC changes every hour to determine cerebral oxygenation.
- Observe for communication difficulties that may indicate increasing edema of laryngeal structures.
- Monitor for dyspnea, stridor, or hoarseness.
- Auscultate breath sounds every hour to detect abnormal sounds, decreased aeration.
- Suction gently as needed using aseptic technique to maintain patent airway.
- Assist with bronchoscopy to determine extent of respiratory injury.
- Monitor arterial blood gas values for acid-base abnormalities and decreased oxygen saturation.
- Monitor carboxyhemoglobin level to determine carbon monoxide poisoning.

- Monitor eschar formation on chest or neck that could compromise respiratory status.
- Administer drugs to support immune response (e.g., GamImmune).
- Administer breathing treatments to prevent alveolar collapse in older children.
- Provide chest physical therapy to maintain patent airway.
- Turn, cough, and deep breathe every 2 hours to mobilize secretions; short periods of crying also encourage aeration.
- Be ready for intubation with an endotracheal tube or tracheostomy; refer to *The Child with a Tracheostomy*, page 280; have emergency tray nearby.

☐ EVALUATION CRITERIA/DESIRED OUTCOMES

The child
- Is free from laryngeal edema, stridor, or hoarseness
- Maintains arterial blood gases within normal limits
- Has no adventitious breath sounds
- Exhibits lucid LOC

NURSING DIAGNOSIS #2
a. **Alteration in cardiac output: decreased** related to evaporative fluid loss, hemorrhage, inadequate fluid resuscitation
b. **Fluid volume deficit** related to inadequate fluid resuscitation, evaporative fluid loss, hemorrhage
c. **Alteration in tissue perfusion: cardiopulmonary, renal** related to fluid loss, edema, thrombosis, stasis, hypovolemia
d. **Alteration in tissue perfusion: peripheral** related to burn ischar formation

Rationale: Capillary destruction in burn injury initiates an initial plasma to interstitial fluid shift causing hypovolemia, which may also result from inadequate fluid replacement. In the absence of adequate fluid replacement, hemolysis of red blood cells and release of myoglobin from damaged muscles leads to decreased renal perfusion. Following the initial plasma to interstitial fluid shift, fluid then begins to leak back into the plasma from the interstitium, causing hypervolemia if fluid resuscitation is not carefully monitored. Circumferential edema or constriction of burn eschar compromises circulation.

☐ GOAL

The child will maintain adequate blood volume, fluid and electrolyte balance; will excrete adequate urinary output; will maintain optimum peripheral circulation.

☐ IMPLEMENTATION

- Record weight of child as soon as possible after admission; weigh daily in same clothes on the same scale, at the same time.
- Monitor vital signs at least every hour and as needed; observe for trends.
- Record accurate fluid intake (e.g., oral, IV) and output (e.g., urine, nasogastric [NG] suction) every hour.
- Observe urine for hematuria or brownish red color indicative of intravascular hemolysis related to thrombosis/hemomyoglobinuria.
- Start IV with large-bore needle.
- Insert Foley catheter utilizing aseptic technique.
- Titrate fluid replacement based on urine output, central venous pressure (CVP), LOC, or other parameters used in your institution.
- Administer crystalloid and/or colloid fluid per hospital protocol; monitor effect.
- Observe hemodynamic parameters for changes in stability caused by fluid overload or hypovolemia.
- Assess for signs/symptoms of inadequate fluid replacement/impending shock (e.g., restlessness, disorientation, excessive thirst, increased pulse, decreased blood pressure, decreased urine output, CVP less than 5 cm water).
- Assess for signs/symptoms of excessive fluid replacement/pulmonary congestion/pulmonary edema (e.g., dyspnea, venous engorgement, moist rales, increased blood pressure, CVP greater than 15 cm water).
- Assess ECG for dysrhythmias that may result from electrical burn injury or hemodynamic instability.
- Monitor laboratory results and report those that directly reflect a fluid and electrolyte imbalance (e.g., hemoglobin, hematocrit, glucose, serum proteins, serum potassium, serum sodium, BUN, creatinine, urinalysis).
- Administer potassium-restricted foods/fluids if child is hyperkalemic.
- Measure circumference of burned areas to determine if edema is increasing; prepare for escharotomy/fasciotomy as necessary.
- Elevate all burned areas if possible to allow for venous return.
- Monitor distal peripheral pulses utilizing a Doppler if necessary; notify physician immediately and prepare for fasciotomy if pulses are unobtainable.

☐ EVALUATION CRITERIA/DESIRED OUTCOMES

The child
- Has body weight change of plus or minus less than 0.25-1 kg/24 hours as appropriate for age
- Maintains CVP between 5 and 15 cm water
- Is hemodynamically stable
- Maintains electrolytes within normal levels
- Excretes at least 0.5-2.0 cc/kg/hour of urine
- Maintains palpable pulse in all extremities

NURSING DIAGNOSIS #3

Alteration in comfort: pain related to tissue edema and destruction, eschar debridement, other treatments

Rationale: Pain receptors left intact will respond to pressure caused by edema or manipulation during treatments resulting in pain. Patients rarely experience total burn anesthesia since deep partial thickness or superficial partial thickness burns are usually peripheral to full thickness injuries.

☐ **GOAL**

The child will maintain an adequate level of comfort.

☐ **IMPLEMENTATION**

- Determine level of discomfort considering depth and extent of injury, areas of involvement, age, other pathology present, and previous treatment.
- Assess the level of discomfort using a 0-10 point self-rating scale or color scale as age appropriate to obtain an objective measure of the pain; refer to *The Child Experiencing Pain*, page 216.
- Maintain an accurate record of amount, time, and type of medication utilized (too much medication too soon can cause respiratory difficulties); chart effect.
- Administer sedation/pain medication IV to increase adequate absorption; give 30 minutes to 1 hour prior to treatments, debridement procedure, and application of topical agents to ensure child comfort and adequate relaxation.
- Administer pain medication cautiously, judiciously, and conservatively, ensuring that child is given adequate relief but is not overmedicated.
- Provide diversional activity to distract child from the pain experience (e.g., sing songs, play music, cartoons, imagery).
- Maintain environmental temperature at approximately 76°-84°F to ensure warmth and comfort of child who is without the protective layer of skin that maintains body heat.

☐ **EVALUATION CRITERIA/DESIRED OUTCOMES**

The child

- Verbalizes decreased pain
- Exhibits behaviors that demonstrate a decrease in pain

NURSING DIAGNOSIS #4

a. **Impairment of skin/tissue integrity** related to loss of protective layer, poor wound healing, decreased nutritional replacement, decreased tissue perfusion
b. **Potential for infection** related to open wounds, poor wound healing

Rationale: Decreased tissue perfusion causes aggregation of cellular debris in the microcirculation, thus preventing adequate blood supply for healing. Decreased nutritional intake, especially of proteins, increases the risk of poor wound healing because insufficient nutrients are provided for tissue repair. Loss of the first line of defense against infection and formation of eschar provides an excellent culture medium for growth of infectious bacteria. In addition, the child with a burn has a compromised immune response. Multiple exogenous factors contribute to the risk of infection (e.g., Foley catheter, IV, CVP) as well as nonadherence to aseptic practices by staff and visitors.

☐ **GOAL**

The child will be free from wound infection.

☐ **IMPLEMENTATION**

- Monitor temperature every hour and as necessary (may have heat loss from impairment in skin integrity or may increase with infection); maintain draft-free room with increased temperature and humidity levels; use heat lamps as needed to maintain temperature.
- Determine the type of isolation techniques to be used; wear gowns, gloves, and masks to help keep the bacterial count to a minimum.
- Maintain an aseptic environment using sterile equipment and supplies.
- Observe for signs and symptoms of infection (e.g., malodorous wound drainage, elevated leukocyte count, elevated temperature).
- Use strict sterile technique when changing dressings.
- Administer antibiotics and observe response.
- Prepare for hydrotherapy treatments and eschar debridement (e.g., tangential excision, enzymatic debridement).
- Apply topical antimicrobials and bacteriostatic agents.
- Prepare for grafting procedures, maintaining asepsis of donor and recipient sites.
- Obtain cultures from wounds, preventing contamination from skin flora.
- Prevent skin surfaces from touching to prevent autocontamination.
- Shave or clip body hair that may harbor bacteria.
- Provide special site care for face, eyes, ears, or perineum.
- Observe for signs and symptoms of septicemia (e.g., positive blood cultures, hemodynamic changes).
- Discourage visits from family or friends with infections.
- Administer tetanus immunization prophylactically.

EVALUATION CRITERIA/DESIRED OUTCOMES

The child

- Has negative wound and blood cultures
- Exhibits evidence of autograft acceptance
- Maintains temperature within normal limits
- Is free from drainage or odor from wound

NURSING DIAGNOSIS #5

a. **Alteration in nutrition: less than body requirements** related to increased caloric requirement, decreased caloric intake, inadequate intake of nutrients, adynamic ileus

b. **Alteration in bowel elimination: constipation/diarrhea** related to adynamic ileus, inadequate intake of nutrients, nasogastric (NG) tube feedings

Rationale: Patients with burns become hypermetabolic, requiring increased caloric intake to maintain nutritional state. Gastric hemorrhage caused by Curling's ulcer and adynamic ileus are results of the gastric dilation that occurs during the stress response to the burn injury.

GOAL

The child will maintain adequate nutrition; will have a routine bowel pattern.

IMPLEMENTATION

- Insert NG tube; attach to low intermittent suction; refer to *The Child Requiring Nasogastric Intubation*, page 194.
- Monitor pH of gastric aspirate for a decrease indicating hyperacidity.
- Administer antacids through the NG tube, clamping tube following administration.
- Weigh child daily or more often as necessary.
- Maintain accurate intake and output records.
- Auscultate bowel sounds every 4 hours.
- Administer hyperalimentation; refer to *The Child Receiving Total Parenteral Nutrition*, page 276.
- Administer tube feedings as ordered after bowel sounds return; refer to *The Child Requiring Tube Feedings*, page 288.
- Assess ongoing nutritional status.
- Monitor bowel evacuation for constipation or diarrhea.

EVALUATION CRITERIA/DESIRED OUTCOMES

The child

- Has intake of 75% of ordered diet
- Maintains weight at least at preburn level
- Is free from paralytic ileus

- Has gastric aspirate negative for occult blood

NURSING DIAGNOSIS #6

a. **Ineffective individual coping** related to perception of body-image changes

b. **Alteration in family process** related to inability to cope with severity of injury, possible death of self or family member, helplessness

c. **Fear** related to physiologic and emotional disruption, perceptions of painful procedures

d. **Grieving** related to actual/perceived loss of body part

Rationale: The burned child and the family are unprepared and may be unable to manage both the internal and external stressors because of compromised resources.

GOAL

The child will verbalize/play out feelings about changes in own body; will cope with the extent and number of losses; the child/family will adapt to hospitalization, changed life-style.

IMPLEMENTATION

- Give as much information as child/family want to help decrease fear and anxiety.
- Encourage to talk about/play out current situation and feelings; provide empathic listening; bandage doll as child has dressings, have doll experience same procedure as child (refer to *The Child Requiring Play Therapy*, page 226).
- Encourage participation and cooperation in care; give child acceptable methods for venting feelings (e.g., "You need to hold still but it's OK to yell") and choices/control over situation as appropriate.
- Assess importance and impact of appearance changes; discuss with child/family.
- Provide careful explanation of procedures to dispel fears.
- Organize care to prevent undue pain and anxiety.
- Inform child/family of any signs of progress.
- Project calm, unhurried attitude while performing procedures.
- Demonstrate respect for child/family.
- Allow for privacy when visitors are with child.
- Provide for financial and spiritual counseling as desired.
- Refer to *The Parent Experiencing Grief and Loss*, page 139, for discussion of the grief process and *The Child Experiencing a Body-Image Disturbance*, page 30.

☐ EVALUATION CRITERIA/DESIRED OUTCOMES

The child/family
- States realistic perception of burn injury
- Expresses fears, grief, anxieties, feelings about self verbally or through play
- Utilizes family for support
- Uses situational support for adaptation

NURSING DIAGNOSIS #7

Knowledge deficit regarding acute phase of burn injury

Rationale: Immediately following an acute burn injury, measures to maintain life will be the priority. Most interventions utilized during this phase will be new to the child. Inadequate preparation may lead to child/family misconceptions of current and future health status.

☐ GOAL

The child/family will demonstrate adequate knowledge of all procedures and their rationale.

☐ IMPLEMENTATION

- Explain all procedures in an age-appropriate manner prior to beginning new and ongoing procedures.
- Encourage verbalization/playing out of questions by child/family; correct misconceptions.
- Discuss child's future with regard to the rehabilitation phase of burn injury.

☐ EVALUATION CRITERIA/DESIRED OUTCOMES

The child/family
- Correctly describes procedures in own words
- Cooperates with health team in all phases of care

The Child with Burns: Convalescent Phase

Definition/Discussion

The convalescent phase following burn injury involves physiologic, emotional, and functional rehabilitation.

Nursing Assessment

☐ **PERTINENT HISTORY**

Medical and surgical history, mechanism of burn injury, medications taken, allergies, loss of function or actual body part, dietary habits

☐ **PHYSICAL FINDINGS**

Vital signs; level of consciousness; depth and extent of burn; fluid status; presence of infection; constipation, diarrhea, bowel sounds; weight; range of motion, level of pain, activity tolerance; sleep patterns

☐ **PSYCHOSOCIAL CONCERNS/ DEVELOPMENTAL FACTORS**

Age, developmental level, regression, child/family interaction, ethnicity, cultural background, financial needs, usual coping mechanisms, acceptance/adaptation to altered body-image status, anxiety, fear, grieving, feelings of powerlessness/loss of control over environment, isolation caused by susceptibility to infection, compliance with health care treatments, peer support/contact

☐ **PATIENT AND FAMILY KNOWLEDGE**

Perception of health status, disease condition, hospital routines; education level; level of knowledge, readiness and willingness to learn

Nursing Care

☐ **LONG-TERM GOAL**

The child will achieve maximum function of any involved body part(s); the child will achieve rehabilitation within the limits of resultant disability; the child will return to former activities in school, sports, activities, hobbies to the extent possible; the child/family will recover emotionally from the burn injury.

NURSING DIAGNOSIS #1

a. **Impairment of skin/tissue integrity** related to increased susceptibility to infection, decreased nutritional replacement, decreased tissue perfusion
b. **Potential for infection** related to open wounds, poor wound or skin graft healing
c. **Hypothermia** related to impaired skin integrity, environmental temperature

Rationale: Decreased tissue perfusion causes aggregation of cellular debris in the microcirculation, thus preventing adequate blood supply for healing, which is necessary for adequate skin grafting. Decreased nutritional intake, especially of proteins, increases the risk of poor wound healing because insufficient nutrients are provided for tissue repair. Loss of skin, the first line of defense against infection, provides an excellent culture medium for growth of infectious bacteria on the original burn wound or skin donor and recipient sites. Loss of skin and wet dressings also predispose to evaporative heat loss. In addition, the child with a burn has a compromised immune response. Multiple exogenous factors contribute to the risk of infection (e.g., Foley catheter, IV, central venous pressure line) as well as nonadherence to aseptic practices by staff and visitors.

☐ **GOAL**

The child will be free from wound infection; will have adequate wound healing for skin grafting; will maintain temperature within normal limits.

☐ **IMPLEMENTATION**

• Maintain temperature of the environment at approximately 76°-84°F (22.2°-28.9°C) to ensure warmth and comfort of child who is without the protective layer of skin to maintain body heat.
• Discuss the importance of hydrotherapy in treatment regimen; encourage child to participate actively as tolerated; balance child's need for control

and tolerance of procedure with the need for debridement.

- Assess the necessity to continue isolation techniques; monitor laboratory data; obtain wound cultures.
- Maintain an aseptic environment using sterile equipment and supplies.
- Prevent child from picking at wound: provide distraction, explain reasons, use rewards, restrain if necessary.
- Observe for signs/symptoms of infection (e.g., malodorous wound drainage, elevated leukocyte count, elevated temperature).
- Use strict sterile technique when changing a dressing.
- Administer antibiotics, medications to support immune response; observe response.
- Apply topical antimicrobials and bacteriostatic agents; evaluate and document effectiveness.
- Prepare for tangential excision, enzymatic debridement by explaining procedures in age-appropriate manner; provide pre-op care as necessary.
- Prepare for grafting procedures by maintaining asepsis of donor and recipient sites; observe viability of donor and recipient sites during dressing changes; discuss concerns and questions regarding the procedure.
- Know about various skin grafts that may be used including
  - *homograft* (allograft): skin taken from another living person or from a cadaver; this type of graft is usually temporary but with the advent of newer immunosuppressant drugs such as cyclosporin A, the graft may be more permanent
  - *heterograft* (xenograft): a temporary graft taken from an animal, usually porcine, or made of synthetic material
  - *autograft:* the child's own unburned skin
- Provide post-op skin graft care
  - elevate grafted extremity or part
  - monitor pulses and capillary refill
  - avoid excessive pressure on area from tight dressings
  - do not use tape on skin
  - observe for excessive bleeding or drainage at sites
  - monitor lifting of graft resulting from edema, which decreases viability of graft
  - observe for decreased viability of recipient site evidenced by darkening of graft edges (i.e., violaceous borders) or purulent drainage
- Observe for signs and symptoms of septicemia (e.g., positive blood cultures, hemodynamic changes).
- Discourage visits from family or friends with infections.

☐ **EVALUATION CRITERIA/DESIRED OUTCOMES**

The child
- Has negative wound and blood cultures
- Exhibits evidence of autograft acceptance
- Maintains temperature within normal limits
- Is free from drainage or odor from wound
- Exhibits no edema or decreased viability of recipient skin graft site

---

NURSING DIAGNOSIS #2
a. **Alteration in nutrition: less than body requirements related** to increased caloric requirement, decreased caloric intake, inadequate intake of nutrients
b. **Alteration in bowel elimination** related to adynamic ileus, nasogastric (NG) tube feedings, inadequate intake of nutrients
c. **Alteration in oral mucous membranes** related to inadequate oral intake or oral hygiene

Rationale: Children with burns become hypermetabolic, requiring increased caloric intake to maintain nutritional state. Even a cooperative child has trouble consuming adequate calories needed for wound healing. Gastric hemorrhage caused by Curling's ulcer and paralytic ileus results from gastric dilatation that occurs during the stress response to the burn injury. Hypertonic tube feedings may cause diarrhea, while inadequate fluid intake may cause constipation and disruption in the oral mucous membranes.

☐ **GOAL**

The child will maintain adequate nutrition; will have a routine bowel pattern; will be free from oral lesions.

☐ **IMPLEMENTATION**

- Maintain NG tube; attach to low intermittent suction until bowel sounds return; refer to *The Child Requiring Nasogastric Intubation*, page 194.
- Monitor pH of gastric aspirate for a decrease indicating hyperacidity.
- Administer antacids per NG tube, clamping tube following administration.
- Weigh child in the same state of undress on the same scale at the same time every day.
- Maintain accurate intake and output records.
- Auscultate bowel sounds every 4 hours.
- Monitor bowel evacuation for constipation or diarrhea.
- Assess ongoing nutritional status; observe oral mucous membranes, assess skin turgor daily.
- Provide oral hygiene every 4 hours.

- Administer total parenteral nutrition as ordered; refer to *The Child Receiving Total Parenteral Nutrition*, page 276.
- Administer high-calorie, high-protein tube feedings or oral diet when tolerated; establish small, frequent feeding interspersed with high-calorie, high-protein snacks; work with child/family regarding food likes and dislikes; consider age-appropriate choices (refer to *Normal Growth and Development*, pages 300–314); refer to dietician as necessary; refer to *The Child Requiring Tube Feedings*, page 288.
- Do not schedule painful procedures immediately prior to meals.
- Provide an environment conducive to eating (e.g., remove soiled dressings, bedpans, and other distractors; eliminate offensive odors; have family/staff eat meals with child, bring in food child likes, have a tea party).
- Know that child may try to exert control over the environment by refusing to eat; do not reinforce behavior by focusing on it; use consistent, firm approach concerning expectations for intake.
- Provide adequate rest to ensure that child is not too tired to eat.

☐ EVALUATION CRITERIA/DESIRED OUTCOMES

The child
- Ingests at least of 75% of diet as ordered
- Maintains weight at least at preburn level and begins to demonstrate consistent weight gain along growth curve
- Is free from adynamic ileus
- Has gastric aspirate negative for occult blood/increasing pH
- Exhibits pink, moist oral mucosa without lesions

NURSING DIAGNOSIS #3

a. **Alteration in comfort: pain** related to treatment protocols and other activities
b. **Sleep pattern disturbance** related to pain, activity

Rationale: Receptors left intact will respond to pressure caused by edema or manipulation during surgery or other treatments resulting in pain. Children rarely experience total burn anesthesia since deep partial thickness or superficial partial thickness burns are usually peripheral to full thickness injuries.

☐ GOAL

The child will maintain an adequate level of comfort; will get sufficient rest and sleep.

☐ IMPLEMENTATION

- Assess the level of discomfort using a 0-10 point self-rating scale or color scale as age appropriate to obtain an objective measure of the pain; consider depth and extent of injury, areas of involvement, age, other pathology present, and previous treatment; refer to *The Child Experiencing Pain*, page 216.
- Maintain an accurate record of amount, time, and type of medication utilized (too much medication too soon can cause respiratory difficulties); evaluate and chart effect.
- Administer sedation/pain medication IV to increase adequate absorption; IM injections may be given when adequate healing has occurred; oral medications may be administered when bowel sounds have returned and there is no evidence of stress ulcers.
- Assist parents in finding ways to comfort child (e.g., help hold in nonpainful position, touching unburned areas, talking in soothing low voice, singing).
- Provide diversional activity to distract child from the pain experience (e.g., music, headphones, TV, self-hypnosis, tapes, imagery).
- Provide an environment conducive to rest and sleep; group nursing care and reduce environmental noise, lights; maintain schedule to provide adequate periods of rest; administer sedatives as necessary; evaluate and chart effectiveness.

☐ EVALUATION CRITERIA/DESIRED OUTCOMES

The child
- Verbalizes/indicates decreased pain
- Increases participation in self-care
- Requires decreased amount of pain medication
- Has at least 4 hours of uninterrupted sleep during night

NURSING DIAGNOSIS #4

a. **Potential for injury** related to contractures and immobility
b. **Self-care deficit** related to immobility, reduced range of motion (ROM)
c. **Diversional activity deficit** related to impaired mobility, decreased self-care ability
d. **Activity intolerance** related to impaired ROM
e. **Alteration in bowel elimination: constipation** related to immobility and pain
f. **Alteration in urinary elimination** related to immobility, decreased fluid intake, renal calculi
g. **Sensory-perceptual alteration** (sensory deprivation) related to immobility, hospitalization

---

Rationale: The burned child is at increased risk for contracture formation as a result of immobilization of a body part. Immobilization of a burn wound encourages formation of hypertrophic scarring, a powerful tightening of skin and underlying structures. The child is at risk for the development of other complications resulting from immobility, including decubitus ulcer formation, constipation, bone demineralization, renal calculi, and sensory alterations. Decreased sensory stimulation, sensory monotony, and sensory deprivation may alter the child's perception of the environment.

☐ GOAL

The child will be free from complications associated with immobility; will participate in age-appropriate diversional activity.

☐ IMPLEMENTATION

- Provide for proper positioning and immobilization of burn wound/graft site (e.g., using splints, traction); consult with physical/occupational therapist to plan adaptive devices for child use; encourage child/family participation in planning.
- Provide active and passive ROM exercises every 4 hours; make into a game, give positive reinforcement for cooperation; ambulate as soon as possible; apply splints as ordered during rest periods and at night; utilize hydrotherapy as necessary; refer to *The Child Requiring Range-of-Motion Exercises,* page 237.
- Turn at least every 2 hours to prevent formation of pressure areas; see *The Child at Risk for Hazards of Immobility,* page 156.
- Provide age-appropriate diversional therapy (e.g., toys, TV, music; tape record parents reading favorite stories, singing songs, family routine at home); encourage visits from family and friends; reorient to surroundings as necessary; refer to *The Child Requiring Play Therapy,* page 226.
- Ensure increased fluid intake to prevent constipation and renal calculi; administer laxatives, stool softeners, or emulsants; evaluate and chart effectiveness.

☐ EVALUATION CRITERIA/DESIRED OUTCOMES

The child
- Performs ROM exercises of all joints every 4 hours while awake
- Participates in activities of daily living to extent possible
- Participates with staff to develop activity/rest schedule as age appropriate
- Has a bowel movement daily

NURSING DIAGNOSIS #5

a. **Ineffective individual/family coping** related to body-image changes, prolonged hospitalization, fear, altered family support, helplessness
b. **Alteration in family process** related to role changes, prolonged hospitalization, helplessness, fear
c. **Spiritual distress** related to body-image changes, helplessness
d. **Fear** related to disfigurement, painful procedures
e. **Grieving** related to actual loss or loss of function of body part
f. **Anxiety** related to imposed hospitalization, uncertain future, loss of social support system and peers
g. **Powerlessness** related to inability to control self-care environment or situation
h. **Social isolation** related to perceived appearance
i. **Noncompliance** with treatment protocols related to perceived hopelessness
j. **Altered growth and development** related to prescribed dependence

Rationale: The burned child/family may continue to demonstrate inability to manage internal and external stressors because of compromised resources. Responses to loss following a burn injury usually include fear of physical discomfort, disfigurement, mutilation, or death. In addition, children will demonstrate regression and concerns regarding abandonment, surgical procedures, and lengthy convalescence. These fears and concerns may be real or unfounded but in any case, resolution may take from several weeks to months or years depending on the severity of burn, course of treatment, and individual response to treatment.

☐ GOAL

The child/family will cope effectively; will achieve a degree of control in management of care; will grieve adaptively; will comply with treatments.

☐ IMPLEMENTATION

- Convey positive attitude about child; reinforce positive aspects of child's appearance and abilities.
- Continue to help to express feelings about current status, fears; accept regressive behavior as appropriate; listen actively; incorporate other health care personnel as appropriate; refer to *The Child Requiring Play Therapy,* page 226, and *The Child with Depression,* page 96.
- Arrange for continued schooling.
- Reinforce use of adaptive coping behaviors while

child/family moves through grieving stages; refer to *The Parent Experiencing Grief and Loss*, page 139.
- Encourage participation and cooperation in care; reward all efforts; give choices/control over situation as appropriate (e.g., "Which leg do you want debrided first?").
- Provide predictability for the child (e.g., do procedures at consistent time and place each day, wear specific object that signifies procedure time, maintain "safe" areas and times).
- Plan experiences for the child to control, manipulate, and succeed in to decrease feelings of powerlessness (e.g., allow to make some decisions regarding own care [e.g., which dressings to remove first, how fast to remove gauze], schedule).
- Provide careful explanations of all procedures to dispel fears.
- Project calm, unhurried attitude while performing procedures.
- Organize care to prevent undue pain and anxiety.
- Inform of all indications of continued progress.
- Provide for financial and spiritual counseling as needed/requested.
- Refer for cosmetic counseling as an enhanced physical appearance may improve child's body image.

☐ **EVALUATION CRITERIA/DESIRED OUTCOMES:**

The child/family
- Verbalizes fears and feelings
- Asks questions indicating adaptive grieving
- Utilizes family/friends and situational support to cope with life-style changes, anxiety
- Complies with treatments, participates in care as age appropriate

---

NURSING DIAGNOSIS #6
Knowledge deficit regarding long-term rehabilitation, home care maintenance program, prevention techniques

Rationale: Inadequate teaching of rehabilitation goals and treatments may lead to child/family misconceptions of current and future health status. Teaching of safety measures may prevent future burns.

☐ **GOAL**
The child/family will identify goals and plans for ongoing rehabilitation and home care; will state safety measures.

☐ **IMPLEMENTATION**
- Discuss impact of returning to home/school/family and peer reaction after a prolonged hospitalization; identify specific physical and emotional qualities necessary to function at home; have school nurse/teacher prepare classmates for child's return to school.
- Monitor child's/family's continuing level of understanding of treatment and home care; teach as necessary.
- Encourage to verbalize/play out questions.
- Explain and demonstrate new procedures that need to be done after discharge; have child/family return demonstration.
- Assist to plan for school, creative, and social needs upon return to home environment; use age-appropriate communication techniques (e.g., play therapy, role playing, story telling, discussion).
- Instruct on medication effects, side effects, dosage, and reportable symptoms of medication overdosage.
- Discuss safety measures (e.g., install smoke detectors, child-proof home, turn water heater thermostat down to 120°, wash clothing in detergent instead of soap, which impairs the flame retardency of children's clothing); tactfully remind family that prevention is the best treatment.
- Assist to make follow-up appointments with physician, clinic, public health nurse, or counseling as necessary.

☐ **EVALUATION CRITERIA/DESIRED OUTCOMES**

The child/family
- Demonstrates procedures correctly
- Outlines specific goals for rehabilitation
- Identifies effects, side effects, dosage, and reportable symptoms of prescribed medications
- States safety measures and methods of implementation
- Plans homebound school, social, and creative activities

The Child Undergoing Cardiac Surgery

Definition/Discussion

Congenital heart disease occurs when there is an embryologic developmental defect in cardiac structure/function resulting in an abnormal opening, obstructive lesions, stricture of a valve, incomplete closure of the ductus arteriosus, or abnormal vessel configuration. Open- or closed-heart procedures may be performed to palliate, correct, or cure the defects. Timing and choice of procedures vary according to the pathophysiologic effects of the defect on the child, as well as the nature of the correction.

Nursing Assessment

☐ PERTINENT HISTORY

Type of cardiac lesion, child's physiologic response to lesion (e.g., cyanosis, activity restrictions), medications, recent exposure to illness (especially upper respiratory infection), any previous palliative/surgical procedures

☐ PHYSICAL FINDINGS

Vital signs, pulses, level of consciousness, presence of murmur/thrill/clubbing, level of hydration, weight, respiratory status (e.g., rate and characteristics of respirations, breath sounds), complete blood count

☐ PSYCHOSOCIAL CONCERNS/ DEVELOPMENTAL FACTORS

Developmental level, coping mechanisms, usual routine of child/family, previous experience with hospitalization, habits (e.g., what comforts child, bedtime routine, favored objects)

☐ PATIENT AND FAMILY KNOWLEDGE

Cardiac lesion, planned surgical procedure, potential complications, convalescent period; level of knowledge, readiness and willingness to learn

Nursing Care

☐ LONG-TERM GOAL

The child will undergo surgery demonstrating adequate knowledge of the procedure and care to assure optimum tolerance; the child will be in a stabilized physiologic and psychologic state prior to surgery and will recover free from preventable complications; the child/parents will adapt to the child's increased level of activity and independence following corrective surgery.

☐ *Pre-op Care*

NURSING DIAGNOSIS #1

Anxiety (moderate) related to hospitalization, impending surgery

Rationale: The child/parents may not have an adequate understanding of hospital procedures, which may make them anxious. They may also have some fear (acknowledged or unrecognized) about the surgery or its outcome, leading to anxiety.

☐ GOAL

The child/parents will verbalize and exhibit a minimal amount of anxiety about hospitalization and impending surgery.

☐ IMPLEMENTATION

- Encourage the child/parents to verbalize feelings and ask questions.
- Refer to *The Child Experiencing Anxiety*, page 11.
- Allow child to express feelings nonverbally through play activities.
- Evaluate the degree of separation anxiety being experienced by the child (refer to *The Child Experiencing Separation Anxiety*, page 258).
- Permit the child to take a favorite toy or security object to the operating room.

☐ EVALUATION CRITERIA/DESIRED OUTCOMES

The child/parents
- Discuss concerns and questions with relative ease
- Identify anxiety and strategies to maintain a minimal level of anxiety and to function appropriately

NURSING DIAGNOSIS #2

Knowledge deficit regarding immediate post-op care requirements

Rationale: *The child/parents may not understand care required during the immediate post-op period.*

☐ GOAL

The child/parents will discuss the important aspects of post-op care.

☐ IMPLEMENTATION

- Allow the preschool or older child to touch equipment to be used; demonstrate equipment (e.g., intermittent positive pressure breathing, IV, chest drainage) utilizing a doll or other aids so the child may visualize more accurately the nature and function of these procedures; show restraints and explain they are not a punishment but for protection.
- Orient the child slowly in a nonthreatening manner, introducing one procedure or aspect of care at a time, so child can assimilate the information more easily and not become overanxious.
- Explain to the child/parents that you will be very busy in the post-op period carrying out protective monitoring and care procedures, so your activities are not interpreted by them to mean that the child is not progressing satisfactorily.

☐ EVALUATION CRITERIA/DESIRED OUTCOMES

The child/parents
- Identify some of the equipment and reasons for its use
- Describe post-op routines/procedures in simple terms

☐ *Post-op Care*

NURSING DIAGNOSIS #1

Alteration in cardiac output: decreased related to post-op dysrhythmias, fluid imbalance, residual cardiac disease

Rationale: *Dysrhythmias (e.g., tachycardia, bradycardia) may occur postoperatively in response to a number of variables (e.g., hypoxemia, electrolyte imbalance, metabolic acidosis, site of surgical correction). The child may not have received adequate fluid replacement and be hypovolemic. Damage to heart muscle from the preexisting condition may be such that the cardiac pump is inadequate. All these causes may lead to decreased cardiac output.*

☐ GOAL

The child will recover from the surgical procedure with good cardiac response.

☐ IMPLEMENTATION

- Observe for cardiac decompensation every 15 minutes until stable, then every hour; monitor heart rate and rhythm, cardiac pressures, peripheral perfusion (pulses and capillary refill), temperature and color of skin and mucous membranes.
- Maintain strict intake and output.
- Monitor all IV lines every hour for patency and rate of infusion, IV sites for redness or swelling (restrain child as needed to protect lines, removing restraints every 1-2 hours to provide range-of-motion); refer to *The Child with an Intravenous Catheter,* page 174.
- Observe for signs of circulatory overload (e.g., dyspnea, orthopnea, restlessness, elevated pulses and blood pressure, weight gain, edema).
- Weigh daily at same time on same scale and in the same clothing; record.
- Measure and record urine output every hour (should not be less than 1 cc/kg/hour) assess urine for specific gravity, blood, and protein every 4 hours.
- Monitor chest tube drainage and record every hour; notify physician if output is equal to or greater than 3 cc/kg/hour or is 5 cc/kg/hour for any 1 hour.

☐ EVALUATION CRITERIA/DESIRED OUTCOMES

The child
- Has cardiac monitoring parameters within normal limits
- Has lab values and urine output within normal limits
- Shows no signs of circulatory overload (e.g., respiratory distress)

NURSING DIAGNOSIS #2

Ineffective breathing pattern related to post-op pain, decreased energy, preexisting pulmonary vascular disease

Rationale: *Post op pain and decreased energy levels may cause the child to hypoventilate, thus providing respiration inadequate to maintain oxygen supply for cellular requirements and possibly causing atelectasis. The child's cardiac condition may have resulted in pulmonary vascular disease with pulmonary hypertension. Children with pulmonary vascular disease are especially at risk for developing post-op complications (e.g., atelectasis, pneumonia, pulmonary vasoconstriction). Infants have thin chest walls so breath sounds are readily transmitted throughout the lung fields making detection of pneumothorax/atelectasis more difficult.*

GOAL

The child will recover from the surgical procedure with good pulmonary function.

IMPLEMENTATION

- Observe respiratory status every 15 minutes until stable, then every hour; monitor rate and depth of respirations, breath sounds (e.g., equality, wheezes), color of skin and mucous membranes, and behavior (restlessness is early indication of hypoxemia).
- Turn, cough, and deep breathe every 2 hours to maintain adequate pulmonary ventilation and drainage; perform chest physical therapy if ordered and monitor effects.
- Monitor and maintain oxygen therapy; restrain/sedate intubated children if necessary.
- Monitor and record arterial blood gases to ascertain adequate ventilation and oxygenation.
- Medicate for pain as necessary to ensure adequate tidal volume; monitor for splinting respirations or resisting cough.

EVALUATION CRITERIA/DESIRED OUTCOMES

The child
- Has normal respiratory rate, breath sounds
- Maintains adequate arterial blood gases
- Demonstrates no pulmonary complications

NURSING DIAGNOSIS #3

Impaired gas exchange related to collapsed lung, mediastinal shift

Rationale: Chest tubes may easily become nonfunctional if they are disconnected, kinked, or occluded by a fibrin clot. An air leak will cause an increased amount of bubbling in the water-seal chamber, which will not fluctuate if the tubing is obstructed. A continued air leak or persistent build up of fluid will result in alterations in intrapleural pressures.

GOAL

The child will have easy, unlabored respirations with rate appropriate for age; will have patent chest tube(s) with no obstruction.

IMPLEMENTATION

- Make certain that all tubing is open and draining; check to see if water is fluctuating in water-seal chamber.
- Milk the chest tube every 15 minutes immediately postoperatively until bleeding is stable or minimal, then at least 3 times daily or as needed; this will help push any clots or fibrin down the lumen, thus assuring patency.
- Check all connections for leaks; tape them securely.
- Assess presence and character of breath sounds, equal chest excursions and signs of respiratory distress (e.g., retractions, grunting, nasal flaring); report adventitious sounds to physician.
- Monitor ABGs for indications of hypoxia suggestive of further respiratory impairment or ineffectiveness of drainage system.
- Check bubbling in water-seal chamber for presence of increased bubbling, suggestive of an air leak; if air leak detected/suspected
  - check for loose connections anywhere within the system
  - retape or reinforce taped connections
  - do not clamp tube as this may put the child at risk of tension pneumothorax
  - notify physician
  - milk tubing, beginning close to insertion site and moving downward until the problem is found
  - if disconnection is not evident and air leak is present, the bubbling will stop when tube is compressed below the air leak
- Check insertion site if unable to find air leak in tubing, put gentle pressure on site; if bubbling stops, seal area with petrolatum gauze; know that the chest tube may be dislodged in the subcutaneous tissue and require reinsertion by physician.
- Replace drainage unit if leak cannot be found at site or in tubing; notify physician if problem is not resolved.
- Use proper safety precautions at all times
  - place collection system in a stand or other device to prevent them from being turned over or broken
  - ensure protection of collection unit (e.g., when transferring child, during portable x-ray, when visitors present)
  - keep at least one clamp large enough to clamp chest tube taped to foot of bed; if collection system should break or fall over, clamp chest tube at once to prevent air from being sucked into pleural cavity; notify surgeon immediately and prepare another set-up
  - ensure collection system is kept below the level of the child's chest if necessary to move child's bed
  - never set collection system on the bed as water may run into child's pleural cavity
  - assist child in ambulating when permitted

EVALUATION CRITERIA/DESIRED OUTCOMES

The child
- Breathes in a normal respiratory pattern, has equal chest excursion, no retractions
- Maintains integrity of water-seal drainage

NURSING DIAGNOSIS #4

Potential for infection related to interruption of skin integrity

Rationale: The surgical wound as well as the placement of invasive monitoring lines (e.g., IV, central venous pressure, arterial) and the insertion of tubes (e.g., chest, Foley catheter, endotracheal) all present potential sources for infection.

☐ GOAL

The child will have a post-op course uncomplicated by wound/skin infection.

☐ IMPLEMENTATION

- Monitor vital signs every 4 hours and as necessary; watch for systemic indications of infection (e.g., elevated temperature, increased pulse and respirations, decreased blood pressure); notify physician of significant findings.
- Maintain aseptic technique when handling IV lines, wound dressings, suctioning.
- Inspect surgical wound, IV lines, chest tube sites for redness, swelling, drainage; report suspicious findings to physician.
- Provide catheter/tube insertion site care as ordered; maintain an occlusive dressing; avoid changing the dressing unless specified by physician or hospital protocol.

☐ EVALUATION CRITERIA/DESIRED OUTCOMES

The child
- Is free from wound/skin redness, swelling, drainage
- Has normal temperature

NURSING DIAGNOSIS #5

Alteration in comfort: pain related to surgical procedure, psychologic discomfort from unfamiliar experiences

Rationale: The surgical procedure is the basis for physiologic post-op pain. The child may also have psychologic pain related to the many procedures and new experiences that occur in the post-op period.

☐ GOAL

The child will experience minimal physical and psychologic discomfort postoperatively.

☐ IMPLEMENTATION

- Use information from parents regarding child's usual behavior when in pain to assess level of pain; refer to *The Child Experiencing Pain*, page 216.
- Observe for use of protective behaviors such as splinting and body positioning.
- Position, use distraction, imagery, music to reduce pain and help child cope.
- Medicate as necessary to keep child comfortable.
- Allow child to express feelings of pain; offer comfort and supportive measures.
- Assess the impact of discomfort on the child's sleep.
- Explain all procedures to child in age-appropriate terms; reinforce that painful procedures are not punishments.
- Encourage parents to participate in care to extent they feel comfortable (child may be more receptive to comfort measures provided by parent).

☐ EVALUATION CRITERIA/DESIRED OUTCOMES

The child
- Shows minimal crying or use of protective behaviors
- Has periods of restful sleep
- Cooperates with most procedures

NURSING DIAGNOSIS #6

Knowledge deficit regarding follow-up care requirements

Rationale: If knowledge deficits exist, the child/parents cannot manage the post-op treatment regimen appropriately at home.

☐ GOAL

The child/parents will verbalize an understanding of needed follow-up care.

☐ IMPLEMENTATION

- Teach parents about medications (e.g., names, actions, dosage, side effects, schedules) and care of incision.
- Explain prescribed exercise/activity regimen and restrictions.
- Provide anticipatory guidance about child's increased ability to be more independent and autonomous in functioning.
- Give parents names and phone numbers of those to call with questions.
- Counsel child/parents re the importance of continued long-term follow-up; need for dental prophylaxis.

☐ EVALUATION CRITERIA/DESIRED OUTCOMES

The child/parents
- Describe child's medications, activity and exercise regimens, incision care
- Describe appropriate post-op activities
- Demonstrate a willingness to allow child some freedom

The Child with a Cast

Definition/Discussion

Casts are applied to immobilize a body part in a specific position to correct or prevent a deformity; to provide rest and healing of a fracture, soft tissue injury, or bone infection; or to permit earlier weight bearing on an injured extremity.

Nursing Assessment

☐ PERTINENT HISTORY

History of present illness, congenital defect, surgery, or trauma including mechanism of injury, type of fracture, and other injuries; past medical history: respiratory/renal problems, peripheral circulatory impairment, neuromuscular or musculoskeletal impairment; elimination patterns; allergies, medications

☐ PHYSICAL FINDINGS

Type and intactness of cast, state of dryness, tightness of cast, signs of drainage or open wounds, other injuries, x-ray findings, pain, color, motion, sensation, temperature and motor ability of extremity distal to cast, capillary refill, pulses, edema, ecchymosis, range of motion (ROM), ability to perform activities of daily living (ADL)

☐ PSYCHOSOCIAL CONCERNS/ DEVELOPMENTAL FACTORS

Age, developmental level, present and past coping patterns, available support systems, interpersonal interactions, body image, adjustment to loss/potential loss of body functioning, previous experience with illness and hospitalization, habits (e.g., what comforts child, usual feeding/bedtime routines, favored objects)

☐ PATIENT AND FAMILY KNOWLEDGE

Understanding of present condition, pathophysiology and relationship of symptoms, current injury, surgical procedures if applicable, treatment modalities, expectations of functional capabilities, mobility aids (e.g., wheelchairs, crutch walking), home care, conditions that require follow-up; level of knowledge, readiness and willingness to learn

Nursing Care

☐ LONG-TERM GOAL

The child will adjust to the confinement and discomfort of a cast; the child will express confidence and independence in providing care; the child will be free from circulatory and nerve impairment.

NURSING DIAGNOSIS #1
a. **Alteration in tissue perfusion: peripheral** related to soft tissue swelling, containment by cast, immobility
b. **Potential for injury** related to tissue swelling, altered circulation, improper cast fit
c. **Alteration in comfort: pain** related to injury/surgery, weight of cast, decreased mobility

Rationale: Trauma, either surgical or accidental, disrupts tissues and the microcirculation resulting in transudation of plasma and bleeding. This causes swelling that may occur within a specific compartment. If swelling is extensive, it may compress blood vessels and further interrupt circulation to the surrounding area and the distal extremity. Swelling occurs as a result of tissue disruption and stimulates nerve endings. As a cast dries, care must be taken to prevent indentations that may compress underlying tissues.

☐ GOAL

The child will maintain adequate peripheral tissue perfusion; will be free from injury; will maintain adequate comfort.

☐ IMPLEMENTATION

• Observe and record circulation and nerve function

every 30 minutes the first 8 hours after cast application, then every 2 hours for the next 24 hours, then every 4–8 hours for the remainder of hospital stay if no complications develop; palpate pulses and compare with unaffected extremity.

- Monitor skin for color (e.g., cyanosis or pallor), temperature, swelling; document capillary refill.
- Observe for changes in sensory/motor function of involved extremity; evaluate sensation in all digits (i.e., fingers, toes) of the affected extremities.
- Check for changes in sensation (e.g., complaints of burning, tingling, prickling, muscle spasm or twitching); signs of discomfort (e.g., movement, facial expression, increased pulse, respiration, blood pressure, crying, irritability).
- Position child utilizing proper body alignment to distribute the weight over a large surface area and to minimize pressures areas.
- Elevate involved extremities at all times (e.g., involved legs may be kept on pillows, arms may be supported in stockinette sling suspended from an IV pole); support child to prevent excessive weight on damp cast, keep heel elevated off mattress or pillow to prevent a flat spot on cast, support upper thigh and hip to prevent external rotation.
- Know that drying time varies with size and type of cast (e.g., plaster of Paris 10–72 hours, synthetic cast 8–10 hours); protect the green/wet cast by handling it with the palms of the hands only; place cast on soft pillows; avoid plastic pillow covers because they inhibit cast drying and cooling.
- Apply icebags to the sides of plaster of Paris cast for the first 24–48 hours supporting them so they do not leave an impression on the cast.
- Promote cast drying by leaving the cast uncovered and turning the child every 2 hours so all sides will dry; a regular fan may be used in the room to assist drying; hair dryers should never be used as they may cause burns from heat conduction through cast and they may dry the outside of the cast while the inside remains wet; replace all damp pillows or linens.
- Monitor and record complaints of pain; refer to *The Child Experiencing Pain*, page 216.
- Notify physician of pain that is increased with passive motion/unrelieved by analgesics/accompanied by loss of active dorsiflexion indicating compartment syndrome; elevate the extremity; prepare to remove or bivalve the cast.
- Administer analgesics as ordered, evaluate for effect after 30 minutes.
- Report any vague abdominal discomfort/pain or pressure resulting in nausea, vomiting, or distension; this may be indicative of the high intestinal obstruction called cast syndrome.
- Prepare to bivalve the cast as needed should any complications occur.

☐ EVALUATION CRITERIA/DESIRED OUTCOMES

The child

- Has skin intact, warm to touch, pink in color
- Has intact sensation, movement above and below cast
- Has pulses present and of equal quality distal to cast
- Is free from indentations in cast
- Demonstrates no restless movements
- Plays happily

NURSING DIAGNOSIS #2
a. **Impairment of skin integrity** related to decreased mobility and casted body part
b. **Potential for infection** related to trauma concealed within the cast

Rationale: Immobility places skin lying over bony prominences at risk for local irritation and ischemic changes secondary to pressure. Inflexible cast material in close proximity to the skin may impinge on blood supply to the dermis. The ulnar/radial styloid, olecranon, and lateral epicondyle are problem areas for upper extremities. The heel, malleolus, perineal nerve, and the shin may be affected in the lower extremities. For children in spica casts, pressure areas may include the coccyx, superior posterior iliac spine, anterior superior iliac crest, trochanteric areas, and ribs. Draining open wounds in the warm, dark environment under the cast are perfect growth media for bacteria.

☐ GOAL

The child's skin will remain intact and free from impairment, irritation, pressure, or infection.

☐ IMPLEMENTATION

- Keep skin clean and dry, cleanse excess plaster from skin, dry well.
- Inspect skin around cast edges for signs of irritation, erythema, rash, or abrasion every 8 hours.
- Pad rough edges of cast; line cast edges with foam padding or pull stockinette lining taut; fold over the edge of cast and tape or petal the cast edge with adhesive tape/moleskin.
- Change moist or soiled linen as needed; keep bed free from wrinkles or cast crumbs.
- Encourage active/passive ROM; refer to *The Child Requiring Range-of-Motion Exercises*, page 237.
- Turn child every 2 hours, observe correct body mechanics and functional alignment; if unable to turn, lift child every 30 minutes and gently massage skin; do not use abduction stabilizer bar between legs of hip spica as a handle.

- Instruct how to turn self; explain importance and encourage to move about as able.
- Keep cast clean and dry at all times; if cast surrounds buttocks and perineum, protect inside from urine and fecal contamination by tucking waterproof material around the perineal edge (e.g., Saran wrap, OpSite); use diapering alternatives for non-toilet-trained child (e.g., sanitary napkin under newborn-size disposable diaper, tucking all edges under edges of perineal opening; use OpSite petaled from cast extending onto skin, encircle perineal opening and apply disposable diaper if cast fits tightly so baby does not move much inside cast.
- Cleanse and dry child's skin thoroughly after each diaper change/use of the bedpan or urinal.
- Remove stains from outer cast with a slightly dampened cloth or scouring powder; rubbing the cast with a piece of dampened plaster will also improve its appearance.
- Inspect cast for intactness, indentations, soiling, or dampness every 8 hours and after each diaper change/use of bedpan; replace wet/soiled sheets, or stockinette.
- Avoid covering cast with polyurethane or varnish as this inhibits evaporation of body moisture.
- Monitor complaints of pain or burning sensations under cast surface.
- Palpate cast over painful area for increased temperature; inspect dependent portions of cast for drainage; smell cast edges to detect foul odor as this may indicate necrosis or infection.
- Instruct child/family not to stick objects inside cast because instruments used for scratching may also break skin integrity; keep small objects away from young child (always important but particularly so here), cover cast with towel during meals to catch crumbs, use lids on glasses to avoid spills, keep child away from sandbox.
- Avoid using lotions or powder that can accumulate under edge of cast and become sticky or cake, causing irritation.
- Rub alcohol on skin under cast edges every 8 hours to keep the skin dry and to toughen it.
- Utilize sheepskin, foam pads, and heel/elbow protectors as necessary to reduce pressure injury.

☐ **EVALUATION CRITERIA/DESIRED OUTCOMES**

The child
- Has intact skin
- Keeps cast clean and intact
- Changes positions frequently

NURSING DIAGNOSIS #3

a. **Impaired physical mobility** related to casted body part
b. **Self-care deficit** related to restrictions imposed by cast

Rationale: Immobilization of any body part will interfere with the child's ability to function independently. Disuse of unaffected muscles and joints may result in muscle atrophy, joint stiffness, and loss of function.

☐ **GOAL**

The child will maintain muscle and joint mobility in the unaffected parts of the body; will perform age-appropriate ADL independently and safely within the restrictions imposed by cast.

☐ **IMPLEMENTATION**

- Place call bell and other frequently used items within easy reach.
- Observe activities child is able to perform independently and reinforce those behaviors.
- Medicate for pain as needed before performing potentially painful ROM exercises; assist with exercises; make exercise into a game.
- Instruct older child to actively exercise those joints above and below cast; instruct to move fingers and toes of affected extremity every hour to stimulate circulation.
- Teach older child to perform active ROM on all unaffected joints and utilize isometric exercises on affected extremity as ordered; refer to *The Child Requiring Range-of-Motion Exercises*, page 237.
- Provide for safe ambulation as soon as permitted; teach crutchwalking and obtain return demonstration; begin activity slowly; stay close to the child initially and reinforce activity.
- Instruct about proper use of ambulatory aids (e.g., crutches, slings).
- Remove all objects blocking the pathway, keep floor clear of obstacles (e.g., toys, throw rugs).
- Use only nonskid soles when ambulating.

☐ **EVALUATION CRITERIA/DESIRED OUTCOMES**

The child/family
- Exhibits full ROM of unaffected joints
- Carries out ADL as able
- Ambulates safely as able

NURSING DIAGNOSIS #4

Ineffective breathing pattern related to immobility imposed by cast, improper cast fit

Rationale: Immobility results in pooling of secretions in dependent areas of lung. Children under 6–7 years of age are primarily diaphragmatic (i.e., abdominal) breathers. Hip spica/body casts limit abdominal movement/chest excursion and impair the child's ability to deep breathe and cough effectively.

GOAL

The child will maintain adequate oxygenation and airway clearance.

IMPLEMENTATION

- Auscultate breath sounds every 4 hours and report any adventitious sounds/productive cough.
- Observe respiratory rate, pattern, patency, and exchange every 4 hours and as necessary; monitor skin color, behavior and mental status, abdominal girth/distension.
- Change position at least every 2 hours; encourage activity to tolerance as ordered.
- Instruct to take deep breaths 10 times every hour; use something the child is familiar with as a reference (e.g., deep breath with every commercial or with every 4 math problems); permit short periods of crying; encourage use of incentive spirometer or games to promote aeration.
- Observe child's ability to fully expand lungs and inform physician of any problem related to restriction by body cast.
- Give small frequent feedings to prevent abdominal distension.

EVALUATION CRITERIA/DESIRED OUTCOMES

The child
- Has unlabored respirations with good air exchange
- Is free from adventitious breath sounds
- Maintains alert mental status

NURSING DIAGNOSIS #5

a. **Ineffective individual/family coping** related to required adaptation to hospital environment
b. **Disturbance in self-concept: body image** related to perceptions of loss of body function/cast as an extension of self
c. **Fear** related to inability to prepare for hospitalization, perceptions of injury, cast removal
d. **Diversional activity deficit** related to impaired mobility
e. **Altered growth and development** related to impaired mobility, reaction to hospital environment

Rationale: Hospitalization disrupts normal routines and practices. Separation from familiar surroundings and loved ones may cause stress, regression, or maladaptation. Injuries resulting in casting are

---

frequently of an emergency nature and the child/family are ill prepared to deal with the imposed changes, affecting resources and the ability to adapt.

GOAL

The child/family will demonstrate positive adaptation to hospitalization and impaired mobility.

IMPLEMENTATION

- Explain all procedures/treatments in age-appropriate way (e.g., apply cast to doll, utilize pictures and coloring book); tell child that cast cutter makes a loud noise and area may feel warm; demonstrate on self/casted doll.
- Discuss rationale for all treatments.
- Describe the injury and relate to symptoms; show child/family the x-rays.
- Allow verbalization/playing out of thought and fears; use drawings, puppets, have favored doll/stuffed animal experience same procedures; refer to *The Child Requiring Play Therapy*, page 226.
- Give the child as much control as possible; place frequently used items within easy reach, provide a trapeze so child can move and turn self when desired; allow realistic choices whenever possible.
- Allow family to remain with child, ask them to bring favorite toys and other diversional hobbies/activities.
- Provide age-appropriate developmental/recreational activities; put child on stretcher or take bed to playroom; use mobiles for infants, encourage holding child if no restrictions on positioning; put child on abdomen surrounded by toys.
- Allow child to play with other children as appropriate.
- Inform parents of effects of hospitalization on development; explain that regressive behaviors are common in children.
- Observe present coping mechanisms; support/guide the child/family to new, more adaptive ones as needed; provide acceptable outlet for frustration (e.g., pounding block, bean bag toss).

EVALUATION CRITERIA/DESIRED OUTCOMES

The child
- Interacts and plays with other children on unit

The child/family
- Participates in care
- Discusses condition, reaction of child to procedures/hospitalization

---

NURSING DIAGNOSIS #6

Knowledge deficit regarding present illness, treatment, cast care, exercise, complications, mobility aids

Rationale: Children/family often harbor misconceptions and misinformation about body functions, illness, and the medical/nursing professions. Conditions and treatments are new and unfamiliar. Casts are usually applied secondary to an emergency situation that does not allow for adequate preparation.

☐ GOAL

The child/family will demonstrate knowledge about the condition, hospitalization, treatments, home and follow-up care

☐ IMPLEMENTATION

- Discuss cast care in the home setting (e.g., elevation, positioning, cleansing of cast, techniques for bathing with a cast, how to properly use mobility aids such as slings, crutches).
- Explain the purpose of the cast and why ROM exercises are important.
- Teach how to care for skin around the cast edges.
- Help parents find ways to position baby for feeding (e.g., astride their leg, in umbrella stroller with wide seat and no firm sides) and ambulation (e.g., place on abdomen on small board with casters and use arms to scoot around).
- Discuss physical limitations of the home environment to identify potential problems on discharge; impress on parents to always restrain child while in a car/auto; discuss car safety (e.g., position child in car seat with shoulder harness and crotch strap if at all possible or put car bed between front and back seats, pad well, and secure baby inside).
- Discuss signs and symptoms of complications (e.g., pain, pulselessness, pallor, swelling, paresthesia, paralysis) and to report these immediately should they occur.
- Explain cast-removal technique and how to care for skin after removal of cast (e.g., cleanse extremity with warm soapy water, do not scrub or rub vigorously, pat dry).
- Discuss restrictions after cast removal; be specific about exercise and mobility.

☐ EVALUATION CRITERIA/DESIRED OUTCOMES

The child/family

- Asks appropriate questions
- Identifies signs/symptoms of complications
- Describes appropriate care after cast is removed

The Child with Cerebral Palsy

Definition/Discussion

According to the United Cerebral Palsy (UCP) Association, cerebral palsy is a group of disabling conditions caused by damage to the central nervous system. "Cerebral" refers to the brain, while "palsy" describes lack of muscle control that is often (but not always) a symptom of nervous system dysfunction. Cerebral palsy can be mild or severe. Types include *spastic* (the most common type): tense, contracted muscles; *athetoid*: constant uncontrolled movements; *ataxic*: poor sense of balance and depth of perception; and *mixed*: a combination of symptoms of all the types of cerebral palsy.

Nursing Assessment

☐ PERTINENT HISTORY

Presence of conditions associated with cerebral palsy (e.g., seizures, problems with vision/hearing/speech, mental retardation, impairments in arm or leg movements); prior hospitalizations; treatments carried out at home/school (e.g., medications); length, characteristics of present illness; usual weight

☐ PHYSICAL FINDINGS

Absence of normal reflexes; irritability; feeding problems; motor development, muscle tones, range of motion (ROM); spasticity; impairments in arm or leg movements; vision/hearing/speech problems; weight, vital signs, level of consciousness, use of adaptive devices

☐ PSYCHOSOCIAL CONCERNS/ DEVELOPMENTAL FACTORS

Developmental level of child; coping mechanisms, habits of child and family; likely impact of hospitalization

☐ PATIENT AND FAMILY KNOWLEDGE

Condition, causes, treatment, prognosis; level of knowledge, readiness and willingness to learn

Nursing Care

☐ LONG-TERM GOAL

The child will develop and maintain abilities to function as independently as possible in activities of daily living, mobility, and communication; the child/family will utilize medical, educational, and social services in order to promote development and prevent complications; the child/family will accept and adjust to the disabilities.

NURSING DIAGNOSIS #1

Self-care deficit (specify) related to physical impairments

Rationale: Cerebral palsy is associated with impairments in muscle control, balance, and coordination that interfere with independent performance of ADL.

☐ GOAL

The child will perform ADL as independently as possible with the use of support measures as needed; will ingest adequate food and fluid to meet body needs.

☐ IMPLEMENTATION

- Adjust hospital routine to child's usual routine as much as possible; provide sameness and consistency in nursing care (e.g., exact schedules, time frames, and same nurse).
- Allow time for child to participate in planning own care as possible; assess strengths and provide help only as needed; utilize adaptive aids (e.g., braces, special hygiene and eating utensils).
- Provide opportunities for child to be as independent as possible with ADL.
- Ensure adequate intake of food and fluid; if child uses special feeding utensils, ensure that they are present at mealtime; allow choice in menu when possible and use supplements as needed; provide

privacy as needed if excessive drooling is a problem at mealtime.
- Preserve skin integrity (e.g., massage bony prominences; use lotions, sheepskins, water mattress); bathe in warm water as cold or hot will trigger spasms.
- Explain and demonstrate use of equipment (e.g., suction machine, IVs) in advance to decrease anxiety and activities.
- Measure and record intake and output, urine specific gravity, to ensure dehydration is not occurring.
- Note stool consistency and frequency, follow usual bowel and bladder training schedule so that child does not regress while in hospital.

☐ EVALUATION CRITERIA/DESIRED OUTCOMES

The child
- Maintains preadmission weight
- Maintains/attains optimal level of independence with ADL
- Retains preadmission bowel/bladder training pattern

NURSING DIAGNOSIS #2

Impaired verbal communication related to inability to articulate/hear spoken words

Rationale: Cerebral palsy is often associated with speech impairments related to motor difficulties/sensoryneural hearing loss. Hearing impairments are most often a complication of kernicterus.

☐ GOAL

The child will utilize a system of communication with family and care givers to express needs, ask questions, and interact with other children in play.

☐ IMPLEMENTATION

- Learn the child's preadmission method of communication; adapt hospital system of communication to meet child's needs.
- Allow time and opportunity for child to communicate thoughts, feelings, and requests.
- Introduce child/parents to speech therapist if appropriate; cooperate with plan of care established by speech therapist.
- Coordinate hearing testing; obtain hearing aids if indicated.

☐ EVALUATION CRITERIA/DESIRED OUTCOMES

The child
- Maintains/improves preadmission communication skills

The child/family
- Demonstrates use of adaptive communication device(s)

NURSING DIAGNOSIS #3
a. **Impaired physical mobility** related to muscle weakness, spasticity
b. **Potential for injury** related to muscle weakness, spasticity

Rationale: Cerebral palsy is associated with impairments in muscle control, balance, coordination, and overall delayed motor development.

☐ GOAL

The child will be free from injury, preventable complications, and deformities; the child/parents will demonstrate measures to promote maintenance of independent motor function and prevent complications/deformities.

☐ IMPLEMENTATION

- Protect from accidents resulting from poor balance and lack of muscle control; be aware that child may not be able to ask for help and may need to rely on nurse's assessment and judgment on what safety precautions are appropriate; do not wait for call light; plan regular frequent checks (e.g., child's condition, safety rails up).
- Use seatbelts in wheelchairs; secure patient in chair and bed as needed for safety.
- Observe for restlessness, agitation, dyspnea; observe for choking or aspiration; remain with child until medications are safely swallowed.
- Prevent contractures; follow usual exercise routine as permitted by physical condition.
- Use passive and active range-of-motion exercises as tolerated; provide rest periods and reduce stimuli to promote calm environment.
- Work with physical therapist to teach parents utilization and maintenance of any new equipment prescribed.

☐ EVALUATION CRITERIA/DESIRED OUTCOMES

The child
- Maintains/improves preadmission range-of-motion and mobility
- Is free from injuries

The parents
- Demonstrate ROM exercises
- Use/maintain adaptive equipment

NURSING DIAGNOSIS #4

Family coping: potential for growth related to adjustment in life-style, caring for chronically disabled member

Rationale: Cerebral palsy is a permanent disabling condition that can create many problems. A child with cerebral palsy poses numerous difficulties requiring adjustments in daily life of the whole family, with constant demands, few rewards, and many frustrations.

☐ GOAL

The child/family will acknowledge the functional limitations caused by cerebral palsy; will discuss feelings and concerns about the disabilities; will implement a plan for independent functioning, prevention of complications and deformities; will utilize extrafamilial resources as appropriate.

☐ IMPLEMENTATION

- Approach child/family in calm, respectful, and unhurried manner; promote trust by expressing acceptance, friendliness, and willingness to listen.
- Be available to listen to feelings/concerns; accept expressed feelings in nonjudgmental way.
- Offer emotional support as child/family go through periods of adjustment/grief/mourning.
- Offer hope that child can learn to be independent in ADL and develop abilities to adapt to limitations; inform family that although damage cannot be cured, new patterns can be established to enhance the quality of life for child and family.
- Allow parent to be the expert on care of child; give acknowledgment and positive reinforcement to efforts to provide a stimulating, healthy environment; reward parent's abilities to assess and provide for child's needs; know that the parent may feel inadequate and overwhelmed.
- Provide time for family members to discuss concerns and problems; find out how long a specific approach has been used, how the approach works and does not work.
- Discuss alternatives with family members *before* giving suggestions or teaching; refer to *Guidelines for Teaching Parents and Children*, page 316.
- Assist family to develop new coping strategies as needed.
- Refer to *The Child with a Developmental Disability*, page 100, if the child has mental retardation.

☐ EVALUATION CRITERIA/DESIRED OUTCOMES

The child/family

- Expresses feelings and concerns regarding limitations of function due to disability

The family

- States and implements plan for care of child

NURSING DIAGNOSIS #5

a. **Diversional activity deficit** related to physical impairment, rigorous therapy schedule
b. **Altered growth and development** related to physical impairment

Rationale: Individuals with cerebral palsy may have normal or superior intelligence or may be mentally retarded. They need stimulation and pleasurable activities to engage in. This may be overlooked because of multiple physical handicaps.

☐ GOAL

The child will be free from boredom; will progress through the stages of development at own rate.

☐ IMPLEMENTATION

- Refer to *The Child Requiring Play Therapy*, page 226, and *Normal Growth and Development*, pages 300–314.
- Offer appropriate play/diversional activities within constraints of physical handicap (e.g., listen to music, movies, TV, have child dictate story and then have child/care giver illustrate/play out story with puppets, use computer adapted with pointer or joystick as indicated, take care of pets, hobbies).
- Incorporate "fun" activities into therapy schedule: rolling on vestibular (i.e., Bobath) ball or riding horseback (helps balance); swimming (may relax muscles, make child feel more graceful).
- Involve child/family in planning activities; teach family to make therapeutic activities fun/enjoyable.

☐ EVALUATION CRITERIA/DESIRED OUTCOMES

The child

- Has no verbal complaints of boredom
- Participates in scheduled activities

NURSING DIAGNOSIS #6

Knowledge deficit regarding measures to promote/maintain independent functioning and prevent complications/deformities

Rationale: If knowledge deficit exists, family cannot appropriately maintain the child's functioning or prevent complications or deformities.

GOAL

The child/parents will verbalize an understanding of cerebral palsy; will state the importance of continuing therapies, and educational/stimulation programs after discharge.

IMPLEMENTATION

- Instruct in technical skills/procedures to be carried out after discharge.
- Teach about maintenance of adaptive equipment.
- Teach about medications (e.g., side effects, dose, when to report to physician).
- Discuss prescribed diet.
- Teach signs and symptoms of dehydration, impaction, and respiratory tract infection.
- Reinforce the importance of follow-up appointments.
- Provide list of community support agencies (e.g., schools, United Cerebral Palsy Association, and centers of independent living).

EVALUATION CRITERIA/DESIRED OUTCOMES

The child/family

- Describes cerebral palsy and appropriate treatment programs
- Demonstrates technical skills
- Uses/maintains adaptive equipment
- Lists signs of dehydration, impaction, and respiratory tract infection
- States the importance of keeping follow-up appointments
- Uses community support services

The Child Receiving Chemotherapy

Definition/Discussion

Antineoplastic drug therapy is used in the treatment of a child with cancer to prevent or reduce the rate of recurrence or to treat metastasis; it may be used alone or in combination with radiation/surgery as part of a multi-modality therapy to prolong tumor-free intervals/to palliate symptoms of cancer/to alleviate complications of cancer.

Antineoplastic drugs fall into 6 categories: alkylating agents, antimetabolites, antibiotics, vinca alkaloids, hormones, and miscellaneous. They are further classified as cell-cycle specific or cell-cycle nonspecific depending upon where in the cell's reproductive cycle they exert their effects. Knowledge regarding the mode of action and the cell-cycle specificity of a particular drug has implications for nursing in terms of timing and sequencing of the drugs, as well as side effects and toxicities.

Methods of administration vary from drug to drug and include oral, intramuscular, intravenous, and intrathecal routes. Frequently, more than one chemotherapeutic drug is used at a time. Drugs used in combination should all have a demonstrated effectiveness against the tumor in question, different modes of action, and different (or minimally overlapping) side effects.

Nursing Assessment

☐ PERTINENT HISTORY

Cancer diagnosis (length, characteristics); previous experience with cancer treatment and side effects encountered

☐ PHYSICAL FINDINGS

Signs and symptoms of primary tumor/metastatic site(s), disability related to disease state, nutritional status, activity level, rest and sleep patterns, resistance to infection, electrolyte balance, bone-marrow function, hygiene, bowel patterns, pain, concurrent medications

☐ PSYCHOSOCIAL CONCERNS/ DEVELOPMENTAL FACTORS

Developmental level, age, child/family support systems, impact on body image (e.g., alopecia), previous experiences with chemotherapy treatment, expectations regarding therapy; cultural beliefs in conflict with prescribed medical regimen (e.g., value of folk or herbal preparations), habits (e.g., usual food/bedtime routines, what comforts child, favored objects)

☐ PATIENT AND FAMILY KNOWLEDGE

Definition of chemotherapy, understanding of the disease and the principles of chemotherapy, expectations of therapy; level of knowledge, readiness and willingness to learn

Nursing Care

☐ LONG-TERM GOAL

The child will continue/complete prescribed course of chemotherapy; the child/parents will manage the common side effects associated with cancer chemotherapy (bone-marrow suppression, nausea and vomiting, alopecia, stomatitis and mucositis, and diarrhea); the child will be free from preventable complications associated with chemotherapy.

NURSING DIAGNOSIS #1

Anxiety related to perceptions of chemotherapeutic regimen, potential side effects

Rationale: The diagnosis of cancer and its treatment (e.g., chemotherapy) bring about fear and anxiety related to changing life-styles and uncertainties about the future. Chemotherapy offers hope against cancer but may have side effects that are life threatening or that disrupt the child's relationships and roles in the family and school environment. The ability to cope with chemotherapy will be influenced by knowledge of the treatment and realistic expectations of side effects as well as the child's/parents' ability to control or manage the side effects.

☐ GOAL

The child/parents will indicate reduced fear/anxiety.

☐ IMPLEMENTATION

- Ask about feelings/concerns regarding chemotherapy; clarify inaccurate perceptions; validate correct understanding; indicate that others have expressed similar feelings.
- Discuss aims and goals of chemotherapy.
- Provide information regarding name, purpose, route, schedule, and dosage of chemotherapy regimen.
- Teach common side effects and signs of toxicity for all drugs being used; provide information regarding interventions to alleviate side effects.

☐ EVALUATION CRITERIA/DESIRED OUTCOMES

The child/parents
- State fear/anxiety is lessened
- Discuss realistic expectations and goals of therapy
- Identify drugs, route, dose, and schedule of chemotherapy regimen

---

NURSING DIAGNOSIS #2

Potential for injury related to infiltration of chemotherapeutic drugs

Rationale: Some chemotherapy agents are caustic (vesicants), causing severe tissue necrosis if drug infiltration (extravasation) occurs during administration. Tissue necrosis can lead to deep, wide ulceration warranting skin grafts. Because chemotherapy causes bone-marrow suppression, drug extravasation can be life threatening if tissue necrosis and infection occur.

☐ GOAL

The child will experience safe administration of drugs; will be free from IV infiltration of a chemotherapeutic drug.

☐ IMPLEMENTATION

- Establish patent IV site for infusion as needed.
- Monitor infusion for signs of infiltration (e.g., stinging, burning, or pain at IV site; lack of blood return; swelling at IV insertion site); monitor continuously if drugs are vesicants (e.g., doxorubicin).
- Teach to recognize and report symptoms of infiltration immediately.
- Have written protocol/physician's prescription for management of extravasation and have necessary antidotes available prior to infusion of any vesicant/irritant drug.
- Initiate management of extravasation as soon as

infiltration is suspected following physician's prescription/institutionally approved protocol.

☐ EVALUATION CRITERIA/DESIRED OUTCOMES

The child
- Maintains patent IV
- Is free from infiltration
- Has any extravasation detected/managed immediately with the approved protocol

---

NURSING DIAGNOSIS #3

Fluid volume deficit related to vomiting

Rationale: Chemotherapy drugs destroy both normal and cancer cells with a rapid proliferation rate. The epithelial lining of the GI tract is affected causing nausea and vomiting.

☐ GOAL

The child/parents will identify factors related to prevention and management of nausea and vomiting; will maintain nutrition and hydration.

☐ IMPLEMENTATION

- Administer antiemetics prophylactically to prevent or minimize nausea and vomiting; continually assess and adjust antiemetic therapy as needed.
- Provide well-ventilated, cool area for infusion.
- Advise/assist child to be well hydrated prior to each course of therapy (e.g., drink extra fluids 24 hours before course).
- Maintain adequate fluid intake during therapy (oral/IV).
- Maintain accurate intake and output during times of vomiting to monitor fluid balance.
- Provide small, easily digested meals prior to chemotherapy.
- Adjust diet during periods of nausea
  - eat cold, bland, dry bulky foods
  - maintain clear liquid intake
  - eat small, frequent meals
- Monitor electrolytes daily if vomiting persists.
- Provide information about distraction and relaxation techniques.
- Provide support by being with child during times of vomiting; closely monitor child for aspiration.

☐ EVALUATION CRITERIA/DESIRED OUTCOMES

The child
- Receives effective antiemetics routinely during chemotherapeutic treatment
- Maintains adequate fluid balance, free from dehydration
- Has normal urine output, electrolyte balance

- Is free from aspiration

The parents

Prepare child appropriately for chemotherapy

NURSING DIAGNOSIS #4

Potential for infection related to bone-marrow suppression

Rationale: Cells produced by the bone marrow have a rapid rate of cellular proliferation. Chemotherapy causes bone-marrow suppression (decreased white blood cell count [WBC]) resulting in an increased potential for infection.

☐ **GOAL**

The child/parents will state signs and symptoms of decreased WBC; will list precautions necessary to avoid complications of infection.

☐ **IMPLEMENTATION**

- Monitor WBC as ordered.
- Assess frequently for signs of infection (e.g., urinary, respiratory, oral, perineal, IV, injection sites).
- Monitor temperature and report any elevation.
- Utilize prevention methods for infection when WBC falls below 1,000 mm³ (e.g., protective isolation).
- Maintain nutritional status.
- Conserve child's energy by alternating rest and activity periods.
- Administer blood component therapy when ordered; refer to *The Child Receiving Blood and Blood-Product Transfusions*, page 24.

☐ **EVALUATION CRITERIA/DESIRED OUTCOMES**

The child
- Has a normal WBC
- Is free from infection

The child/parents

List signs/symptoms of infection and precautions to take if they appear

---

NURSING DIAGNOSIS #5

Potential for injury (hemorrhage) related to bone-marrow suppression

Rationale: Bone-marrow suppression with impaired platelet production and platelet destruction places the child at risk for hemorrhage.

☐ **GOAL**

The child/parents will state signs and symptoms of thrombocytopenia; will list precautions necessary to avoid hemorrhage and steps to take if hemorrhage occurs.

☐ **IMPLEMENTATION**

- Monitor platelet count as ordered; watch for decreases.
- Observe for bleeding (e.g., hematuria, bleeding gums, bruising, epistaxis, hemoptysis, bloody stool, bleeding from puncture sites).
- Teach child not to engage in rough contact activities.
- Administer blood component therapy when ordered and monitor for complications (refer to *The Child Receiving Blood and Blood-Product Transfusions*, page 24).
- Provide emotional support while waiting for blood parameters to return to normal.

☐ **EVALUATION CRITERIA/DESIRED OUTCOMES**

The child
- Is free from bleeding
- Has lab values within normal limits

The child/parents

List signs of hemorrhage and actions to take in case of hemorrhage

---

NURSING DIAGNOSIS #6

Disturbance in self-concept: body-image related to loss of hair

Rationale: Hair follicle cells multiply rapidly accounting for the hair loss associated with some chemotherapy agents. Hair loss may be confined to hair on head or may include other body hair (e.g., pubic hair, eyebrows).

☐ **GOAL**

The child will manage problems related to hair loss; will experience only minor disturbance in body image related to alopecia.

☐ **IMPLEMENTATION**

- Inform child/family of expected initiation, degree, and duration of hair loss
  - begins 1–2 weeks after chemotherapy
  - amount of hair loss depends on chemotherapy drug
  - hair will regrow after cessation of chemotherapy but may be different color/texture
- Utilize scalp hypothermia techniques if permitted (not suitable for leukemia or if scalp metastasis is suspected) and if child can tolerate them.

- Minimize the psychologic impact of hair loss by allowing verbalization of feelings related to loss and by giving support; refer to *The Child Experiencing a Body-Image Disturbance*, page 30.
- Identify alternative head coverings: encourage child to obtain a wig, attractive scarves, or hats in advance of hair loss.
- Suggest the option of cutting hair prior to loss for children with long hair.

☐ EVALUATION CRITERIA/DESIRED OUTCOMES

The child
- Utilizes resources to minimize the psychologic impact of hair loss
- Verbalizes feelings about changed body-image

NURSING DIAGNOSIS #7

Alteration in oral mucous membranes related to inflammatory response to chemotherapy

Rationale: The epithelial cells of the GI tract proliferate rapidly. Chemotherapy causes an inflammatory response that results in mucositis and stomatitis.

☐ GOAL

The child will be free from oral discomfort; the child/parents will identify activities to prevent/manage mucosites and stomatitis.

☐ IMPLEMENTATION

- Assess oral mucosa (cheeks, palate, tongue, gums, throat) twice daily.
- Document child's complaints of oral pain or changes in sensation, taste.
- Utilize gentle oral hygiene after eating and every 4 hours while awake; use soft toothbrush.
- Maintain adequate hydration.
- Minimize trauma to mucous membranes by having child eat soft, bland foods and by avoiding temperature extremes in food and drink.
- Utilize topical and systemic antibiotic/antifungal medications as ordered.
- Instruct in the use of oral anesthetics PRN for mouth pain.

☐ EVALUATION CRITERIA/DESIRED OUTCOMES

The child
- Exhibits no irritation or ulceration in oral mucosa
- Is free from signs of infection/pain
- Has pink, moist mucosa
- Maintains normal dietary and fluid intake

NURSING DIAGNOSIS #8

Alteration in bowel elimination: diarrhea related to effects of chemotherapeutic drugs on bowel mucosa

Rationale: Diarrhea is the result of the effects of chemotherapy on the rapidly dividing epithelial cells lining the GI tract.

☐ GOAL

The child will prevent or manage alterations in bowel elimination.

☐ IMPLEMENTATION

- Assess usual pattern of bowel elimination.
- Monitor character and frequency of stools.
- Adjust diet to reduce stool consistency
  - eat low-residue diet, high in protein and calories
  - eliminate foods and beverages that irritate or stimulate the GI tract
  - eat small, frequent meals
  - avoid extremely hot or cold foods
- Monitor fluid and electrolyte balance; maintain adequate hydration.
- Weigh daily.
- Medicate with antidiarrheal agents as needed; monitor effectiveness.
- Maintain perineal skin integrity with thorough cleansing and drying after each bowel movement; provide information regarding skin care to child/parents.
- Encourage child to exercise if possible after each meal.

☐ EVALUATION CRITERIA/DESIRED OUTCOMES

The child
- Maintains normal body weight, fluid and electrolyte balance
- Has intact perineal skin
- Has normal bowel sounds and bowel movements of normal frequency and consistency

---

NURSING DIAGNOSIS #9

Knowledge deficit regarding self-care, follow-up activities during home care

Rationale: Following the administration of chemotherapy, the child/parents must continue to observe for side effects. The child must receive follow-up care to monitor effects of the drugs, and in some cases the child will continue taking oral preparations at home, necessitating clear instructions regarding administration schedules.

GOAL

The child/parents will carry out activities that minimize side effects of treatment, promote an optimum level of health, and prevent further complications of treatment; will state signs and symptoms of anemia, thrombocytopenia, infection; will understand precautions necessary to avoid infection or bleeding.

IMPLEMENTATION

- Reinforce rationale behind the overall treatment plan.
- Outline drug protocol; provide a calendar of drug administration times.
- Discuss expected side effects of drugs and define methods to minimize potential side effects.
- Instruct about signs and symptoms of life-threatening side effects and when to notify the physician.
- Stress the importance of follow-up appointments to monitor blood counts and disease process.
- Review interventions to maintain/regain optimal nutrition.
- Encourage adequate rest and activity periods.
- Allow verbalization of fears and concerns related to body-image and life-style changes; ensure that child/parents can describe strategies for adjustments needed.
- Provide information on available resources if needed.

EVALUATION CRITERIA/DESIRED OUTCOMES

The child/parents

- List route, dosage, and frequency of ordered chemotherapy drugs
- State common side effects of drugs to be taken and common methods for prevention/minimization of side effects to be expected
- Identify appropriate times to call physician
- Discuss plans for optimal nutritional intake and hydration
- Comply with appointments for follow-up check/blood counts with physician/clinic

The Child/Family Adapting to Chronic Illness

Definition/Discussion

Chronic illness refers to a physical disorder with a protracted course (usually longer than 3 months) that can be progressive and fatal, or associated with a relatively normal life span despite impaired functioning. Such an illness frequently has acute exacerbations requiring intensive medical attention, followed by a long period of supervision, observation, and care at home; usually it is the child and family who must manage the illness on a day-to-day basis. The most common chronic illnesses are asthma, cardiac conditions, and diabetes mellitus. It is estimated that 7%–10% of children are affected with a serious chronic illness.

Nursing Assessment

☐ PERTINENT HISTORY

Course of illness (e.g., time since diagnosis, characteristics of acute exacerbations requiring hospitalization, number of days in hospital and absent from school during past year); treatment strategies (e.g., medical management, teacher or school nurse management); academic achievement; use of community and social support systems

☐ PHYSICAL FINDINGS

Physical growth; physical limitation from the illness itself, or from prescribed treatments; pain or discomfort; other handicapping conditions (e.g., mental retardation, cerebral palsy); physical/behavioral symptoms indicating episodic illness or acute exacerbation of the chronic condition

☐ PSYCHOSOCIAL CONCERNS/ DEVELOPMENTAL FACTORS

Cognitive/social/emotional/developmental level of functioning including academic achievement and peer relationships; coping mechanisms, including use of support systems, daily routine at home; impact of hospitalization(s) and school absence(s); changes in child's development as a result of illness/treatment; parental attitudes towards the child's illness; impact of treatment regimen on the child/family

☐ PATIENT AND FAMILY KNOWLEDGE

Previous educational efforts; need for compliance with therapeutic regimen; knowledge of treatment plan, ability to perform plan and give medications, as well as readiness (emotionally and financially) to manage the child's health at home; level of knowledge, readiness and willingness to learn

Nursing Care

☐ LONG-TERM GOAL

The parents will manage and will help the child manage the complex treatment procedures at home; the parents will work to prevent the illness from disrupting normal family functioning or the family's involvement in the community; the child will cope with the realities of the illness while continuing to attend school and participating in age-appropriate activities as much as possible; the family will encourage achievement of age-appropriate developmental tasks by the child.

NURSING DIAGNOSIS #1

Alteration in health maintenance related to chronic disease process with its remissions and exacerbations, need for a lifelong period of medical treatment

Rationale: *A chronic illness is usually treatable but not curable, and requires a lifelong commitment to complex, expensive, and sometimes painful procedures for managing the illness and maintaining optimal level of health. Treatment regimen may be beyond the child's cognitive capabilities, or it may be too time consuming for parents to supervise the child's daily illness-related tasks.*

☐ GOAL

The child/parents will perform the necessary home treatments and procedures to manage the illness and maintain the child at home; the child will perform necessary treatment procedures under parental supervision as age and condition permit.

☐ IMPLEMENTATION
- Recognize the primary role of the parents as care givers.
- Discuss which aspects of the management of the illness should be the child's responsibility, which the parents', and how the physician, nurse, and other health professionals will remain involved.
- Plan discussions at regular intervals as the illness changes over time and as the child becomes capable of greater responsibilities.
- Encourage the child's involvement in age-appropriate health promotion and illness management tasks (at home and in the hospital).
- Provide educational sessions and materials that will enable the child/parents to learn day-to-day illness management tasks.
- Identify community health providers who can reinforce health teaching/procedures and assist with health maintenance activities at home; encourage parents to communicate with these providers (including school nurse) to describe ongoing treatments, report observations and the results of daily tests relevant to the child's condition.
- Evaluate roles of all family members (especially the child) in the management of the child's health on a regular basis.

☐ EVALUATION CRITERIA/DESIRED OUTCOMES
The child
- Is maintained at home
- Participates in illness-management tasks as able

The child/parents
- Establish an efficient daily routine for ongoing home treatments.
- Perform home treatments and procedures appropriately

NURSING DIAGNOSIS #2
Family coping: potential for growth related to impact of the child's disease on the family's functioning

Rationale: A family with a chronically ill child must exert a great deal of effort to effectively manage the child's disease while encouraging normal development in the child. Preventing the illness from disrupting normal family functioning is an important goal to work toward.

☐ GOAL
The family will cope with and master the stress of the illness; will increase sharing, support, and heighten self-esteem.

☐ IMPLEMENTATION
- Support parents with reassurance, realism, and repetition, as family members come to grips with the reality of the child's illness and treatment.
- Help parents develop strategies to adjust to the crisis of chronic illness.
- Encourage parents to expect age-appropriate behavior and set realistic limits for their child.
- Analyze support systems and use of community resources (medical, financial, social) that help in the process of long-term adjustment to chronic illness.
- Recognize the need for additional supports and refer for services in the community.
- Coordinate services and help family and health care team to communicate effectively with one another.

☐ EVALUATION CRITERIA/DESIRED OUTCOMES
The family
- Communicates effectively with one another and with other family members to function as a stable family system
- Establishes and maintains healthy relationships with friends and effective relationships with community resources
- Assists all members of the family unit to achieve developmental tasks

---

NURSING DIAGNOSIS #3
Disturbance in self-concept: body image/self-esteem/role performance/personal identity related to impact of specific illness characteristics (e.g., visibility, prognosis, treatment requirements, functional capabilities)

Rationale: In some cases, the severity of the illness and the child's generally poor health may limit functioning so that the child is deprived of critical experiences resulting in poor social skills, lowered self-esteem, and greater dependence on parents than is developmentally appropriate.

☐ GOAL
The child will participate in school programs, family and peer activities; will be as independent from parents as developmentally appropriate.

☐ IMPLEMENTATION
- Assess the child's attitude toward the illness and treatment.
- Encourage compliance with treatment regimen.
- Encourage school attendance (educational continuity is of vital concern).
- Communicate regularly with teachers and com-

munity health providers when homebound/hospital teaching is needed.

- Help parents to think of creative ways to revise/adapt treatment routines allowing for play time with peers and other normalizing experiences in the community.
- Recommend participation in discussion, activity, or support groups (counseling) that can provide peer support and decrease social isolation.
- Teach the child to perform developmentally appropriate self-care activities and illness management tasks; counsel parents to encourage the child's independence in these areas.

☐ EVALUATION CRITERIA/DESIRED OUTCOMES

The child

- Performs developmentally appropriate self-care activities
- Participates in age-appropriate recreation with peers
- Expresses feelings

NURSING DIAGNOSIS #4

Social isolation related to the parents' gradual withdrawal from friends and community resources after diagnosis of chronic illness in their child

Rationale: Decreased energy, decreased financial resources, embarrassment or shame about their child's condition, and anger that others were spared the pain of a chronically ill child can lead to self-imposed social isolation.

☐ GOAL

The parents will develop and maintain social relationships with family members, friends, and neighbors; the family will utilize community resources appropriately.

☐ IMPLEMENTATION

- Assist parents in the identification of possible activities that promote enjoyable family and community interactions.
- Involve family in parent/sibling/family support groups, or in social/recreational activities sponsored by disease-related foundations or organizations.
- Promote the child's participation in school and after-school social activities.

☐ EVALUATION CRITERIA/DESIRED OUTCOMES

The family

- Participates regularly in social activities

NURSING DIAGNOSIS #5

Anxiety related to unpleasant treatments, prognosis, loss of control, and the variable course of the illness

Rationale: The child/parents experience anxiety when faced with learning and carrying out complex, often painful treatments; children and parents worry about what the future holds for them; parents' anxieties about their child's health may influence child-rearing patterns.

☐ GOAL

The child/parents will be supported while adjusting to the diagnosis of chronic illness; will express feelings and concerns to health care professionals; the parents will be motivated and comfortable in the daily care and decision making regarding their child.

☐ IMPLEMENTATION

- Assess child, parents, and sibling(s) for behaviors reflecting anxiety.
- Listen and give emotional support; refer for counseling if indicated or requested.
- Encourage child/family to learn about the illness and treatment.
- Prepare child for procedures or consequences of the illness in an age-appropriate manner.
- Give parents positive reinforcement for cooperation with treatment plan, learning new skills, and realistic child-rearing practices.
- Maintain sensitivity towards families who are battling with feelings of anxiety and may be angry with health care providers; consider mental health referral if appropriate.

☐ EVALUATION CRITERIA/DESIRED OUTCOMES

The child/parents

- Express feelings to the health care team
- Respond positively to the support and encouragement of team members
- Carry out treatments at home while maintaining positive family functioning
- Identify community resources that provide emotional support or services during the variable course of the child's illness

---

NURSING DIAGNOSIS #6

Activity intolerance related to illness and exacerbation of symptoms or treatment complications, with accompanying loss of functioning

---

☐ GOAL

The child will engage in daily care activities to the fullest extent possible as well as participate in developmentally appropriate recreation/social activities.

☐ IMPLEMENTATION

- Encourage the child to do as much daily personal care as the chronic illness will allow.
- Teach parents behavioral management techniques to reinforce the child's participation at home.
- Set up a schedule with consultation from health care team (physician, occupational and physical therapists) for participation in recreation activities and exercise programs; give praise and attention for the child's progress with the program.
- Assist the child to acquire and use self-help devices as well as adaptive equipment if recommended by health care team.
- Communicate the child's functional potential and recommended activity level (including rest periods if necessary) to school personnel; reassess functional potential periodically and communicate results to parents and school.

☐ EVALUATION CRITERIA/DESIRED OUTCOMES

The child
- Performs developmentally appropriate activities of daily living within limits of disability
- Participates in exercise program and/or recreational activities with peers on a regular basis

The parents
- Communicate regularly with health care team regarding child's functional potential and activity level

---

NURSING DIAGNOSIS #7

Knowledge deficit related to measures to promote maintenance of independent functioning, prevent complications, exacerbation of symptoms, deformities

---

☐ GOAL

The child/parents will verbalize an understanding of the chronic illness, treatment plan, use of medications, home care responsibilities, and available support services.

☐ IMPLEMENTATION

- Instruct in technical skills/procedures to be carried out at home; help parents decide what aspects of the management of the disease should be the child's responsibility (according to developmental/cognitive abilities).
- Teach how and when to communicate with the physician between clinic appointments, to describe ongoing management behaviors, personal observations, and the results of daily tests relevant to the child's condition.
- Refer to community health nurse to provide reinforcement of health teaching at home; help parents to communicate relevant information with school nurse.
- Teach about maintenance of medical or adaptive equipment to be used at home or school.
- Teach signs and symptoms of illness complications, including crisis situations and how to obtain emergency care.
- Reinforce importance of regular communication and follow-up appointments with health care team, community health nurse, and school nurse.
- Provide written information (if available) published by disease-specific foundations or associations, including educational programs sponsored by these organizations.

☐ EVALUATION CRITERIA/DESIRED OUTCOMES

The child/parents
- Describe the chronic illness and prescribed treatment program
- Demonstrate home management skills and use of medical or adaptive equipment
- Communicate concerns and information with health care providers at appropriate times
- Keep follow-up appointments
- Use community support services

The Child with
Chronic Renal Failure (CRF)

Definition/Discussion

Chronic renal failure is a progressive, irreversible deterioration of renal function leading to end-stage renal disease, which usually results in fatal uremia unless interventions of dialysis or kidney transplant are performed. The stages of CRF are
- *diminished renal reserve:* reduced renal function without the accumulation of metabolic wastes in the blood
- *renal insufficiency:* metabolic wastes begin to accumulate in the blood resulting in elevated BUN, serum creatinine, uric acid, and phosphorus levels
- *uremia:* excess amounts of nitrogenous wastes accumulate in the blood since the kidneys can no longer maintain homeostasis

Onset of CRF is usually slow with mild, intermittent symptoms.

Nursing Assessment

☐ PERTINENT HISTORY

Known renal disease, primary or secondary to trauma; surgery; metabolic disorders, especially diabetes mellitus and liver failure; family history of renal disease

☐ PHYSICAL FINDINGS

Refer to *The Child with Acute Renal Failure,* page 7; in addition, bronzing of skin; dry, brittle hair; uremic frost (i.e., whitish crystals on skin from waste products being excreted through perspiration); short stature, osteodystrophy, joint pain; amenorrhea; metabolic acidosis; hepatitis B, non-A and non-B (from multiple blood transfusions); condition of access site

☐ PSYCHOSOCIAL CONCERNS/ DEVELOPMENTAL FACTORS

Age, developmental level, compliance with the treatment protocol, support system, depression, powerlessness, social isolation, grieving, motivation, regression, habits (e.g., what comforts child, bedtime routines, favored objects)

☐ PATIENT AND FAMILY KNOWLEDGE

Options for treatment, participation in decision making, level of knowledge, readiness and willingness to learn

Nursing Care

☐ LONG-TERM GOAL

The child will maintain predialysis status as long as possible, living within restrictions imposed by the disease; the child/parents will deal with the possibility of long-term dialysis or renal transplant if feasible.

NURSING DIAGNOSES #1 to #3

Refer to Nursing Diagnoses #1, #2, and #3 in *The Child with Acute Renal Failure,* page 7.

NURSING DIAGNOSIS #4
a. **Grieving** related to loss of renal function, required life-style changes, poor prognosis
b. **Fear** related to unknown events, painful procedures, separation from family and friends, and anticipated death
c. **Ineffective individual/family coping** related to diagnosis, life-style changes, necessary decision making

Rationale: It is normal for a child with a chronic, disabling diagnosis to experience the stages of the grieving process (i.e., denial, anger, depression, bargaining, acceptance) as one perceives the loss of a normal bodily function, and changes in body image and normal life-style. The younger child has fears related to the separation from family and friends that are experienced with each hospitalization. Also, many painful procedures occur during hospitalization that increase the child's level of anxiety and inability to cope. Fear of dying is a normal reaction to CRF in the school-age child and adolescent. Many complications of CRF are life threatening and it is realistic to expect that the disease process will shorten the child's life span.

GOAL

The child will accept/adjust to body and role changes brought about by restrictions imposed by CRF; the child/parents will express feelings about life-style changes, concerns and fears about CRF.

IMPLEMENTATION

- Plan nursing care to allow for time each day to discuss specific aspects of the disease process, prescribed therapy, and treatment options; ask the child/parents to describe what this information means.
- Allow expression of feelings, limiting only those that are destructive; observe behaviors of the younger child for a more accurate assessment of feelings (e.g., crying, play activities).
- Structure interventions according to the stage in the grieving process; refer to *The Parent Experiencing Grief and Loss*, page 139.
- Arrange for the child/parents to confer with the nephrology nurse specialist, transplant coordinator, or dialysis nurse for detailed information about options being considered.
- Discuss goals and ability to meet the desired goals; focus on short-term rather than long-term expectations.
- Support adaptive coping mechanisms; assist child in finding alternatives if present strategies are not effective (e.g., if child is throwing things, then provide soft indoor ball, or encourage other energy-consuming activity).
- Utilize developmentally appropriate techniques to explain procedures (e.g., allow to insert needle into dolls, pre-op teaching).
- Make appropriate referrals if the child/parents are not adapting (e.g., express hopelessness, refuse to adhere to prescribed regimen), crisis intervention may be necessary; refer to *The Family Requiring Crisis Intervention*, page 85.
- Include parents and other family members in discussion; inform of support groups available in the community; initiate referrals for family therapy as necessary; confer with social services department to initiate referrals for financial assistance.
- Encourage self-care as appropriate for child's age and developmental level; encourage independence; provide realistic options and choices.

EVALUATION CRITERIA/DESIRED OUTCOMES

The child/parents
- Demonstrate verbal and nonverbal behaviors reflecting understanding and acceptance of the chronic course of renal failure

- Describe implications of life-style changes
- Verbalize feelings about death as appropriate for age and circumstances

---

NURSING DIAGNOSIS #5

Alteration in comfort: pain related to osteodystrophy

Rationale: *Inability of the kidneys to maintain electrolyte balance may result in disturbance of the calcium-phosphorus ratio; when the calcium-phosphorus product (i.e., serum calcium multiplied by serum phosphorus) exceeds 40, calcium phosphate crystals precipitate into soft tissue, and blood vessels. Bone deformities may develop.*

GOAL

The child will be free from joint pain; will maintain normal serum calcium and phosphorus levels.

IMPLEMENTATION

- Administer medications to regulate calcium/phosphorus balance.
- Monitor serum calcium and phosphorus levels; report elevated calcium-phosphorus product.
- Initiate comfort measures (e.g., heat, support, analgesics) when joint pain is present.
- Medicate for relief of pain as needed; avoid analgesics that are detoxified by the kidneys; monitor effects.

EVALUATION CRITERIA/DESIRED OUTCOMES

The child
- Maintains/regains normal serum calcium and phosphorus levels
- Is free from joint pain

NURSING DIAGNOSIS #6

Alteration in comfort (pruritus) related to uremic frost

Rationale: *In end-stage renal disease the kidneys are unable to excrete metabolic wastes so alternate routes of excretion are used by the body in an effort to compensate for the failure of this vital function. The child's perspiration will contain end products of metabolism, leaving an irritating whitish powder on the skin called uremic frost.*

GOAL

The child will be free from pruritus.

IMPLEMENTATION

- Bathe child at least daily and as needed; use minimal soap, to remove accumulated wastes; apply lubricating lotion (without additives) to prevent dryness.
- Turn at least every 2 hours if bedridden; massage back and coccyx with each turn; use sheepskin and other standard decubitus prevention measures for bony prominences.
- Use a solution of 2 tablespoons vinegar to 1 pint warm water to dissolve uremic crystals once they have developed; rinse with warm water.
- Explain that dialysis removes the metabolic wastes and thus decreases the likelihood of uremic frost developing.
- Explain the importance of not scratching skin surfaces; use mittens on infants and young children as appropriate; evaluate the need for medications to mnimize itching.

EVALUATION CRITERIA/DESIRED OUTCOMES

The child

- Reports decrease in or absence of pruritus
- Is free from uremic frost
- Does not scratch skin

NURSING DIAGNOSIS #7

Potential for injury related to motor, cognitive, and sensory deficits secondary to uremic encephalopathy

Rationale: Elevated serum ammonia levels are toxic to central nervous system tissues. In end-stage renal disease, decreased cognitive functioning may be evidenced. Problems with control of skeletal muscles may result in impaired physical mobility.

GOAL

The child will be free from physical injury; will be oriented to time, place, and person as appropriate for age and developmental level.

IMPLEMENTATION

- Monitor blood pH, BUN, serum creatinine, and ammonia.
- Assess neurologic status at least every 2–4 hours; observe for decreased interest in toys/games, tremors, peripheral numbness or loss of muscle strength, asterixis, convulsions, or decreased levels of consciousness.
- Utilize parents to assist with assessment of changes in LOC as much as possible.
- Inspect room for environmental hazards; discuss safety precautions with staff and child/parents.
- Orient child to unfamiliar surroundings; be sure to leave personal items and call button within reach prior to leaving room.
- Assist with ambulation as tolerated; if child requires a walker, or wheelchair, stress the importance of calling for assistance before getting out of bed or chair.
- Orient to time, place, and person as necessary; encourage conversation to maintain mental alertness and active participation in activities of daily living.

EVALUATION CRITERIA/DESIRED OUTCOMES

The child

- Is oriented to time, place, and person with no change in neurologic status
- Is free from injury

NURSING DIAGNOSIS #8

Knowledge deficit regarding treatment regimen

Rationale: An understanding of the disease process of CRF, including effects on each body system, potential complications, and life-style changes required can increase compliance with treatment. This knowledge is essential to support the highest quality of life within the constraints of the individual's condition.

GOAL

The child/parents will understand the progression of CRF, expected symptomatology, avoidable complications, prescribed diet, fluid restrictions, medications (e.g., toxic effects to be reported to physician), and treatment of choice for end-stage renal disease.

IMPLEMENTATION

- Establish a teaching plan according to specific learning needs of child/parents.
- Explain normal kidney function and the extent of renal function present; discuss how laboratory studies reflect ongoing renal status; identify signs and symptoms that might indicate changes in fluid and electrolyte balance; instruct to contact physician should problems develop.
- Instruct about the importance of daily weight as an indication of fluid retention; schedule conference with physician and parents to discuss amount of weight gain or loss to be reported.
- Review the signs and symptoms of infection and bleeding, stressing the importance of immediately informing the physician of their occurrence.
- Provide a list of prescribed medications; establish a daily schedule of administration with the child/parents; plan for specific medications to be given

on an empty stomach or with milk or meals; if antibiotics are ordered, explain why constant blood levels are desirable; ensure that toxic effects to be reported to physician are clearly understood.

- Discuss prescribed dietary regimen; explain why protein, sodium, potassium, and fluid are restricted; have dietician assist parents plan menus consistent with child's preferences as much as possible; reinforce information; provide a list of foods to be included and avoided; stress the importance of reading labels, especially on diet for sodium and potassium content.
- Establish a plan for providing continuing emotional support via individual, family, or group sessions in the community.

☐ **EVALUATION CRITERIA/DESIRED OUTCOMES**

The child/parents

- Describe disease course and acceptance of diagnosis
- List significant signs and symptoms, including toxic effects of prescribed medications, to be reported to physician
- Verbally commit to comply with prescribed diet and fluid restrictions
- Make arrangements for follow-up laboratory studies on an outpatient basis

The Child with a Cleft Lip/Cleft Palate

Definition/Discussion

Cleft lip is a failure of fusion of the primary palate ranging from just a small notch in the lip to a nonunion extending up to the floor of the nose. Cleft palate is a failure of fusion of the secondary palate and may involve only the uvula or extend through the soft and hard palates. These defects are congenital, bilateral or unilateral and occur separately or together.

Nursing Assessment

☐ PERTINENT HISTORY

Prenatal history, familial history of clefts; birth weight/length; growth patterns; weight gains/loss; feeding history; type of formula/breast milk, method, time involved; history of otitis media, upper respiratory infections; presence of oral prosthesis; previous surgeries; involvement of other disciplines (e.g., dentist, speech therapy, and audiology)

☐ PHYSICAL FINDINGS

Characteristics of cleft(s), respiratory status, hearing, presence of additional congenital defects, nutrition/hydration status, speech pattern

☐ PSYCHOSOCIAL CONCERNS/DEVELOPMENTAL FACTORS

Developmental level of child, habits at home; behaviors when upset and what provides comfort; self-esteem/coping methods of child/parents; observed interaction between family members and child, guilt or blaming behaviors

☐ PATIENT AND FAMILY KNOWLEDGE

Understanding of condition and therapies, level of knowledge, readiness and willingness to learn

Nursing Care

☐ LONG-TERM GOAL

The child will grow and develop normally; the parents will resolve feelings of producing a less-than-perfect newborn; the parents will love and adequately care for the child; the parents will adapt to the need for years of treatment of the child's defect.

NURSING DIAGNOSIS #1

Grieving related to the birth of a child with a congenital defect(s)

Rationale: Parents anticipate the birth of a perfect baby, not one with defects. Cleft lip is particularly visible and disfiguring, making it hard to accept. Cleft palate is not as visible but more serious.

☐ GOAL

The parents will accept the child and nurture appropriately.

☐ IMPLEMENTATION

- Allow parents to express their negative feelings toward the child; give them support; do not make judgments.
- Refer to *The Parent Experiencing Grief and Loss,* page 139.
- Schedule time with the parents; be an attentive listener; introduce the fact that with surgery and over time the child's defect can be corrected.
- Stress that child has the same needs as others (e.g., to be fed, held, kept warm and dry); encourage both parents to change, hold, and feed their child.
- Be a role model for the parents; show acceptance for the child as an individual.
- Praise parents for care-giving achievements.
- Point out positive aspects of infant (e.g., color of hair, eyes, turning towards parent's voice).
- Encourage parents to make realistic plans as to the necessity for future surgery, medical/psychologic follow-up, speech therapy.
- Encourage parents to have others (e.g., grandparents, babysitter) learn child's routine so they can have own time away from infant.

The parents
- Verbalize acceptance of child
- Demonstrate love of the child
- Stroke, touch, feed, play with, nurture baby appropriately

NURSING DIAGNOSIS #2

Alteration in nutrition: less than body requirements related to inability to suck effectively

Rationale: The child with a cleft lip/palate usually does not have an effective suck. As a result the child may aspirate and take a longer than normal time to feed. Feeding can become a frustrating experience for both child and parent.

□ **GOAL**

The child will gain weight/length along normal growth curve; parents will develop a successful, individualized feeding plan for child.

□ **IMPLEMENTATION**

- Explain to parents that the baby has trouble sucking because of the cleft(s); demonstrate feeding techniques to them and supervise them feeding baby.
- Help parents to find feeding method best suited to their child; if mother wishes to breastfeed, teach her to manually extend nipple and place it in child's mouth; use soft, regular cross-cut or premature nipples with the hole slightly enlarged, or cleft lip/palate nipples, or feeders from formula companies; if sucking methods are unsuccessful, use a large syringe with rubber tubing at the tip to squirt formula slowly in the side of the mouth.
- Assist parents to develop techniques to facilitate nipple use and sucking; make sure nipple is in normal feeding position, not in cleft; encourage sucking by stroking cheek or moving jaw; place index finger lengthwise over cleft in lip to help create suction.
- Feed the child in an upright position at all times; feed slowly, burp frequently, and rinse baby's mouth with water after every feeding.
- Praise parents for their efforts at feeding; encourage the holding and feeding of the baby in a relaxed manner (babies are very responsive to parental anxiety).
- Position the child in an infant seat or on side after feeding, not abdomen.
- Remove and clean maxillary prosthesis every day.
- Introduce post-op feeding method (e.g., rubber-

tipped syringe) a few days before lip repair so infant can become accustomed to it.
- Use a paper cup or side of plastic spoon for feeding after palate repair; do not use metal utensils or straws.

□ **EVALUATION CRITERIA/DESIRED OUTCOMES**

The child
- Takes feedings with no excessive stopping, crying, gasping, choking
- Shows weight/length increase along growth curve

The parents
- Verbalize satisfaction with feeding routine
- Take an acceptable amount of time, are not frustrated with feeding

---

NURSING DIAGNOSIS #3

Potential for infection related to malfunctioning eustachian tubes, aspiration, or surgery

Rationale: Children with cleft lip/palate are at risk for developing otitis media due to the high incidence of malfunctioning or malpositioned eustachian tubes; upper respiratory infection or aspiration are possible because of the direct connection between the nasal cavity and oropharynx.

□ **GOAL**

The child will be free from respiratory/ear infection; the parents will report signs of infection.

□ **IMPLEMENTATION**

- Monitor for and teach parents to notify health team when child has signs of infection (e.g., fever over 101°F [38.3°C], excessive mucus, coughing, rubbing ears, diarrhea, irritability).
- Keep child away from persons with upper respiratory disease.
- Reinforce good feeding techniques to prevent aspiration.
- Change position every 2 hours.

□ **EVALUATION CRITERIA/DESIRED OUTCOMES**

The child
- Is free from respiratory/ear infection

The parents
- Report signs of infection to health team

NURSING DIAGNOSIS #4

Alteration in oral mucous membranes related to surgical intervention

Rationale: Cleft lip/palate are a disruption in the oral cavity. Corrective surgery results in a further break in integrity. The suture line in the lip needs meticulous care to promote optimum cosmetic effect. Care for the palate suture line is difficult in the young child, but the suture line must be kept clean to ensure healing.

☐ GOAL

The child's suture lines will remain intact free from infection.

☐ IMPLEMENTATION

- Review appropriate post-op feeding techniques and oral hygiene preoperatively.
- Apply elbow restraints to prevent the child from putting hands or toys in mouth.
- Keep child from crying and putting tension on the suture line by anticipating needs (e.g., feeding, comforting, holding, rocking).
- Evaluate need for analgesics; evaluate effects after administration of medication.
- Keep catheter away from suture line when suctioning; avoid touching sutures during feeding or suctioning.
- Reposition at least every 2 hours in infant seat; move from side to side, but do not position on abdomen after lip repair; do not let baby rub face on sheets or on shoulders.
- Use distraction with an older child who is playing with suture lines with tongue (e.g., introduce new activities, divert attention).
- Feed infant with a rubber-tipped syringe to prevent sucking.
- Feed older child a liquid diet using a cup; do not allow child to suck or use a straw.
- Advance to a pureed diet for 6 weeks after palate repair.
- Clean incisions after each feeding; cleanse suture line of inner and outer lip gently with 1:1 water and hydrogen peroxide solution and sterile swabs, rinse with sterile water or saline; apply thin layer antibiotic ointment.
- Provide suture care for palate by rinsing mouth gently with water after each feeding.

☐ EVALUATION CRITERIA/DESIRED OUTCOMES

The child
- Has well-healed incision
- Has no disruption, redness, purulent drainage, fever

NURSING DIAGNOSIS #5

Ineffective airway clearance related to laryngeal and/or incisional edema

Rationale: Post-op laryngeal edema may occur as a result of intubation during surgery. Incisional edema may also cause respiratory compromise. After palate repair, the child must learn to breathe through smaller nasal passages. Clots may fall off the incision and block the airway. Either of these situations can cause respiratory distress.

☐ GOAL

The child will not experience respiratory compromise.

☐ IMPLEMENTATION

- Maintain patent airway; observe carefully for signs of respiratory distress (e.g., tachycardia, tachypnea, irritability, restlessness, retractions, nasal flaring, cyanosis, grunting).
- Observe for bleeding and excess mucus in the mouth and report to physician as necessary.
- Suction only when necessary using soft catheter, low suction; avoid suture lines.
- Monitor child's response to high-humidity oxygen tent if ordered.
- Position in infant seat or on side (may place on abdomen if only palate has been repaired).

☐ EVALUATION CRITERIA/DESIRED OUTCOMES

The child
- Appears comfortable
- Is afebrile
- Has no signs of respiratory distress

NURSING DIAGNOSIS #6

a. **Impaired physical mobility** related to restricted activity
b. **Altered growth and development** related to impaired mobility

Rationale: The use of restraints is necessary to prevent disruption of the suture line by the child. Restraints limit movement and exploration of the environment, may cause skin breakdown, altered muscle and nerve function, or developmental delay.

☐ GOAL

The child will be free from alteration in muscle or nerve function; will maintain age-appropriate developmental behavior.

☐ IMPLEMENTATION

- Introduce child and parents to elbow restraints before surgery; explain reason for use; explain

that hands are still free, just cannot bend elbows to get to mouth; have parents apply restraints periodically in the week prior to surgery.
- Send restraints to OR with child; ensure that they are applied correctly.
- Remove restraints one at a time, every hour, to allow range of motion; watch child carefully so hand does not go near mouth.
- Reinforce the importance of keeping restraints on until sutures are healed (e.g., usually 2 weeks for a lip repair and 6 weeks after palate repair).
- Encourage safe age-appropriate activity (e.g., holding, cuddling, singing to child, looking at books, touching different textured objects, picking up small objects and putting them in container, puzzles, clay, walkers, swings, wagon rides, walking).
- Allow child to express frustration at having restraints on, providing the expressions do not disrupt the suture line (e.g., excessive crying).

☐ EVALUATION CRITERIA/DESIRED OUTCOMES

The child
- Has no skin excoriation around restraints
- Has good pulses, sensation, movement, temperature of upper extremities
- Performs age-appropriate skills

NURSING DIAGNOSIS #7

Impaired verbal communication related to impaired muscle development, insufficient palate function, or hearing loss

Rationale: Children with cleft palate often have a hypernasal quality to their speech, have inadequate function of palatal and pharyngeal muscles, and are prone to recurrent ear infections that may lead to hearing loss. All of these may interfere with the acquisition of normal speech patterns. Children with cleft palates should not have tonsillectomies or adenoidectomies since this tissue is thought to aid in forming a seal between naso- and oropharynx during swallowing or phonation and removal often exacerbates speech defects.

☐ GOAL

The child will have understandable speech patterns; will have otitis media promptly recognized and treated.

☐ IMPLEMENTATION
- Know that the best speech outcome correlates with early palate repair (3–6 months of age).
- Coordinate referrals (e.g., speech therapist, psy-chologist, dentist/orthodontist, audiologist) and follow-up to ensure consistency of care.
- Teach parents symptoms of otitis media (e.g., irritability, pulling at ear, withdrawn or inactive) and to note child's response to voices/noise.
- Actively listen to child when speaking, be a role model for good speech patterns.

☐ EVALUATION CRITERIA/DESIRED OUTCOMES

The child
- Speaks in an understandable, age-appropriate manner
- Hears others speaking
- Uses hearing aid if needed

The parents
- List signs of otitis media

NURSING DIAGNOSIS #8

Disturbance in self-concept: self-esteem related to facial deformity and speech impediment

Rationale: Children with cleft lip/palate, having obvious deviations from normal regarding appearance and speech, are often stared at and teased by others. These children often feel abnormal and need extra assistance in developing and maintaining a positive self-concept.

☐ GOAL

The child will develop a positive self concept; will be free from adverse psychologic effects of facial deformity.

☐ IMPLEMENTATION
- Encourage parents to discuss their feelings so they can support the child.
- Explain to parents that encouraging child to accomplish age-appropriate developmental tasks will encourage mastery and a sense of achievement.
- Be a good role model by showing acceptance of child.
- Use age-appropriate techniques to encourage child to verbalize feelings about defect and response of others; refer to *The Child Requiring Play Therapy*, page 226; discern how child handles feelings of inadequacy, sadness.
- Role play with child how to handle situations where others tease.
- Read books with child and discuss stories of others with deformities/handicaps.
- Provide parents with information on dolls available with cleft lip/handicaps.
- Encourage endeavors in which the child has demonstrated success.

- Provide opportunity for child's class to visit the hospital.
- Initiate mental health referrals if indicated.

☐ EVALUATION CRITERIA/DESIRED OUTCOMES

The child
- Verbalizes that others like/love him/her, likes self
- Plays with peers
- Demonstrates affection; hugs/kisses others
- Smiles, laughs, plays appropriately
- Demonstrates no signs of depression; sleeps well, does well in school, has appropriate appetite

The parents
- Demonstrate love, approval, support, acceptance of child

NURSING DIAGNOSIS #9

Knowledge deficit related to condition, feeding and suctioning techniques, surgical site care, risks of otitis media

Rationale: In order to provide optimal care, child/parents must have adequate knowledge and understanding of condition and complications.

☐ GOAL

The child will be free from preventable complications; the child/parents will verbalize an understanding of the condition and treatment.

☐ IMPLEMENTATION

- Explain condition to parents as they are able to cope with information; include information about cause, anatomy, complications (e.g., otitis media, malocclusion, need for speech therapy) and infant needs for love and security.
- Be present when physician discusses plan for corrective surgeries; reiterate and clarify information as needed.
- Demonstrate proper feeding and suctioning techniques; have parents return demonstrate.
- Have parents do return demonstrations on care of surgical site(s).
- Discuss with parents reasons for minimizing crying, sucking, laughing, or blowing after surgery; explain rationale for positioning.
- Assist parents to provide child's teacher with information about cleft lip/palate as needed.
- Give parents written instructions for care; phone number to call for questions/assistance.

☐ EVALUATION CRITERIA/DESIRED OUTCOMES

The child
- Is free from complications

The parents
- Verbalize need for corrective surgery and possible later revisions
- Verbalize need for speech therapy; probablility of need for orthodontia
- Demonstrate appropriate feeding, suctioning, and restraint techniques, and care of surgical site(s)

The Child with a Common Communicable Disease

Definition/Discussion

Communicable diseases are those caused by a specific agent or its toxic products, transmitted either by direct contact or indirectly through contaminated articles. Encephalitis may be a complication of systemic viral illness in mumps, rubella, chickenpox, and especially measles. There is some evidence that Reye's syndrome may be linked with some viral illnesses, especially chickenpox. Table 4 details the wide variety of communicable diseases; some are more frequently seen than others. Appropriate childhood immunizations have resulted in a significant decrease in the incidence of many of these diseases.

The nursing care presented in this guide pertains to the commonly encountered communicable diseases: chicken pox, measles, and mumps.

Nursing Assessment

☐ **PERTINENT HISTORY**

Recent exposure to communicable disease, recent travel, anyone ill at home, immunization status of child and family, treatment of symptoms

☐ **PHYSICAL FINDINGS**

Vital signs, weight (present and healthy), review of systems for symptoms pertinent to each disease (see table 4).

☐ **PSYCHOSOCIAL CONCERNS/ DEVELOPMENTAL FACTORS**

Age, developmental level, previous coping mechanisms, extended family support, use of community resources, use of folk remedies for treatment, habits (e.g., what comforts child, eating/bedtime routines, favored objects)

☐ **PATIENT AND FAMILY KNOWLEDGE**

Disease pathology, treatment, acceptance of/need for compliance with treatment, ability to accept/enforce measures to decrease communicability; level of knowledge, readiness and willingness to learn

Nursing Care

☐ **LONG-TERM GOAL**

The child will remain free from communicable disease OR will regain optimal health, free from complications; the child will resume former roles in home, family, and society; the child will not pose a threat to the health of others.

NURSING DIAGNOSIS #1

Potential for infection related to susceptibility of exposed individual, virulence of organism

Rationale: There are many variables affecting the communicability of disease from carrier to person, including immunization/health status, age, maturity/ functioning of immunologic system of exposed individual, and virulence/innoculating dose of infecting organism. A natural active immunity may occur when the child has experienced/been exposed to a disease (e.g., measles, mumps). Occasionally, however, recovering from the disease does not ensure adequate immunity and immunizations are still required (e.g., diphtheria).

☐ **GOAL**

The child will receive appropriate immunizations; the child/parents will take steps to limit exposure of others if disease is present.

☐ **IMPLEMENTATION**

• Recommend appropriate immunization schedules using the current American Academy of Pediatrics guidelines as prevention is the best treatment (see table 5).
• Teach signs of immunization reactions

DPT (diphtheria, pertussis, tetanus): local reaction at site (e.g., induration, redness, nodule, mild temperature elevation, irritability)

TOPV (trivalent oral polio vaccine): reportedly none

MMR (measles, mumps, rubella): fever, rash (symptoms usually occur 5–12 days after vaccination); transient arthritis and arthralgia (1–3 weeks after vaccination)

- Report severe reactions (e.g., fever of 105°F [40.5°C] or greater, severe swelling of injection site, shock-like episode, seizures, persistent/unusual crying lasting greater than 3 hours).
- Give Haemophilus influenza, type B (HIB) vaccine in single dose to all children between the ages of 2 and 6 years, and in children, aged 18–24 months who are in day care; inform parents that vaccine is unlikely to be completely effective in the 18- to 24-month-old group; discuss side effects (usually only local reaction at site and occasional fever) and alternative of vaccination (high risk of developing some type of HIB disease in early childhood); administer rifampin prophylaxis to household contacts of HIB cases as ordered.
- Give yearly immunization against influenza to high risk (e.g., chronically ill) children.
- Teach child/family with communicable diseases to avoid contact with previously noninfected persons, pregnant women (especially with rubella and chickenpox), immunocompromised, debilitated, and elderly individuals; exclude from day care children who develop acute diarrhea.
- Notify day care centers, schools, parents, and public health department of communicable disease cases as appropriate.
- Exclude immunocompromised children from school/day care during epidemics.
- Teach necessary isolation techniques as appropriate.

☐ **EVALUATION CRITERIA/DESIRED OUTCOMES**

The child/family
- Is immunized appropriately for age
- States specific measures to limit exposure to others

NURSING DIAGNOSIS #2
a. **Impaired gas exchange** related to disease process
b. **Ineffective airway clearance** related to disease process
c. **Ineffective breathing pattern** related to neurologic damage

Rationale: Bronchopneumonia, one of the chief complications of measles, may be caused by the measles virus itself or due to secondary bacterial invasion; refer to *The Child with Pneumonia*, page 228.

NURSING DIAGNOSIS #3
a. **Alteration in comfort: pain** related to disease process
b. **Alteration in comfort** (pruritus) related to rash
c. **Impairment of skin integrity** related to rash

Rationale: Fever, chills, headache, myalgia, and malaise occur with influenza. Mumps is characterized by painful swelling of the parotid gland(s); in postpubertal males orchitis may occur. Individuals with rubella, especially older females, may have arthralgia, tenderness and swelling of the joints. The rash of chickenpox is characteristically pruritic, occasionally severe. The rashes of measles and rubella may or may not produce mild pruritus. Secondary bacterial infection is a potential complication when there is any break in skin integrity; it is the most common complication of chickenpox.

☐ **GOAL**

The child will experience minimal pain, discomfort; will be free from secondary bacterial infection of skin lesions.

☐ **IMPLEMENTATION**

- Refer to *The Child Experiencing Pain*, page 216.
- Treat symptomatically: maintain bedrest as appropriate; suggest acetaminophen for fever/discomfort; teach not to give aspirin with viral disease because of the possible association with Reye's syndrome.
- Educate postpubertal mumps patients to remain in bed until afebrile; suggest a soft, nonacidic diet, support scrotum if orchitis occurs; apply ice packs to relieve parotid discomfort.
- Clip child's nails and keep hands clean; put mittens on young child to prevent scratching; teach older child to apply pressure to pruritic area instead of scratching.
- Give tepid baths, apply topical antipruritic/anesthetic.
- Administer oral antihistamine as ordered; monitor for desired effect.
- Bathe child often with mild soap and water to prevent infection.
- Refer child to primary health care provider for treatment of infected vesicles with oral antibiotics (topical antibiotics are sensitizing and should not be used).

EVALUATION CRITERIA/DESIRED OUTCOMES

The child
- Has pain controlled with nursing interventions
- Has no verbal complaints or nonverbal indicators of pain
- Obtains adequate rest
- States itching is under control, appears comfortable
- Obtains uninterrupted sleep periods
- Is free from secondary bacterial infection

NURSING DIAGNOSIS #4

Fluid volume deficit related to disease process

Rationale: If basal metabolic rate and insensible water loss are increased (e.g., with fever, diaphoresis, tachypnea) and/or fluid intake is decreased because of anorexia, the child is at risk for dehydration.

GOAL

The child will maintain proper fluid balance.

IMPLEMENTATION

- Refer to *The Child with a Fever*, page 128.
- Monitor intake and output carefully; maintain proper fluid and electrolyte intake/replacement.
- Assess for signs of dehydration (e.g., dry mucous membranes, poor skin turgor, decreased urine output, increased heart and respiratory rates, decreased blood pressure [later sign in child], plus depressed eyeballs, sunken fontanel in young child).

EVALUATION CRITERIA/DESIRED OUTCOMES

The child
- Has vital signs within normal limits for age
- Maintains good skin turgor and urine output

NURSING DIAGNOSIS #5

Diversional activity deficit related to isolation from peers

Rationale: Once diagnosed and until the period of communicability has elapsed, the child will be isolated from individuals at risk. This usually includes peers in school and day-care settings and siblings. Often the child with a mild form of a communicable disease may not feel ill and can become easily bored and restless.

GOAL

The child will engage in selected age-appropriate activities while maintaining isolation from peers, family members.

IMPLEMENTATION

- Provide age-appropriate quiet activities (e.g., artwork, records, TV, board games).
- Know that children with measles may be photosensitive; restrict reading, bright lights, TV, close work, if troublesome.
- Introduce new quiet activities (e.g., knitting, building models, listening to recorded books).
- Allow child to rest in an area where s/he can observe others.
- Provide attractive meals, colorful fluids to increase intake and vary stimuli.
- Rotate nonsusceptible caregivers to vary contacts; avoid heavy burden on one person.
- Involve child in planning daily schedule, choosing activities.
- Provide school work if appropriate; encourage phone calls to friends if desired.
- Provide bathtub play, especially if child has pruritis, rash.

EVALUATION CRITERIA/DESIRED OUTCOMES

The child
- Plays quietly
- Offers no expressions of boredom
- Participates in a variety of quiet activities

NURSING DIAGNOSIS #6

Knowledge deficit regarding disease process and goals of treatment

Rationale: Insufficient knowledge about the disease process could result in decreased ability to prevent the disease, increased chances of spreading the disease, and lack of appropriate care and treatment measures.

GOAL

The child/family will be knowledgeable about the disease process.

IMPLEMENTATION

- Teach the importance of active immunization early in life with boosters at appropriate intervals to maintain immunity status and to keep a permanent record of family immunizations.
- Review the description of disease, methods of control, and action needed for the health and education of the child, contacts, and community, including environmental control.

- Give specific guidelines regarding day care, school attendance.
- Urge immediate medical care for exposed children, particularly those who have not been actively immunized or who are immuno-compromised; refer all contacts of confirmed cases for medical examination and surveillance according to health department policy.
- If a communicable disease is diagnosed, instruct regarding comfort measures, isolation requirements, signs of complications.

☐ **EVALUATION CRITERIA/DESIRED OUTCOMES**

The child/family

- States importance of obtaining/keeping up to date with immunizations and immunization schedule
- States how specific disease is transmitted and methods to decrease communicating it to others
- States appropriate care measures for specific disease
- Describes appropriate dosage, schedule, and side effects of any medications administered
- Lists signs of complications and states when and to whom to report them

Table 4
Communicable Diseases

Disease	Incubation Period	Communicability	Symptoms
Chickenpox (Varicella)	11–21 days	Few days prior to onset of symptoms until all vesicles have crusted over	Moderate fever, headache, malaise, occasional sore throat, discrete lesions characterized by macules, papules, vesicles, and crusting
Diphtheria	1–4 days	Variable until virulent bacilli have disappeared from discharges and lesions (usually 2 wks)	Tough, fibrinous, grayish membrane, usually on the tonsils or nasopharynx; sore throat, dysphagia, fever, nausea, vomiting, chills, enlarged and tender cervical lymph glands, edema of the neck (severe cases)
German Measles (Rubella)	14–21 days	7 days prior to 5 days after onset of rash	Malaise, fever, headache, rhinitis, postauricular and suboccipital lymphadenopathy, rash for 3 days, stiff joints
Giardiasis	Possibly years	Via fecal-oral route, contaminated water; cysts are able to service from hours to weeks on environmental surfaces	Nausea; flatulence; epigastric pain; abdominal cramps; distension; watery, foul-smelling diarrhea; weight loss
Haemophilus Influenza, Type B (HIB)	Within 2–4 days	Length unknown, probably as long as organisms are present in upper respiratory tract, even without a nasal discharge	Fever, headache, rhinitis, coughing, lethargy, decreased appetite often progressing to anorexia, ear infections, epiglottitis, upper and lower respiratory tract infection, cellulitis, arthritis, osteomyelitis, carditis, septicemia, meningitis
Influenza	48 hours	Probably 3 days from clinical onset	Chills and fever, rhinitis, cough, headache, malaise, inflamed respiratory mucous membranes, generalized aches and pains

Table 4
Communicable Diseases, Cont.

Disease	Incubation Period	Communicability	Symptoms
Measles (Rubeola)	8–18 days	4 days prior to 4 days after appearance of rash; most infectious just prior to onset of rash; spread is person to person via respiratory droplets; airborne and fomite transmission are possible	Koplick's spots, fever, rhinitis, cough, conjunctivitis, photophobia, mild pruritus, leukopenia
Mumps	14–24 days	7 days before to 9 days after onset of parotid swelling; height of infectiousness just before and after onset of swelling	Painful enlargement of the salivary glands, usually the parotids; chills and fever, headache, anorexia, malaise, dysphagia
Whooping Cough (Pertussis)	6–20 days	Early catarrhal stage after paroxysmal cough, gradually decreasing over 4 weeks	Paroxysmal or spasmodic cough that ends in a prolonged, high-pitched, crowing inspiration; anorexia, listlessness, copious amounts of viscid mucus, vomiting
Poliomyelitis	3–5 days (minor illness) 7–14 days (major illness)	Not known precisely; virus found soon after infection, persists about 1 week in throat, 4–6 weeks in feces	Fever, headache, stiff neck and back, malaise, sore throat, deep muscle pain, sometimes flaccid paralysis of various muscle groups
Salmonella	8–48 hr after ingestion of contaminated food	Via fecal-oral route, water, food, especially milk, flies; antibiotic therapy of uncomplicated salmonella gastroenteritis can increase symptoms, prolong carrier state, and lead to the emergence of resistent strains	Fever, nausea and vomiting, cramping, abdominal pain, diarrhea; incubation period: 8–48 hr after ingestion of contaminated food
Shigellosis	1–4 days	Via fecal-oral route, contaminated food, and inanimate objects; organism does not survive well outside the human host, but the number of organisms required to produce illness is very small; person-to-person transmission is most common mode of spread	Fever, irritability, drowsiness, anorexia, nausea, vomiting, diarrhea, tenesmus

Table 5
Recommended Immunization Schedule

Age/ Immunization	Side Effects	Contraindications	Nursing Implications
			Inform parents of benefits/risks of all vaccines; obtain informed consent.
2 Months DPT	Mild: tenderness, induration, nodule at site; irritability, fever Serious (report to physician): fever > 105°F, convulsions, prolonged screaming longer than 3 hours, severe alteration in LOC, shocklike episode, allergic reaction	Previous reactions, developing or progressive CNS disease	Rotate injection sites during primary series, warm compresses to site, acetaminophen as ordered.

Table 5
Recommended Immunization Schedule, Cont.

Age/ Immunization	Side Effects	Contraindications	Nursing Implications
TOPV	Serious: Paralytic disease in vaccines or unimmunized contact	Live virus vaccine: do not give if immunosuppressed or immunodeficient	Assess for immunodeficiency or unimmunized contacts in home; check with physician to arrange for them to be immunized with inactivated polio vaccine; if OPV given, educate about strict handwashing techniques (virus shed through stool).
4 Months DPT TOPV			
6 Months DPT (TOPV)			TOPV optional, may be given in areas with increased risk of exposure to polio.
15 Months MMR	Measles: mild transient rash, fever 5–12 days postvaccination Serious: rarely encephalopathy, allergic reaction in those hypersensitive to eggs (vaccine grown in chick embryo cultures) Mumps: mild fever, rarely parotitis	Live virus vaccines: do not give if immunosuppressed or immunodeficient	Assess for history of anaphylactic reaction to eggs; give SQ
	Rubella: rarely: rash, low-grade fever, lymphadenopathy; transient arthritis and arthralgia 1–3 weeks postvaccination, persists 1–3 days (rare in those under 12 years, frequent in older)	Pregnant women	
18 Months DPT TOPV			HIB given now if in daycare; better "take" if given at 24 months.
24 Months HIB	Tenderness, induration at site, fever, irritability		Give SQ
4–6 Years DPT TOPV			Should be given before entering school.
14–16 Years Td			Repeat every 10 years.

DPT = diphtheria, pertussis, tetanus
TOPV = trivalent oral polio vaccine
MMR = measles, mumps, rubella
HIB = Haemophilus b polysaccharide vaccine
Td = tetanus, diphtheria (adult dose)

The Child with Congenital Heart Disease: Medical Management

Definition/Discussion

Congenital heart disease occurs when there is an embryologic developmental defect in cardiac structure/function resulting in an abnormal opening, obstructive lesions, stricture of a valve, incomplete closure of the ductus arteriosus, or abnormal vessel configuration.

Nursing Assessment

☐ **PERTINENT HISTORY**

Type of cardiac defect, physiologic response to defect (e.g., cyanosis, activity restrictions), medications, recent exposure to illness (e.g., especially upper respiratory infection), previous palliative/surgical procedures

☐ **PHYSICAL FINDINGS**

Tachycardia, blood pressure (comparison of upper and lower extremities), tachypnea, dyspnea, retractions, skin color, pulses, presence of murmur/thrill/clubbing, feeding pattern, pattern of weight gain, complete blood count

☐ **PSYCHOSOCIAL CONCERNS/DEVELOPMENTAL FACTORS**

Developmental level, coping mechanisms, usual routines of child/family, previous experience with hospitalization

☐ **PATIENT AND FAMILY KNOWLEDGE**

Understanding of diagnosis, knowledge/acceptance of prognosis, medication regimen, future plans for care; level of knowledge, readiness and willingness to learn

Nursing Care

☐ **LONG-TERM GOAL**

The child will have the cardiac defect detected and the cardiopulmonary status will be stablized; the child will develop physically and psychosocially within the limitations imposed by the defect; the parents will be assisted to cope with the child's diagnosis and prognosis.

NURSING DIAGNOSIS #1
a. **Alteration in cardiac output: decreased** related to heart malformation
b. **Fluid volume excess** related to alteration in cardiac output
c. **Potential for injury** related to cardiac catheterization

Rationale: The child with congenital heart disease may experience decreased cardiac output due to the malformation, which in turn may lead to congestive heart failure (CHF) characterized by fluid volume excess. After a cardiac catheterization to diagnose the nature and severity of the defect, hemorrhage/infection may occur at the insertion site.

☐ **GOAL**

The child will remain free from complications associated with the treatment of cardiac defect.

☐ **IMPLEMENTATION**

- Observe quality and strength of apical and peripheral pulses, color and warmth of the skin.
- Establish baseline degree of cyanosis (e.g., circumoral, digital, mucous membranes, degree of polycythemia, clubbing).
- Monitor for symptoms of CHF (e.g., irritability, tachycardia, tachypnea, dyspnea, fatigue when feeding, anorexia, periorbital edema, oliguria, hepatomegaly).
- Prepare child/parents for cardiac catheterization and other diagnostic procedures (e.g., x-rays) as needed.

Pre-cardiac catheterization
- Teach parents purpose of test.
- Keep child NPO 4–6 hours pretest.
- Give infant pacifier and offer comfort.
- Obtain baseline vital signs including brachial and pedal pulses.

Post-cardiac catheterization
- Maintain pressure dressing at insertion site.
- Monitor catheter insertion site for bleeding every hour (e.g., watch for blood oozing around the dressing, any area blood may accumulate as a result of gravity).
- Monitor pulses and skin warmth, color distal to insertion site every hour.
- Monitor vital signs every 2 hours.
- Monitor for signs of infection; keep site clean and dry; change diapers frequently.

☐ **EVALUATION CRITERIA/DESIRED OUTCOMES**

The child
- Maintains vital signs within normal limits
- Is free from bleeding/infection at catheter insertion site
- Is free from dyspnea, cyanosis, edema

NURSING DIAGNOSIS #2

Impaired gas exchange related to pulmonary congestion

Rationale: In some congenital heart defects large amounts of blood may pool in the lungs resulting in pulmonary vascular congestion and compromised pulmonary compliance. This makes the child more susceptible to recurrent respiratory infections.

☐ **GOAL**

The child will be free from pulmonary congestion; will have signs of respiratory infection recognized and treated promptly.

☐ **IMPLEMENTATION**
- Monitor quality and rate of respirations; listen to lung sounds; report diminished breath sounds, rales, rhonchi, cough, or retractions.
- Encourage coughing and deep breathing if able.
- Position child upright to allow maximal diaphragmatic excursion.

☐ **EVALUATION CRITERIA/DESIRED OUTCOMES**

The child
- Shows improvement of respiratory status
- Has improved breath sounds

NURSING DIAGNOSIS #3

Alteration in nutrition: less than body requirements related to fatigue during eating and increased caloric requirements

Rationale: Infants with CHF tire easily during feedings and may be able to take only small amounts. However, caloric requirements are increased due to the hypoxemia caused by respiratory distress. Decreased intake and increased caloric needs result in inadequate nutrition.

☐ **GOAL**

The child will ingest adequate food and fluids to maintain normal weight and support growth.

☐ **IMPLEMENTATION**
- Weigh every morning without diaper on same scale, at the same time, and record.
- Record intake and output accurately; weigh diapers (subtract dry weight from wet weight; 1 gram = 1 cc).
- Provide small, frequent feedings to reduce fatigue associated with the work of eating.
- Feed cyanotic infant in knee-chest position; use a soft, "preemie" nipple, allow frequent rests and burping; use blow-by oxygen to decrease respiratory distress caused by the work of sucking.
- Adjust concentration of formula to increase calorie content per ounce if ordered (may add Polycose or MCT oil).
- Know that children on diuretics are very thirsty; diuretic dosages are usually adjusted so fluids do not have to be restricted.
- Provide sodium-restricted diet as necessary and when age appropriate.

☐ **EVALUATION CRITERIA/DESIRED OUTCOMES**

The child
- Shows steady weight gain along growth curve
- Increases tolerance of feedings

NURSING DIAGNOSIS #4

a. **Ineffective family coping** related to diagnosis/prognosis of child
b. **Alteration in parenting** related to hospitalization, fears of child's illness

Rationale: The parents of a child with congenital heart disease have many feelings as they grieve for the "lost" perfect child. Dealing effectively with these feelings will allow the parents to move ahead and assume care for the child and make responsible decisions concerning future treatment. Not dealing with feelings may lead to ineffective coping and altered parenting skills.

☐ GOAL

The parents will express feelings regarding the birth of an imperfect child; will discuss fears of the unknown and concerns over proposed treatment plan; will express a belief that they have important roles in successful treatment plan.

☐ IMPLEMENTATION

- Explore parents' concerns and feelings of fear, guilt, anger, grief, and inadequacy.
- Reduce parents' fears and anxieties by giving information and comforting support.
- Refer to *The Parent Experiencing Grief and Loss*, page 139.
- Support and reassure parents to enable them to effectively comfort the child.
- Involve the parents in the child's care; provide/ reinforce simple explanations and demonstrations.
- Explain to parents the reality of the diagnosis (e.g., if problems are more likely to develop gradually than suddenly).
- Provide access to parent-support groups if available.
- Answer parents' questions honestly about prognosis, future surgery as necessary; see *The Child Undergoing Cardiac Surgery*, page 43.
- Encourage parents to include others (e.g., grandparents, sitters) in child's care to prevent exhaustion.
- Assist parents to obtain religious consultation, baptism for infant if requested.

☐ EVALUATION CRITERIA/DESIRED OUTCOMES

The parents
- Discuss concerns and seek help appropriately
- Assist in formulating a treatment plan
- Demonstrate improved ease and competence in caring for their child

---

NURSING DIAGNOSIS #5

a. **Altered growth and development** related to congenital heart disease
b. **Alteration in family processes** related to the adjustments necessitated by child's condition

Rationale: The child's condition may necessitate adjustments in family routines, resulting in difficulty meeting the normal developmental needs of the child as well as meeting needs of other family members. Family functions also may be disrupted.

☐ GOAL

The child's physical, motor, cognitive and social development will be maintained at near normal levels; the parents will express strategies for fostering normal growth and development, maintaining near normal family life.

☐ IMPLEMENTATION

- Initiate the process of helping the parents cope with child's age-related developmental needs (e.g., discipline, self-esteem, play); refer to *Normal Growth and Development*, pages 300–314.
- Reinforce that most children with cyanotic heart disease can tolerate short periods of crying despite increased cyanosis.
- Emphasize the importance of treating the child normally to avoid overdependency; model this behavior for parents.
- Prepare parents for the possibility of developmental delays or activity intolerance as child grows; counsel them regarding appropriate age-related physical activities.
- Remind parents that child has all the needs of a normal child and must be followed by a pediatrician (e.g., to monitor noncardiac health status, receive immunizations).
- Help parents develop strategies to avoid exaggerated sibling rivalry or resentment of the increased attention given to the child with heart disease.

☐ EVALUATION CRITERIA/DESIRED OUTCOMES

The child
- Progresses toward normal developmental milestones
- Receives routine pediatric care (unrelated to cardiac problems)
- Has appropriate sibling and family interactions

The parents
- Describe methods to set limits without being overprotective
- Identify strategies for maintaining near normal family life

---

NURSING DIAGNOSIS #6

Knowledge deficit regarding follow-up care and necessary medications

Rationale: The parents need to understand plan of care and medications so they can contribute to the plan, follow the child's progress closely, monitor effectiveness/side effects of medications, and report any adverse signs immediately.

GOAL

The parents will verbalize an understanding of the congenital heart defect, the child's condition, treatment aims, and anticipated outcomes of the selected therapeutic regimen; will administer cardiac medications with accuracy and safety; will demonstrate understanding of indications and possible side effects.

IMPLEMENTATION

- Instruct parents regarding signs of CHF, diet, and activities.
- Teach parents interventions to conserve child's energy and relieve frightening symptoms.
- Teach parents appropriate dosages, schedule, methods of administration, and side effects of each medication ordered
  - allow infants to suck medications through a nipple; use dropper or syringe for older infants/children
  - give medications 1 hour before or 2 hours after feedings; do not mix with foods or formula for administration
  - consult with physician for guidelines regarding missed or possibly vomited doses of drugs
  - keep all medications out of reach of all children in the family
- Teach parents that children with congenital heart disease are more seriously affected by diarrhea or prolonged vomiting when they occur; tell parents to notify physician immediately at first signs of diarrhea or vomiting (child may require hospitalization for parenteral doses of medications or temporary dosage adjustment).
- Teach parents to keep child from being exposed to others with upper respiratory infections.
- Explain signs that indicate complications and discuss where and whom to contact for help.
- Provide the names and phone numbers of persons to contact should problems develop.

EVALUATION CRITERIA/DESIRED OUTCOMES

The parents
- Verbalize treatment aims
- Demonstrate competence in special techniques used in caring for child
- Demonstrate accurate administration of medications
- Describe medication names, actions, dosages, side effects, and schedule
- State when and whom to contact in case of questions/problems

The Family Requiring Crisis Intervention

Definition/Discussion

Crisis intervention refers to those approaches used to restore someone to a state of emotional equilibrium, from one of disequilibrium (the crisis state), that is equal to or better than the functioning at the precrisis level.

Nursing Assessment

☐ **PERTINENT HISTORY**

Recent illness or loss; stresses of the past year; transitions; trauma, catastrophic illness or accident; job, family stability; decreased ability to carry out activities of daily living (ADL); current threatening event

☐ **PHYSICAL FINDINGS**

Altered vital signs, anxiety (e.g., moderate, severe, panic), decreased concentration, somatic complaints, agitation, tension, neglect in self-care

☐ **PSYCHOSOCIAL CONCERNS/ DEVELOPMENTAL FACTORS**

Developmental level, normal coping methods, supportive or dysfunctional family history, ego strengths, dependency patterns, apathy, distorted perceptions, regression to lower levels of functioning, habits/routines at home

☐ **PATIENT AND FAMILY KNOWLEDGE**

Previous experiences; perception of the problem, severity of disruption; internal and outside support or agencies; ability to decrease anxiety; socialization, interpersonal, and communication skills; level of knowledge, readiness and willingness to learn

Nursing Care

☐ **LONG-TERM GOAL**

The child/family will achieve adaptive resolution of the crisis; the child/family will return to usual roles with a realistic perception of what has occurred and with adequate coping mechanisms.

NURSING DIAGNOSIS #1

Ineffective individual/family coping related to perceived inability to deal with problem, distorted perception of the problem

Rationale: Usual coping mechanisms may not prevent increased stress when a threatening event occurs. The child/family may have a distorted perception of the problem and may feel unable to deal with it. The inability to manage the stress situation results in disequilibrium.

☐ **GOAL**

The child/family will state perception of stressful situation and develop coping mechanisms effective in the crisis state.

☐ **IMPLEMENTATION**

* Assess feelings regarding the stressful event and what the perception of the problem is; remember child's/family's perception is what is important and may differ from yours.
* Allow to respond at length and in detail to your questions; do not challenge any statements; try to determine exactly what is most threatening; listen and encourage child/family to keep talking.
* Determine the real/anticipated loss(es) involved; assess behavior in light of the grief and mourning process.
* Determine usual coping strategies and how successful these methods are.
* Encourage verbalization about supportive individuals or agencies and whether or not they would be of value in the present situation.
* Ask what you could do to make child/family feel better right now; if at all possible, provide it.
* Provide basic needs; if child becomes very dependent in ADL, allow this dependency to occur for the immediate time.
* Help child to gradually increase independence in ADL; involve in self-care, slowly at first, then gradually add more activities.

- Provide opportunities for child/family to make decisions about daily care; give some control over own situation; praise them for making decisions, for coping with current stress, for helping self/selves to feel better.
- Ask for child's/family's ideas on what can be done next to improve the situation; incorporate your ideas with theirs to give a sense of control.
- Support and reinforce reality when behavior indicates that child/family is beginning to adapt or cope (e.g., asking questions, focusing on reality); share with them how you see it; ask them to clarify or validate your perceptions.
- Incorporate into the nursing care plan suggestions for new methods of coping with the crisis state; enlist the cooperation of staff in assisting the child/family with these.

☐ EVALUATION CRITERIA/DESIRED OUTCOMES

The child/family
- Appraises situation realistically
- Verbalizes feelings regarding the threatening event
- Identifies usual methods of coping with problems
- States need for new ways to handle the disequilibrium
- Identifies at least 2 effective strategies

NURSING DIAGNOSIS #2

Anxiety related to feelings of being overwhelmed by threatening event

Rationale: Situations perceived as threatening produce increased anxiety that can result in inability to manage situation, which leads to feeling overwhelmed.

☐ GOAL

The child/family will identify causes of threat; will achieve skill in managing the anxiety.

☐ IMPLEMENTATION

- Refer to *The Child Experiencing Anxiety*, page 11.
- Ask what the child/family is feeling at this time (e.g., scared, anxious, panicky) and what occurred to cause these feelings (e.g., new diagnosis, new roommate, new equipment).
- Encourage verbalization of all feelings of anxiety and discern those that are the most threatening; listen actively and with empathy.
- Make any environmental changes that are possible to decrease the impact of the threat (e.g., change room, allow family to stay for additional support).
- Share information regarding tests, procedures,

etc.; tell what to expect and how orders are carried out.
- Enlist the help of other personnel in planning for care that will decrease anxiety; share your perceptions and information with them.
- Teach simple relaxation techniques (e.g., deep breathing) to use whenever needed to keep anxiety from increasing.
- When leaving room, tell when you will be back; return at the appointed time.

☐ EVALUATION CRITERIA/DESIRED OUTCOMES

The child/family
- Identifies causes of threat and describes threatening event
- Makes realistic requests to keep anxiety manageable
- Uses relaxation techniques
- Requests staff assistance appropriately

NURSING DIAGNOSIS #3

Grieving related to an actual or perceived loss

Rationale: An individual's grief is affected by many factors, including personality, previous losses, intimacy of relationship, and personal resources. Unresolved grief is a pathologic response of prolonged denial of the loss or a profound psychotic response that leads to problems in coping. Dysfunctional grieving is evidenced by loss of self-esteem, depression, excessively strong dependency needs, and ambivalent feelings for the lost person or object. Such unresolved grief leaves the individual susceptible to further psychologic trauma that can in turn lead to crisis, depression, and suicide.

☐ GOAL

The child/family will describe loss and the meaning of the loss; will express and share grief with others; will resolve the loss in an adaptive manner.

☐ IMPLEMENTATION

- Refer to *The Parent Experiencing Grief and Loss*, page 139, for review of the grief process.
- Assess for any contributing/causative factors that may delay the grief work.
- Listen and encourage expression of feelings (e.g., fear, despair, anger, sadness).
- Develop a relationship of trust through one-to-one interactions.
- Give support and reassurance by accepting feelings and experiences.
- Explore, if indicated, what it is that makes child feel hopeless, worthless, that life is not worth living.

- Provide support by discussing feelings and coping mechanisms.
- Encourage to share grief and provide support for each other.
- Discuss new coping mechanisms; encourage to practice them.
- Involve in the decision-making process.

☐ EVALUATION CRITERIA/DESIRED OUTCOMES

The child/family
- Expresses feelings
- Shares feelings and concerns with family members
- Participates in decision making for the future

NURSING DIAGNOSIS #4

Alteration in family process related to situational or pathophysiologic stressor

Rationale: When the normally supportive and adaptively functioning family experiences a stressor, the family's previously effective functioning ability may be challenged. Common factors that contribute to an alteration in family process include illness of a family member, trauma, loss of a family member or valued object, gain of a new family member, disaster, economic crisis, change in family roles, conflict, psychiatric illness, and social deviance. When the child's/family's usual problem-solving methods are inadequate to resolve the situation, a crisis may occur. In response to crisis, the child/family will either return to precrisis functioning, develop a higher level of functioning, or develop an ineffective (lower) form of functioning.

☐ GOAL

The family will return to the precrisis level of functioning; will verbalize feelings to nurse and to each other on a regular basis; will maintain a functional system of mutual support for each other.

☐ IMPLEMENTATION

- Help identify feelings of stress, past and current methods of coping, strengths and weaknesses.
- Encourage to share thoughts and feelings with each other, to interact and communicate daily.
- Encourage recognition and verbalization of feelings including guilt, anger, hostility, and blame.
- Help to make realistic appraisal of the situation.
- Urge to list choices, available resources.
- Assist to reorganize roles as needed at home and to set priorities to maintain family integrity and to reduce stress.

☐ EVALUATION CRITERIA/DESIRED OUTCOMES

The family
- Shares feelings and concerns
- Sets priorities and implements adaptive coping strategies
- Reorganizes home roles as needed
- Maintains or returns to precrisis level of functioning

NURSING DIAGNOSIS #5

Knowledge deficit regarding utilization of support systems, problem-solving techniques needed to avert a crisis state

Rationale: A crisis will not develop if situational supports are sufficient, perception of the problem is realistic, and effective coping solutions are available.

☐ GOAL

The child/family will identify available support; will develop alternative coping to solve current problem.

☐ IMPLEMENTATION

- Give information as needed (e.g., hospitalization, treatment therapy); ask for feedback to ensure understanding.
- Teach to brainstorm alternate solutions to current problem, to look at the pros and cons of each one; do not tell them what to do, but ask if one of the solutions could possibly work; role play alternative solutions.
- Check the effectiveness of new coping options by asking what actions they would take if confronted with a situation similar to the one just experienced; reinforce positive adaptation and coping; teach as necessary.
- Help to identify support systems available.
- Refer to outside support or agency to correct family or individual dysfunction once crisis is resolved.

☐ EVALUATION CRITERIA/DESIRED OUTCOMES

The child/family
- Has a realistic perception of what occurred
- Fosters situational supports in the form of family, friends, job
- States at least 3 options available to use to cope with stress
- Lists community resources to go to if another threatening situation occurs

The Child with Croup: Laryngotracheobronchitis or Epiglottitis

Definition/Discussion

Croup is a term used to describe a symptom complex of respiratory manifestations: a barking cough, hoarseness, inspiratory stridor, and respiratory distress from edema in the laryngeal area. Laryngotracheobronchitis (LTB) is a viral infection of the larynx, trachea, and bronchi. Epiglottitis is a bacterial infection (usually Hemophilus influenza type B) of the epiglottis and surrounding area.

Nursing Assessment

☐ PERTINENT HISTORY

Previous hospitalizations, *LTB*: barky cough, low-grade fever, upper respiratory infection; *epiglottitis*: high fever, muffled voice, sore throat, difficulty swallowing, excessive drooling, refusal of foods and fluids, upper respiratory infection

☐ PHYSICAL FINDINGS

LTB: inspiratory stridor, tachypnea, tachycardia, restlessness, cyanosis, use of accessory muscles (e.g., suprasternal, substernal retractions); *epiglottitis*: sitting up, neck extended, breathing through mouth, inspiratory stridor, tachypnea, tachycardia or signs of obstruction (e.g., listlessness, cyanosis, bradycardia, bradypnea, decreased breath sounds)

☐ PSYCHOSOCIAL CONCERNS/ DEVELOPMENTAL FACTORS

Age, developmental level, ability to understand rationale for interventions, experience with separation from parents, habits (e.g., what comforts child, bedtime routine, favored objects), coping methods

☐ PATIENT AND FAMILY KNOWLEDGE

Prior experiences with respiratory illnesses, understanding of need for immediate attention, level of knowledge, readiness and willingness to learn

Nursing Care

☐ LONG-TERM GOAL

The child will recover free from preventable complications; the child will return to normal daily activities after a short convalescence.

NURSING DIAGNOSIS #1

Ineffective airway clearance related to inflammation and obstruction of the upper respiratory tract

Rationale: Inflammation of the upper airway or epiglottis causes obstruction of the movement of air into and out of the lower respiratory tract. Stimulation of the epiglottis with a tongue blade, throat swab, or just opening the mouth may cause a sudden obstruction if the child has epiglottitis.

☐ GOAL

The child will breathe without difficulty; will have a normal respiratory rate and color.

☐ IMPLEMENTATION

- Monitor vital signs closely every hour and as necessary; observe pattern, rate, and characteristics of respirations; note and record clinical features of child's condition (e.g., color, wheezing, nasal flar-

ing, hoarseness, drooling, cough characteristics, location and type of pain).
- Be especially vigilant and report immediately signs of increasing airway obstruction (e.g., tachycardia, tachypnea, sitting up or head thrust forward for mouth breathing, retractions or stridor at rest, pallor, listlessness, circumoral or circumoral cyanosis, anxiety, restlessness [sign of hypoxia], and diminution of breath sounds).
- Have emergency equipment closely available (e.g., intubation tray, tracheostomy supplies, Ambu bag); refer to *The Child with a Tracheostomy*, page 280, if appropriate.
- Avoid visualizing the epiglottis.
- Monitor effects of humidified oxygen at ordered flow rate.
- Place child who has LTB in a croup tent with *cool* mist; avoid *cold* mist as it may precipitate bronchoconstriction; monitor oxygen concentration (FiO_2) in tent every 2 hours.
- Assist child to maintain an upright position; place infant in infant seat with head supported, or raise head of crib mattress.
- Maintain a quiet, calm environment; minimize crying (increases oxygen needs).
- Monitor effects of medications; (e.g., LTB: bronchodilators such as racemic epinephrine per nebulizer; epiglottitis: antibiotics).
- Keep child sedated (carefully, so as not to further depress respiration) and properly restrained if intubated.

☐ **EVALUATION CRITERIA/DESIRED OUTCOMES**

The child
- Has normal respiratory rate and effort, normal color, no cyanosis
- Has clear breath sounds with free movement of air

NURSING DIAGNOSIS #2

Fluid volume deficit related to inadequate oral intake, tachypnea, and fever

Rationale: Fever increases metabolic rate, thus increasing the body's need for water; tachypnea causes increased insensible water loss; the dysphagia associated with epiglottitis inhibits adequate oral intake of fluids.

☐ **GOAL**

The child will ingest adequate fluids for age/weight.

☐ **IMPLEMENTATION**
- Calculate maintenance fluid requirement for weight; add fluids to compensate for increased in-

sensible losses and fever; monitor intake and output carefully.
- Maintain IV at ordered rate; decrease IV rate as oral intake increases; protect IV from infiltration or dislodgement; refer to *The Child with an Intravenous Catheter*, page 174.
- Monitor temperature every 4 hours and as necessary, every hour if febrile.
- Weigh daily in the same clothes, at the same time, on the same scale.
- Check urine specific gravity on each voided specimen.
- Monitor mucous membranes and skin turgor every shift and as necessary.
- Dilute antibiotics in appropriate amount of fluid to prevent phlebitis.
- Ascertain fluids preferred by child; offer hourly when awake in order to meet daily fluid requirement; utilize novel approaches to drinking (e.g., playing tea party, using funny straws); offer fluids at room temperature or warm (cold fluids may increase respiratory distress).

☐ **EVALUATION CRITERIA/DESIRED OUTCOMES**

The child
- Has urine output of at least 1–2 ml/kg/hour
- Has urine specific gravity of 1.003–1.020
- Has moist mucous membranes
- Has good skin turgor
- Maintains/regains preillness weight
- Has patent IV until no longer needed

NURSING DIAGNOSIS #3

Anxiety related to dyspnea, unfamiliar environment, interventions, and equipment (e.g., croup tent, endotracheal tubes)

Rationale: Anxiety and agitation will increase child's need for oxygen.

☐ **GOAL**

The child will cooperate with interventions in an age-appropriate manner; parents will assist child to deal with hospital-related stressors.

☐ **IMPLEMENTATION**
- Orient child to time, place, and physical status using concepts appropriate to cognitive level.
- Allow parents to remain with child; provide them with breaks as needed; assure them that child will be observed closely in their absence.
- Explain to child/parents rationale for use of croup tent or nasotracheal tube; encourage child/parents to verbalize concerns; use age-/developmentally appropriate communication techniques (e.g., play,

story telling); refer to *The Child Requiring Play Therapy*, page 226.

- Obtain croup tent, if required, that covers entire bed so that child feels less restricted; check sheets frequently for dampness; change linen to decrease discomfort.
- Arrange communication methods if child is intubated (e.g., bell at bedside, picture chart depicting needs, paper and pencil for child able to write).
- Plan care so that child receives uninterrupted rest/sleep periods; disturb child as infrequently as possible.

☐ EVALUATION CRITERIA/DESIRED OUTCOMES

The child
- Smiles, talks, plays
- Cooperates with procedures
- Has adequate rest/sleep pattern
- Expresses feelings/concerns in a developmentally appropriate manner

The parents
- Comfort child

NURSING DIAGNOSIS #4

Diversional activity deficit related to respiratory isolation, bed rest

Rationale: The child with LTB or epiglottitis will be restricted from performing usual activities while hospitalized. Additionally, the child may be isolated for protection of self/others.

☐ GOAL

The child will cope with the stresses related to hospitalization; will have access to age-appropriate activities.

☐ IMPLEMENTATION

- Provide age-/developmentally appropriate diversions within constraints of environment; refer to *The Child Requiring Play Therapy*, page 226, and *Normal Growth and Development*, pages 300–314.
- Ascertain child's favorite activities and make them available within the constraints imposed by isolation/croup tent; provide toys that can be gas autoclaved or cleaned with bacteriocidal agents upon removal from room; do not use mechanical toys that may spark and cause a fire when oxygen is in use.
- Provide appropriate visual, auditory, and tactile stimulation; arrange crib/bed so child can observe activities going on outside of room.
- Remember that intubated infant cannot cry to alert others to needs and should never be left alone.

- Assign a volunteer to spend time in room with child when parents are absent.
- Allow siblings to enter room if permitted and there is no current illness or exposure to communicable disease in past 3 weeks; provide masks and gowns; ensure siblings are adequately prepared for what they will see.
- Enter child's room frequently in order to assess needs and to assure child that s/he is not being ignored; spend time playing with child every 2 hours as feasible.

☐ EVALUATION CRITERIA/DESIRED OUTCOMES

The child
- Has no excessive crying, agitation, or irritability related to lack of stimulation
- Participates in age-appropriate activities

NURSING DIAGNOSIS #5

Knowledge deficit regarding home care

Rationale: Recurrence of epiglottitis is rare; however, recurrence of croup is relatively common and may, if it is not severe, be managed at home when parents have adequate knowledge.

☐ GOAL

The child will return to normal daily activities; parents will be comfortable with home management of mild croup; will seek assistance in a timely manner if croup becomes severe.

☐ IMPLEMENTATION

- Instruct regarding home management of mild croup
  - use cool humidifier or take child into bathroom with shower running when breathing difficulties occur
  - provide additional oral fluids
- Instruct regarding administration of antibiotics if child had epiglottitis; include side effects to observe for and importance of completing entire prescription.
- Assure that a temporary loss of mastery of recently acquired developmental skills is a normal response to hospitalization; encourage parents to assist child to deal with feelings about the experience through books, drawings, or having child verbalize experience.
- Provide with phone numbers of persons to contact if they have questions or concerns; ensure they have a return appointment.

☐ EVALUATION CRITERIA/DESIRED OUTCOMES

The child

- Returns to normal activities

The parents

- Manage recurrence of mild croup at home
- Identify need for immediate health care assistance
- State appropriate administration of antibiotics if ordered and potential side effects
- Keep follow-up appointment

The Child with Cystic Fibrosis

Definition/Discussion

Cystic fibrosis is a chronic dysfunction of the exocrine glands transmitted as an autosomal recessive trait. It is characterized by abnormal mucus secretion that causes obstruction of the airways, the pancreatic ducts, the gallbladder, the intrahepatic bile ducts, and the reproductive tract. Eventually, fibrosis of the affected organs occurs.

Cystic fibrosis occurs most frequently in Caucasians. It is diagnosed by a sweat test that shows increased levels of sodium and chloride. Life expectancy in cystic fibrosis has increased to the extent that most patients will live to adulthood.

Nursing Assessment

☐ PERTINENT HISTORY

Frequent episodes of pneumonia; persistent cough; loose, foul-smelling stools; poor weight gain; family history of cystic fibrosis; "salty" taste to child's skin

☐ PHYSICAL FINDINGS

Tachypnea, productive cough, barrel chest, clubbing of nailbeds, shortness of breath, failure to gain weight, cyanosis, steatorrhea, meconium ileus in infant or meconium ileus equivalent (i.e., intestinal obstruction due to hardened inspissated stool) in child; decreased pO_2, increased pCO_2; elevated sweat chloride; chest x-ray, pulmonary function studies

☐ PSYCHOSOCIAL CONCERNS/ DEVELOPMENTAL FACTORS

Age, degree of participation in developmentally appropriate activities; self-image; degree to which parents foster child's independence and involvement in normal activities, family's acceptance of disease, child's/family's coping mechanisms and ability to problem solve

☐ PATIENT AND FAMILY KNOWLEDGE

Understanding of disease and strategies for minimizing complications; community, supportive, and financial resources; genetic transmission of disease; ability to deal with a chronic, eventually fatal disease; level of knowledge, readiness and willingness to learn

Nursing Care

☐ LONG-TERM GOAL

The child will experience no complications or only minimal complications of the disease; the child/family will maximize coping skills required in order to live with a chronic, eventually fatal, disease.

NURSING DIAGNOSIS #1
a. **Ineffective airway clearance** related to increased pulmonary secretions
b. **Impaired gas exchange** related to increased pulmonary secretions

Rationale: Abnormal mucus production causes obstruction of the bronchi and bronchioles, preventing normal flow of air into and out of the alveoli.

☐ GOAL

The child will be free from dyspnea and tachypnea, will effectively clear the airways of mucus; will participate in usual activities; will be free from respiratory infections; will maintain arterial blood gases at near normal levels.

☐ IMPLEMENTATION

- Assess respiratory status (e.g., rate, depth, and ease of respirations; breath sounds; skin color) every 4 hours, as well as with treatments and activity.
- Observe and document amount, color, and quality of sputum; obtain sputum for culture and sensitivity as ordered.
- Ensure that ordered antibiotics are diluted in adequate fluid (if given IV) and administered over the recommended period of time.
- Initiate percussion and postural drainage (PD) as needed (usually once daily to every 4 hours during hospitalization)

- review procedure with parents/child
- auscultate breath sounds prior to and following PD
- perform PD prior to meals (to prevent vomiting) and at bedtime
- administer nebulized mist prior to PD to moisten and thin secretions
- concentrate on areas with the greatest amount of secretions
- Teach/review breathing exercises; have child cough at end of expiration for greatest effectiveness.
- Know that the age of the child can determine ability and willingness to cough (e.g., child younger than 2 years cannot expectorate; school-age children and adolescents are often embarrassed to cough in school or in public).
- Administer oxygen at low flow (no greater than 2 liters/minute) per cannula or mask as needed.

☐ **EVALUATION CRITERIA/DESIRED OUTCOMES**

The child
- Has improved breath sounds and arterial blood gases
- Participates in normal activities
- Has no cyanosis

NURSING DIAGNOSIS #2

Alteration in nutrition: less than body requirements related to interference with enzyme secretion, compromised respiratory status

Rationale: The pancreas normally secretes trypsin, lipase, and amylase, which digest protein, fats, and carbohydrates respectively. The child with cystic fibrosis is, therefore, unable to adequately digest and absorb fats and proteins (carbohydrate metabolism is affected to a much lesser degree), or absorb fat-soluble vitamins (A, D, E, K). In addition, the work of breathing often interferes with ingestion of adequate nutrients while requiring additional energy sources.

☐ **GOAL**

The child will ingest adequate nutrients for normal growth; will increase height and weight along a normal growth curve; will have stools of normal consistency, frequency, and color.

☐ **IMPLEMENTATION**
- Assist child/parents to plan well-balanced, high-protein, high-carbohydrate, low-fat meals that incorporate the child's food preferences; place in-

fants with cystic fibrosis on a partially digested formula such as Pregestimil or Portagen.
- Administer pancreatic enzymes with meals and snacks; titrate the amount of replacement enzyme with the fat or protein content of the meal or snack; teach child to swallow capsules or sprinkle enzyme powder over nonfat, nonprotein foods such as applesauce; do not mix powder with foods containing tapioca or other starches.
- Note color, consistency, and frequency of stools; increase the amount of pancreatic enzymes if steatorrhea occurs, decrease if constipation or diarrhea occur.
- Administer water-miscible vitamins and iron supplements (pancreatic enzyme supplements interfere with the absorption of iron).
- Supplement diet with sodium chloride (salt) tablets in hot weather or if child has a fever.
- Administer liquid nutritional preparations through the night if child has a gastrostomy.

☐ **EVALUATION CRITERIA/DESIRED OUTCOMES**

The child
- Ingests diet sufficient in calories/nutrients for age and activity level
- Increases height and weight along own growth curve
- Is free from steatorrhea

NURSING DIAGNOSIS #3

Ineffective individual/family coping related to chronic illness and the risk of life-threatening complications

Rationale: Chronic illness disrupts the normal lifestyle of the entire family. Periods of crisis (e.g., the hospitalization of the child for pneumonia) may cause the parents to focus on the ill child and lose sight of the needs of well siblings. The financial expenditures associated with the treatment of cystic fibrosis can quickly upset the family's financial stability. All family members experience grief at the loss of a healthy family member, but will probably demonstrate it in different ways.

☐ **GOAL**

Family members will verbalize feelings about the illness and its impact on their lives; will identify community informational, support resources and utilize them appropriately; siblings will receive adequate attention from the adults in the family; parents will focus on their roles as spouses in addition to their roles as parents.

IMPLEMENTATION

- Talk to each family member (this may also include grandparents, close friends, etc.) in order to assess the impact of the illness on their lives and the ways in which they are coping.
- Help to develop new coping mechanisms where existent ones are ineffective.
- Encourage discussion of feelings about the illness/loss of a family member.
- Encourage parents to obtain relief from the heavy responsibilities of caring for their child by training extended family, friends, or babysitters to do daily treatments to give parents a break.
- Arrange for parents/children to meet other families who have a member with cystic fibrosis.
- Identify available community informational, supportive, and financial resources for the family.

EVALUATION CRITERIA/DESIRED OUTCOMES

The child/family
- Communicate openly with one another concerning feelings, needs
- Use resources appropriately
- Feel they are receiving adequate attention from each other

NURSING DIAGNOSIS #4

Disturbance in self-concept related to alteration in appearance, limitations on activities

Rationale: The child with cystic fibrosis is likely to be smaller than peers and less able to participate in strenuous physical activities. The cough associated with cystic fibrosis is often a source of embarrassment. The young adolescent usually develops sexual characteristics later than the peer group.

GOAL

The child will have a positive self-concept and value personal strengths; will be comfortable expressing feelings regarding the disease and any limitations it might impose; will demonstrate accomplishments in areas of interest.

IMPLEMENTATION

- Assist child to express (e.g., verbally, through play, drawings) feelings about self as an individual.
- Assist child to recognize strengths and accomplishments.
- Suggest ways in which child can excel despite limitations imposed by illness (e.g., swimming, art).
- Provide information to teachers/peer group so that child's illness has minimal impact on school and extracurricular activities; ask parents to visit school to discuss child's needs (e.g., pancreatic enzymes with meals and snacks, respiratory care, limitations in sports activities, school work, and letters, phone calls, visits from friends when hospitalized or house-bound) with appropriate personnel.
- Encourage child to take an active role in planning and implementing the treatment regimen.
- Introduce child to other children who are coping effectively with cystic fibrosis.
- Encourage parents to allow the child independence in some choices and activities.
- Provide child with accurate information regarding possible future occurrences; discuss career choices, developing intimate relationships, and having children with the adolescent.

EVALUATION CRITERIA/DESIRED OUTCOMES

The child
- Expresses feelings about the illness
- States strengths and accomplishments
- Makes realistic plans for the future

NURSING DIAGNOSIS #5

Anticipatory grieving related to shortened expected life span

Rationale: Approximately 50% of children with cystic fibrosis die before the age of 18. The child's understanding of and feelings about death will depend upon the developmental level and experiences with the deaths of others. The fear of death will arise each time the child experiences a serious exacerbation of clinical signs.

GOAL

The child/family will express their feelings about the anticipated death and participate in decisions for the future.

IMPLEMENTATION

- Refer to *The Parent Experiencing Grief and Loss*, page 139, and *The Child who is Dying/Terminal*, page 116.
- Note the response of child/family members to the potential early death of the child.
- Utilize age-appropriate tools (e.g., drawings, stories, play) to elicit the feelings and concerns of children unable to articulate them.
- Answer questions honestly, listen openly, and follow through with commitments to establish a trusting relationship with the child/family members.

- Allow each family member to move through the grieving process at own pace.
- Assist the child/family to identify and use support systems.
- Identify for the child/family members feelings they may be having at any point; assure them that in most cases those feelings are a normal part of grieving.
- Identify potential pathologic grief reactions (e.g., suicidal ideation, agitation, inability to make decisions); refer for counseling if appropriate.

☐ EVALUATION CRITERIA/DESIRED OUTCOMES

The child/family
- State feelings about anticipated death of child
- Make realistic plans for the future
- Participate in normal daily activities
- Utilize support systems

NURSING DIAGNOSIS #6

Knowledge deficit regarding prevention of complications and need for compliance with treatment regimen

Rationale: Progression of lung deterioration can be slowed through vigorous pulmonary therapy. Optimum nutritional status will help to forestall serious infections and enhance normal growth and development. The family that is knowledgeable about cystic fibrosis will be better able to anticipate potential problems and develop successful coping strategies.

☐ GOAL

The child/parents will comply with the prescribed treatment regimen to minimize the incidence of respiratory infection and maintain optimal nutrition status; the family will successfully incorporate management of the illness into daily activities.

☐ IMPLEMENTATION

- Provide information regarding the pathophysiology of the disease and its effect on body systems.
- Teach/review postural drainage and percussion, use of equipment, diet, and administration of enzymes, vitamin and iron supplements.
- Teach/review signs of pulmonary infection and encourage child/parents to seek health care assistance immediately; remind child to avoid contact with persons with respiratory infections.
- Provide time for the child/parents/family members to ask questions and express concerns.
- Remind parents that well siblings will have questions and concerns about their own health as well as the health of the sibling with cystic fibrosis.
- Provide parents with phone numbers of persons to contact if they have questions, problems with equipment, or trouble obtaining medications.

☐ EVALUATION CRITERIA/DESIRED OUTCOMES

The child/family
- Describes and implements the treatment regimen
- Asks questions and expresses feelings
- Identifies sources of information, support, and financial assistance

The Child with Depression

Definition/Discussion

Depression is a reaction to one's inability to adapt to change/loss/separation. Depression in children is a constellation of factors characterized by sadness, low self-esteem, and internalization of anger/aggression, which interfere with the child's day-to-day activities. Manifestations vary according to the developmental level of the child, risk factors, and family interactions; however, symptoms of depression may include boredom, restlessness, fatigue, difficulty concentrating, behavioral changes/problems, "acting out," accident proneness, sighing, somatic complaints, sleep disturbance.

Nursing Assessment

☐ **PERTINENT HISTORY**

Duration and characteristics of symptoms; incidence of situational or maturational loss, chronic or terminal illness, trauma, physical/sexual abuse; alcohol/chemical dependency

☐ **PHYSICAL FINDINGS**

General appearance, sleep patterns, elimination, nutrition, activity patterns

☐ **PSYCHOSOCIAL CONCERNS/ DEVELOPMENTAL FACTORS**

Interactional patterns, developmental level, expression of affect, school functioning, peer/family relations, level of thought disruption; habits (e.g., what comforts child, eating/bedtime routines, favored objects)

☐ **PATIENT AND FAMILY KNOWLEDGE**

Child's self-evaluation, parental perception of child's behavior; awareness of existence of a problem and willingness to work toward a solution

Nursing Care

☐ **LONG-TERM GOAL**

The child will express feelings of increased self-esteem and hope; will demonstrate increased positive social interactions.

NURSING DIAGNOSIS #1
a. **Hopelessness** related to inability to feel positive about present life situation
b. **Powerlessness** related to feeling overwhelmed by events or emotions
c. **Ineffective individual coping** related to life events
d. **Altered growth and development** related to depressed mood

Rationale: Hopelessness and powerlessness characterize depression and may result in passivity and despondency. This is debilitating to a child striving to achieve age-appropriate developmental tasks. Depression may be a response to traumatic life events (e.g., natural disasters, unexpected deaths, rape, physical/sexual abuse). A severely depressed child may experience reality disorientation, or an inability to problem solve even the simplest of motor tasks, speak cohesively and intelligibly, or comprehend conversation.

☐ **GOAL**

The child will express feelings in age-appropriate ways; will perform age-appropriate developmental tasks.

☐ **IMPLEMENTATION**

- Ask child how s/he sees things, whether anything helps him/her feel better, and what might help improve situation.
- Use play therapy/role playing to assist the child in gaining mastery over the event; refer to *The Child Requiring Play Therapy,* page 226.
- Support disclosure of painful memories.
- Praise ability to share feelings whether it be through play therapy or verbalization.
- Administer prescribed antidepressants as ordered; note effectiveness.
- Assist child to engage in small structured social encounters.
- Praise child's efforts to participate.
- Familiarize self with age-appropriate developmen-

tal tasks; refer to *Normal Growth and Development,* pages 300–314.

- Engage child in activities that match or are slightly below developmental level; provide opportunities for success; avoid activities that set the child up for failure.
- Advance to increasingly higher-level tasks; praise and reinforce accomplishments.
- Allow child to make decisions concerning care (e.g., when to brush teeth) if appropriate; keep decisions simple; restrict choices so as not to overwhelm child.

☐ **EVALUATION CRITERIA/DESIRED OUTCOMES**

The child

- Expresses fears, concerns
- Demonstrates age-appropriate developmental tasks
- Makes simple decisions regarding care
- Participates in play therapy

NURSING DIAGNOSIS #2

a. **Self-care deficit: hygiene/grooming** related to inability to make decisions, feelings of hopelessness/worthlessness
b. **Disturbance in self-concept: body image/self-esteem** related to distorted perception
c. **Alteration in bowel elimination: constipation/encopresis** related to lack of exercise, poor-quality intake, withholding
d. **Alteration in nutrition: more than body requirements** related to perceived comfort value of food
e. **Alteration in nutrition: less than body requirements** related to perceived negative connotations of food

Rationale: The depressed child may be immobilized to the point of not bathing, brushing teeth, combing hair, eating, sleeping, or dressing appropriately (e.g., too warm for hot days or vice versa, or not changing clothes, wearing unkempt clothing). This contributes increasingly to depression, distorted body image, and decreased self-esteem. Children may experience depressive symptoms as a result of internalized anger. This often presents itself psychologically as withholding attention and affection. It may further progress to the physical withholding of stool as the child attempts to gain control over these feelings. Lack of exercise and poor nutritional intake because of depression may also result in constipation. Regressive behavior (e.g., wetting during the day) may be seen. Children may use food as a comfort mechanism or avoid food altogether.

☐ **GOAL**

The child will take an active role in self-care; will resume a normal elimination pattern; will ingest a diet appropriate for nutritional needs.

☐ **IMPLEMENTATION**

- Assist child with hygiene and grooming; praise positive aspects of child's appearance.
- Praise and reinforce independent attempts at completing even small daily tasks.
- Reinforce (e.g., visually with star chart) efforts to participate in self-care, play/school work.
- Assist child in planning new, more effective skills for coping; practice mastery of coping skills via play therapy/role playing.
- Provide appropriate diet with increased roughage (e.g., fresh fruit, vegetables, high-fiber cereals).
- Encourage and reinforce participation in exercise.
- Administer stool softener, mineral oil as ordered; monitor for effectiveness.
- Set aside consistent toilet-time (e.g., after meals, before bedtime); praise and reinforce toilet use.

☐ **EVALUATION CRITERIA/DESIRED OUTCOMES**

The child

- Participates successfully in self-care, play activities, and school
- Eats an appropriate diet
- Stays dry during the day if age appropriate
- Passes soft stool at least every 2 days

NURSING DIAGNOSIS #3

a. **Sleep pattern disturbance** related to fears, anxiety, inactivity or sleeping during the day
b. **Diversional activity deficit** related to inactivity

Rationale: The depressed child may be restless, have nightmares, or be fearful of being left alone. The child who withdraws from activity during the day or who is allowed to sleep for prolonged periods in the day may not be able to sleep at night.

☐ **GOAL**

The child will maintain/regain a normal sleep pattern; will actively participate in games, conversation, helping others.

☐ **IMPLEMENTATION**

- Explore child's fears and anxieties related to nighttime, being alone, sleeping through play therapy or conversation.

- Follow a consistent bedtime routine (e.g., drink of water, trip to bathroom, bedtime story, hug and a kiss).
- Provide a nightlight.
- Sit at child's doorway if necessary to keep child in room and as reassurance until child falls asleep.
- Choose activities, games, and possible playmates that are developmentally appropriate.
- Elicit activities/interests from child; encourage and praise the child's participation.
- Encourage physical activity from the child (e.g., running, tag, jump rope).
- Monitor the child's social interactional patterns.
- Assist the withdrawn child to tolerate brief periods of contact with another child (e.g., sit with child); increase gradually the group size as tolerated by the child.
- Structure activities with another higher functioning child to serve as a role model and help the withdrawn child participate.

☐ **EVALUATION CRITERIA/DESIRED OUTCOMES**

The child
- Sleeps restfully without waking through the night
- Participates in bedtime routine
- Interacts appropriately with peers

NURSING DIAGNOSIS #4

Potential for injury related to self-abusive behavior, accidents

Rationale: The depressed child may engage in self-abusive behaviors (e.g., biting, hitting, scratching, head-banging), or appear very clumsy and accident prone (e.g., falling while climbing, running out into the street, touching a hot oven, falling down during play).

☐ **GOAL**

The child will redirect energies toward developmentally appropriate and safe behavior and play activities.

☐ **IMPLEMENTATION**
- Identify child's abusive/accidental tendencies.
- Prevent child physically from completing abusive/accident-potential behavior.
- Engage child in an activity that distracts the child so that abusive/accidental behavior cannot be continued when the new activity is begun.

- Praise child's participation in the new safe behavior.
- Stress your desire to keep child safe.
- Reinforce safe behavior (e.g., with star chart, hugs, praise, pats).

☐ **EVALUATION CRITERIA/DESIRED OUTCOMES**

The child
- Engages in no self-abuse
- Verbalizes a safe behavior versus an unsafe behavior
- Does not participate in any unsafe behaviors

NURSING DIAGOSIS #5
a. **Ineffective family coping** related to failure to comprehend severity of depression (meanings of behavioral changes)
b. **Alteration in family processes** related to inability to cope with a child member experiencing depression
c. **Knowledge deficit** regarding childhood depression

Rationale: Parents and others may underestimate the importance of behavioral symptoms, or may deny that the behavioral change exists. The normal supportive environment of the family is challenged when the child experiences depression. The family must be allowed to verbalize their feelings and receive external support when needed.

☐ **GOAL**

The family will recognize and effectively manage depressive changes in the child's behavior; will return to its functionally supportive state; will increase communication and understanding regarding the child's experience with depression.

☐ **IMPLEMENTATION**
- Assess family's understanding of the child's status.
- Assess level of disruption in family functioning.
- Point out changes in behavior (subtle or blatant) as they relate to depressive symptoms (e.g., withdrawal, increased motor activity, decreased appetite, increased appetite, decreased attentiveness, increased aggression); demonstrate and role play with family ways to manage these behaviors.
- Encourage family to express their feelings regarding the changes in the child.

- Encourage and allow family members to verbalize feelings to nurse and to one another.
- Assist family members in maintaining mutual support of one another.
- Encourage family to seek professional help when needed.

☐ EVALUATION CRITERIA/DESIRED OUTCOMES

The family
- Demonstrates recognition of a symptom and effective management techniques by role playing
- Is mutually supportive of one another and of the child

The Child with Developmental Disability

Definition/Discussion

Developmental disability, also known as mental retardation, refers to a subaverage general intellectual functioning that originates during the developmental period and is associated with impairment in adaptive behavior. Children with developmental disabilities need the same basic services that other human beings need for normal development, including education, vocational preparation, health services, and recreational opportunities. In addition, many moderately, severely, and profoundly retarded children need specialized services such as diagnostic evaluation centers, early intervention programs, special education services, and residential living.

Nursing Assessment

☐ PERTINENT HISTORY

Present complaints, course of illness or accidental injury (e.g., length, characteristics); home treatment for illness or injury; presence of chronic health impairments; number/length of prior hospitalizations; physical setting in which the child resides (e.g., home, residential, institutional); special services/procedures required by the child's developmental disability; previous level of function

☐ PHYSICAL FINDINGS

Vital signs; level of consciousness; weight; presence of other handicaps such as cerebral palsy, epilepsy, blindness, or deafness; presence of physical/behavioral symptoms indicating pain/discomfort; functional capabilities

☐ PSYCHOSOCIAL CONCERNS/ DEVELOPMENTAL FACTORS

Level of intellectual functioning; adaptive behavioral skills; overall developmental level; coping mechanisms/habits of child and family; impact of normal routine on child/family; stressors/concerns of family; support systems available

☐ PATIENT AND FAMILY KNOWLEDGE

Developmental program needs of child, adaptation/ acceptance of child's level of functioning/prognosis; level of knowledge, ability, readiness and willingness to learn

Nursing Care

☐ LONG-TERM GOAL

The developmentally disabled child will learn, develop, and grow at own rate to become a productive participant in society.

NURSING DIAGNOSIS #1

Self-care deficit: feeding, bathing/hygiene, dressing/grooming, toileting related to physical/mental deficit

Rationale: *The child with a developmental deficit may be unable to perform/communicate basic needs; therefore, parents, nurses, and other care providers may have to assist the child and be responsible for ensuring that basic needs are met.*

☐ GOAL

The child will ingest adequate food/fluids to meet body's needs; will have a normal bowel pattern.

☐ IMPLEMENTATION

- Maintain consistency and establish a routine; schedule meals, naps, medications, and treatments at the same time every day.
- Follow the child's normal routine as closely as possible.
- Assist the child in development of a communication system to express needs (e.g., make felt board with specific pictures [toilet, cup, wheelchair] and have child point to what is desired; teach sign language).
- Ensure adequate intake of food and fluid; use supplements when necessary and allow choice of food when possible; if child uses special feeding utensils, ensure they are present in advance.
- Attend to activities promoting good hygiene/oral

care; brush teeth after meals and upon rising; keep child clean; establish a routine bathing pattern; preserve skin integrity (e.g., massage, lotions, sheepskins, water mattress); support the child's efforts to perform self-care activities.
- Provide experiences that promote self-sufficiency in self-care skills; allow as much independence as possible in activities of daily living.
- Ambulate as much as possible; use active and passive range-of-motion as appropriate; refer to *The Child Requiring Range-of-Motion Exercises*, page 237.
- Monitor normal pattern of bowel/bladder elimination; clean perianal area of stool/urine immediately.

☐ **EVALUATION CRITERIA/DESIRED OUTCOMES**

The child
- Maintains/regains admission weight and level of hydration
- Maintains good skin condition
- Maintains adequate level of personal hygiene

NURSING DIAGNOSIS #2

Anxiety related to hospitalization, separation from family, disruption of daily routines

Rationale: Developmentally delayed children have intellectual/emotional limitations that increase difficulties in adapting to hospitalization, or changes in caregivers and routines; in understanding the reason for hospitalization and related restrictions; and in communicating feelings of anxiety. Children with a developmental disability frequently are less anxious and more cooperative when schedules and time frames are exact.

☐ **GOAL**

The child will adjust to the hospital/altered environment; will exhibit behavioral indicators of trust and security; will maintain relationship with family.

☐ **IMPLEMENTATION**
- Encourage and allow time for child to express feelings/understanding in own way.
- Accept expressed feelings with nonjudgmental words and actions.
- Provide consistency in nursing care; assign one nurse per shift to do all care.
- Adjust hospital procedures to child's usual routine as much as possible.
- Follow through on promises made to child (e.g., if you say you will return at a specific time, do so).
- Provide diversions (e.g., toys, games) that are ap-

propriate to level of functioning; tell family to bring in favorite toys and to stay with child if possible.
- Encourage interaction with child's peers, family members, or care providers so child maintains significant relationships; ask for assistance in correctly interpreting communication and behavior; allow them to provide care when possible.
- Allow child to participate as much as possible in decision making regarding care.

☐ **EVALUATION CRITERIA/DESIRED OUTCOMES**

The child
- Maintains admission level of functioning within limits imposed by physical illness

---

NURSING DIAGNOSIS #3

Altered growth and development related to mental/emotional/cognitive deficit

Rationale: Developmental disabilities are associated with impairments in adaptive behaviors; adaptive behavior refers to the child's adjustment to everyday life; children with developmental disabilities learn more slowly than others and reach a lower overall level of functioning.

☐ **GOAL**

The child will function at a level consistent with his/her cognitive skills and adaptive abilities.

☐ **IMPLEMENTATION**
- Discuss and promote the concept of "normalizing" experiences to promote self-sufficiency, adjustment, and mental growth (e.g., eating meals with others, music therapy in groups).
- Permit the child to express feelings, but at the same time do not allow unacceptable behavior (e.g., temper tantrums); reinforce appropriate behavior.
- Provide toys, games, equipment, educational supplies, and teaching that will enable the child to increase cognitive, social, motor skills.
- Communicate and interact with the child in an age-appropriate fashion; maintain dignity in all interactions with the child.
- Allow and encourage family members, siblings, and nondisabled peers to visit and interact with the child.
- Foster self-worth; provide personal space so child's belongings are accessible; encourage child to care for the physical environment if appropriate.

EVALUATION CRITERIA/DESIRED OUTCOMES

The child

- Maintains/improves level of function
- Participates in "normalizing" experiences, with family, sibling, nondisabled peers

---

NURSING DIAGNOSIS #4

Potential for injury related to developmental disability

Rationale: Cognitive and physical limitations associated with developmental disability may preclude the child's understanding of dangers, use of safeguards, and requesting help appropriately in dangerous situations. Because the child adapts slowly to new activities/situations/environments (e.g., the hospital), the developmentally delayed child is at risk for injury.

GOAL

The child will cooperate with hospital rules and regulations regarding safety as able; will be free from preventable accident or injury.

IMPLEMENTATION

- Institute safety precautions as appropriate (e.g., check safety rails frequently; restrain only if necessary; stay with anxious child; make frequent checks; do not underestimate child's strength).
- Plan for mobility aids as needed (e.g., wheelchair, walker, other special equipment).
- Observe for mouthing of nonfood items.
- Do not wait for call light; plan regular checks so child expects you.
- Remain with child until medications are swallowed safely; be alert to medication side effects that interfere with function/safety.
- Explain/demonstrate procedures and equipment (e.g., suctioning, gavaging) in advance so when used, will not cause fear or be removed by child.

EVALUATION CRITERIA/DESIRED OUTCOMES

The child

- Is free from accidents
- Complies with hospital rules
- Does not swallow toxic/nonedible items

NURSING DIAGNOSIS #5

a. **Family coping: potential for growth** related to having a child with a permanent disability
b. **Ineffective family coping** related to having a child with a permanent disability
c. **Alteration in family processes** related to having a child with a permanent disability

Rationale: The developmentally disabled child's inability to perform age-appropriate tasks and need for specialized training, as well as "normalizing" experiences, forces the family into an adjustment process that includes developing alliances with professionals. The family struggles with adapting to life with a handicapped child in a world of nondisabled persons.

GOAL

The parents will express an understanding of developmental disabilities; will facilitate the child's development; family members will express their feelings/concerns; will interact positively with the child.

IMPLEMENTATION

- Provide opportunities for parents/family members to discuss feelings (e.g., anger, guilt, hostility); accept these expressions in a nonjudgmental manner by both words and actions.
- Provide information about changes in child's level of function, strengths and weaknesses.
- Include child/parents/family members in planning individual programs and routines for the child.
- Support families through the times when they are separated from the child.
- Provide opportunities for families of children in residential programs to discuss their feelings about home visits; assist them in planning for visits to prevent/avoid problems.
- Provide opportunities for families to interact with other families with developmentally delayed children, to share experiences and information.
- Be alert to indications of ineffective coping such as abuse or neglect of child and refer to counseling/appropriate agencies as necessary; refer to *The Child with Nonaccidental Trauma*, page 209.

EVALUATION CRITERIA/DESIRED OUTCOMES

The family members

- Express feelings about the child's disabilities and level of function
- Develop an alliance with care givers who are seen as supportive and helpful
- Participate in decision making about child's program

NURSING DIAGNOSIS #6

Knowledge deficit regarding deficit, treatment, skills necessary to care for child at home/other setting

Rationale: If knowledge deficit exists, the child's health problems/behaviors cannot be appropriately

managed, nor can individualized educational/so-cial/recreational experiences be planned to meet the child's special needs.

☐ GOAL

The child will maintain/improve current levels of function; family members will verbalize an understanding of the child's specific needs.

☐ IMPLEMENTATION

- Allow the child to participate as much as possible in the decision making process.
- Assist the family members to learn technical skills as well as behavioral techniques that are necessary in caring for the child (e.g., scheduling, routines, and equipment).
- Correct any misunderstandings and provide health teaching; refer to the appropriate nursing care planning guide for current medical diagnosis.
- Teach skills that may need to be employed after discharge (e.g., dressing changes).
- Review/teach about medications (e.g., dosage, time, method of administration, side effects).
- Visit the home or other transfer site to assess needs (e.g., additional equipment, supplies), or consult with home health nurse prior to discharge.
- Provide time for child/family members to practice necessary home care (e.g., dressing changes, soaks).
- Provide information regarding community agencies/resources; provide telephone numbers of physician, clinic, day treatment/residential programs.
- Ensure that family realizes that options (e.g., home care, residential care) may change as the child's/family's situation changes.

☐ EVALUATION CRITERIA/DESIRED OUTCOMES

The child
- Maintains/improves functioning

The family members
- Describe child's care needs accurately
- Demonstrate skills/procedures to be carried out after discharge
- Schedule follow-up appointments with physician/clinic/program
- List community support services available

The Child with Diabetes

Definition/Discussion _____

Diabetes mellitus is a chronic metabolic disorder that affects the body's ability to manufacture/utilize insulin, the hormone produced by the beta cells of the pancreas. Insulin is required for the body to utilize carbohydrates and store fat. There are two major classifications of diabetes
- *Insulin-dependent* (IDDM or Type I): Most frequently manifests in children and adolescents and accounts for 10% of all persons with diabetes. Its onset is rapid; etiology is thought to be a genetic predisposition with perhaps a viral component mediating the onset. Because of the growth requirements of children and adolescents, control is often difficult.
- *Noninsulin-dependent* (NIDDM or Type II): occurs most often in persons over the age of 40, especially those who are overweight.

Nursing Assessment _____

☐ PERTINENT HISTORY

Age, behavior (e.g., irritable, very tired), usual dietary pattern/activity level, medications (e.g., type of insulin, dose, time); glucose monitoring techniques being used

☐ PHYSICAL FINDINGS

General condition, vital signs; height; current weight, recent loss; serum glucose levels: random, fasting, before meals (ac); abdominal pain; blurred vision; excessive thirst (polydipsia) or hunger (polyphagia); changes in amount or pattern of urination (e.g., frequent voiding [polyuria], enuresis in a previously toilet-trained child)

☐ PSYCHOSOCIAL CONCERNS/ DEVELOPMENTAL FACTORS

Developmental level, grade if in school, interests, hobbies, identified stressors, usual coping patterns, and supportive family members or friends; habits (e.g., what comforts child, favored objects, usual routines)

☐ PATIENT AND FAMILY KNOWLEDGE

Reason for hospitalization; pathophysiology of disease; dietary planning; insulin and insulin administration, especially during an illness/infection; recognition and management of hypo/hyperglycemia, life-long nature of disease, long-term complications, glucose monitoring/urine testing techniques, foot care, exercise, stress management, follow-up care, community resources, level of knowledge, readiness and willingness to learn

Nursing Care _____

☐ LONG-TERM GOAL

The child will reach and maintain the optimum level of performance possible; the child will live within the limits of the disease and treatment regimen, to prevent, as much as possible, the pathologic changes and complications of diabetes; the child will accept and integrate successfully the diabetic life-style into self-concept; the child will achieve self-confident control; the child will resume normal home, school, family, social, and community roles with necessary adaptation.

NURSING DIAGNOSIS #1
a. **Alteration in nutrition: more than body requirements** related to intake in excess of activity expenditure
b. **Alteration in nutrition: less than body requirements** related to insufficient caloric intake to promote growth, maintain development; inability of the body to utilize nutrients available

Rationale: Nutritional alterations are expected because of the nature of diabetes. When an individual cannot manufacture/utilize insulin, that person's metabolic processes are necessarily altered. "More than body requirements" may pertain to a child whose weight is 10% or more above the ideal for height and frame, to a child with observed or expressed undesirable eating patterns, as well as to a child with sedentary activity patterns. "Less than body requirements" is appropriate for a child

---

whose weight is 10%–20% below ideal for height and frame, for a child whose reported/observed intake is less than the minimum daily requirement, or for a child whose actual or potential metabolic needs are in excess of intake. Additionally, a child with diabetes may appear to take in sufficient amounts of food but continue to loose weight because the body is unable to utilize nutrients available.

☐ GOAL

The child/parents will adjust nutritional intake to meet metabolic needs.

☐ IMPLEMENTATION

- Give all meals and snacks on time, encouraging full consumption; record and measure amounts left and give replacement (e.g., carbohydrate, fat, protein) feedings.
- Encourage to eat meals/snacks at about the same times daily; discourage between-meal snacking unless prescribed.
- Monitor serum glucose levels before meals, at bedtime snack, and as necessary; provide supplementary feedings or insulin as indicated by glucose and activity levels.
- Test urine for sugar/acetone; check specific gravity; record/report all abnormal findings.
- Monitor for signs and symptoms of hypoglycemia (i.e., insulin reaction or insulin shock) and hyperglycemia (i.e., diabetic coma, diabetic ketoacidosis, or DKA); initiate appropriate measures to correct either complication (see Table 6).
- Administer insulin as prescribed; review specific actions and precautions to be taken.
- Administer vitamin/mineral supplements as ordered.
- Encourage physical activity regularly as tolerated; balance activity with rest.

☐ EVALUATION CRITERIA/DESIRED OUTCOMES

The child
- Adheres to prescribed diet
- Eats prescribed amount of food daily at same times
- Remains free from hypoglycemic/hyperglycemic reactions

NURSING DIAGNOSIS #2
a. **Potential for infection** related to hyperglycemia
b. **Impairment of skin integrity** related to slow healing process, increased susceptibility to infection

---

Rationale: Increased serum glucose levels in the peripheral vascular vessels provide a medium for bacterial growth, predisposing the child to the development of infections. Children with impaired skin integrity are at highest risk for developing infection, but the potential is there for all children with diabetes. Vascular changes, uncommon before puberty, usually occur in those who have had diabetes for more than 10 years. Thus, foot care is not quite as important for the younger child as it is in the adolescent with diabetes, but certain aspects of preventive care should be discussed.

☐ GOAL

The child will be free from infections; will maintain healthy intact skin.

☐ IMPLEMENTATION

- Obtain/record baseline vital signs, check lab values, and monitor for significant changes that might indicate the presence of infection (e.g., elevated temperature, pulse, respirations; decreased blood pressure).
- Inquire about itching or burning on urination, diminished urinary output, frequency, cloudy or foul-smelling urine, or pneumaturia (i.e., bubbly voided urine due to the action of bacteria on glucose in the urine).
- Observe/report lesions of the mouth, gums, and perineal areas.
- Encourage good oral hygiene practices and refer to dentist if appropriate.
- Inspect child's skin every 8 hours; record subjective and objective data about skin lesions, skin wounds, ulcers, and pressure areas.
- Ensure that bedridden diabetic child changes position at least every 2 hours to maintain adequate circulation to all pressure points.
- Ensure skin is dried thoroughly after bathing; apply lotion to roughened or very dry areas; avoid using alcohol on skin.
- Prevent the chafing and irritation caused by perspiration by powdering skin and encouraging wearing of loose-fitting cotton garments next to the skin.
- Eliminate pressure areas (e.g., tight shoes/clothing).
- Tell to avoid, as much as possible, thongs and sandals, and not to go barefoot, even on the beach or swimming pool decks.
- Advise to wear properly fitting, well constructed shoes (e.g., leather or canvas), and supportive slippers; suggest checking for nail points, roughly stitched areas, or other lumps that may cause irritation; avoid vinyl or rubber shoes that do not allow feet to "breathe"; break in new shoes gradually for

short periods; alternate pairs of shoes to allow them to air out and regain strength.
- Teach basic first aid for minor injuries; tell the child/parents to cleanse the area promptly, apply alcohol and a dry, sterile dressing; discourage applying any medication without first checking with the physician.

☐ EVALUATION CRITERIA/DESIRED OUTCOMES

The child
- Is free from infection
- Maintains intact skin

NURSING DIAGNOSIS #3

a. **Grieving** related to reaction to, perceptions of chronic illness
b. **Disturbance in self-concept: body image** related to perceptions of chronic illness, being different than peers
c. **Altered growth and development** related to illness, restrictions on life-style

Rationale: Parents may be unable to cope with feelings of guilt that they "transmitted" the disease or grieve over the loss of the "perfect" child. Maintaining good diabetic control entails time/energy expenditures and changes in life-style. The child/parents may feel unable to cope with all of the changes and demands placed on them; may be required to achieve disease control, which may or may not pose developmental problems. Children, particularly adolescents, are intolerant of body imperfections and being different from peers; having diabetes may accentuate these feelings. Denial of the disease will be less likely if all family members accept its presence and the child is aided in expressing rather than keeping thoughts within.

☐ GOAL

The child will have a positive self-image; the child/family will cope effectively with feelings about diabetes.

☐ IMPLEMENTATION

- Encourage to identify/express (e.g., verbally, through drawings, play) feelings and concerns about diabetes; be an empathic listener.
- Help build on previously successful coping strategies; assist child/parents to look at alternative solutions but avoid choosing the answer for them.
- Refer to *The Parent Experiencing Grief and Loss*, page 139, and *The Child Experiencing a Body-Image Disturbance*, page 30.
- Be alert to signs that may indicate rebellion against disease (e.g., noncompliance, acting out).
- Arrange for participation in peer group discussions; refer for counseling as necessary; assist

child (particularly adolescent) to see that everyone is special although different and diabetes is only one of many particular differences.
- Help fearful/uncooperative child cope with daily injections; discuss parents' feeling of ambivalence about giving the injection.
- Assist child/parents to realize that insulin administration is an expected daily routine just as tooth brushing.
- Make management flexible so it can accommodate to individual life-styles; encourage child/family to maintain normal activity patterns.
- Spend time with child not associated with diabetic management; teach parents to do likewise.
- Stress the importance of the child's participation in age-appropriate activities; suggest sending child to camp for diabetic children.
- Encourage parents to teach another caretaker child's routine/care needs so they can feel comfortable leaving the child.
- Encourage family activities that do not stress/focus on diabetes.
- Assist parents to slowly give up the caretaker role as the child becomes increasingly capable of caring for self.

☐ EVALUATION CRITERIA/DESIRED OUTCOMES

The child/family
- Expresses positive self-image and coping abilities
- Verbalizes feelings about diabetes
- Identifies own coping strategies and support systems

NURSING DIAGNOSIS #4

a. **Powerlessness** related to lack of knowledge about diabetes, perceived lack of personal control
b. **Ineffective individual/family coping** related to perceptions of disease, restrictions on life-style, feelings of guilt

Rationale: When confronted with a chronic disease such as diabetes, the child/parents may at times feel overwhelmed, whether it be at the initial diagnosis, during a situational or maturational crisis, or when new complications or other disease processes are present. These nursing diagnoses may be appropriate for the child/parents with diabetes who express feelings of being unable to control the situation or who refuse to participate in decision making, deferring instead to health care providers. Emotional upsets, other illnesses, and normal growth patterns may increase the child's need for insulin. If the child can be helped to adjust to these situations, diabetic control will be enhanced.

GOAL

The child/parents will identify those aspects of diabetes that are possible to control; will participate in making decisions related to the treatment of diabetes.

IMPLEMENTATION

- Review psychosocial assessment for data regarding individual patterns of coping and supportive persons.
- Observe family relationships to estimate the degree of support available; include supportive persons in interventions.
- Allow expression of fears and concerns; listen attentively without minimizing feelings; offer suggestions without directly telling the child/parents what to do; when possible, offer alternative solutions to current problems.
- Assess the need for home health care.
- Encourage to keep regularly scheduled appointments for follow-up care, pointing out how such visits are crucial to maintaining control.

EVALUATION CRITERIA/DESIRED OUTCOMES

The child/parents
- Express increased feelings of control
- Discuss diabetes, treatment, possible complications
- Participate in the decision-making process regarding treatment of diabetes

---

NURSING DIAGNOSIS #5

Knowledge deficit

Rationale: *When diabetes is newly diagnosed, it may be expected that the child/parents will not have information about diabetes necessary to achieve and maintain control. The following diagnoses are not limited to the newly diagnosed child, but may apply to those who request specific information or who, on the basis of observed behavior, require teaching.*

a. **Knowledge deficit** regarding dietary planning

Rationale: *Diet therapy is the cornerstone of the management of diabetes. The dietary prescription represents the number of grams of carbohydrate, protein, and fat to be used in the daily food plan. It is calculated to provide an adequate intake of vitamins and minerals to meet the caloric requirements of the person depending on the nutritional state, growth needs, the normal activity needs, and the ideal body weight as determined by sex, height, age, and bone structure. The number of calories prescribed is based on the child's calculated caloric needs, hunger, and activity level.*

Foods having approximately the same amounts of carbohydrate, protein, and fat have been

---

grouped together into exchange lists. Within a group, foods may be substituted/exchanged for each other in the amounts given.

The daily insulin requirements are based on the planned dietary prescription and blood sugar values. To successfully manage diabetes, the child/parents must be familiar with the prescribed plan and make adaptations during illness or if child is having difficulty swallowing. The child/parents need to be taught how to manage the dietary plan when traveling or eating in restaurants.

GOAL

The child/parents will plan a well-balanced daily menu, consistent with prescribed dietary plan and recommended methods of preparation; will modify the usual dietary plan if ill or unable to swallow solid food.

IMPLEMENTATION

- Ensure that the child and the primary food preparer have a copy of the prescribed dietary plan; schedule appropriate number of meals/snacks (e.g., 3 meals and 2–3 snacks/day), use quantitative measuring (e.g., ½ cup, 1 slice).
- Read through the plan with the family; allow time for the family to read through it again and to ask questions.
- Use a kitchen scale, measured containers and serving pieces to assist in learning portion sizes.
- Provide practice sessions to ensure that the child/parents are able to correctly measure desired portions.
- Arrange for child/parents to make food selections cafeteria-style if possible; reinforce appropriate choices and correct inappropriate ones.
- Review exchange lists with the child/parents; have them choose which foods may be substituted for others in various situations.
- Provide guidelines for adjusting the dietary plan when the child is ill, unable to chew, or has missed/failed to finish a complete meal
  - the need for insulin continues and may even increase during illness; therefore, unless specifically directed otherwise, the child should continue to take insulin
  - caloric needs may be increased during illness, therefore, it is important to replace carbohydrate foods in the dietary plan
  - when solids are poorly tolerated, take fluids containing 10–15 gm carbohydrates every hour or 50 gm carbohydrate for every meal missed
- Encourage to use the usual meal plan as much as possible during illness, selecting exchanges that are appealing and easily digested.
- Advise that fluid and mineral needs are increased when diarrhea, vomiting, or fever are present; en-

courage to take sips of water, bouillon, or tea in addition to liquids that provide carbohydrates; monitor blood sugars more frequently; notify physician immediately if unable to tolerate any food or liquids.
- Explain how to use glucagon IM when child is unable to swallow.
- Provide travelling tips (e.g., do not carry emergency supplies in luggage; prearrange diabetic meals on airplanes).
- Offer suggestions for eating out in restaurants/at school/in friends' homes (e.g., avoid fried or creamed foods, gravies; ask for margarine and diet salad dressings).

☐ **EVALUATION CRITERIA/DESIRED OUTCOMES**

The child/parents
- Select well-balanced meals/appropriate snacks, using prescribed dietary plan and exchange lists
- List foods allowed and those to be avoided
- Adapt usual dietary plan if ill or unable to swallow solid foods
- State when to notify physician
- Modify usual dietary plan appropriately for traveling/eating in a restaurant

---

b. **Knowledge deficit** regarding medication management

Rationale: Because the pediatric diabetic patient is insulin dependent, daily administration of the hormone is necessary for life. Insulin may be injected by single injection or insulin pump (a battery-powered device that works like a syringe to continuously or intermittently inject the desired amount of insulin into the child through a catheter into the abdomen). Before attempting to teach the child/parents, the nurse should be familiar with the various types of insulin preparations, their sources, times of onset of action and peak activity (i.e., the time at which a hypoglycemic reaction is most likely to occur), and recommendations for storing and handling.

☐ **GOAL**

The child/parents will become familiar with the type of insulin prescribed; will correctly store insulin, prepare and administer injections; will care for equipment safely; will recognize side effects and notify the physician of their occurrence.

☐ **IMPLEMENTATION**
- Explain that the specific amount of insulin prescribed is determined by serum glucose levels.
- Teach that most insulin preparations are U-100

(i.e., the solution contains 100 units of insulin in every cc); store insulin for daily use at room temperature; extra vials should be stored in refrigerator.
- Provide several different vials of insulin, asking the child/parents to examine them carefully, to look at their appearances and at the labels to distinguish one from another; be sure to include modified as well as purified preparations; point out the cloudy appearance of the modified preparations.
- Teach to check expiration dates.
- Stress importance of using the correct insulin syringe (e.g., if the dose prescribed is less than 50 units, it is advisable to use the 0.5-cc syringe to reduce the margin of error; if the dose is greater than 50 units, it is advisable to use the 1cc insulin syringe).
- Demonstrate how to withdraw the desired dose from the vial; supply written step-by-step instructions.
- Demonstrate how to give an injection, explaining the steps as you go along; supply written step-by-step instructions.
- Show how to mix insulins if indicated; supply written step-by-step instructions.
- Instruct where to give insulin injections and how to change the sites to prevent pitting of the skin and lipohypertrophy (i.e., spongy thickening of the subcutaneous tissue), which can interfere with the blood supply to the area and may cause delayed absorption of insulin; use a site-rotation sheet and encourage the child/parents to keep a record of injection sites.
- Have the child/parents practice giving injections of insulin while in the hospital; practice on an orange first, then move to actual injections; observe the practice sessions to reinforce good technique and offer encouragement.
- Review the instruction manual for an insulin pump when one is in use.
- Review the signs, symptoms and treatment for insulin reaction/hyperglycemia (Table 6); have child/parents list them for you; teach parents that for both hypo/hyperglycemia, younger children cannot tell them how they feel or express symptoms very easily; teach assessment for visible signs; emphasize the importance of blood sugar monitoring.
- Tell adolescents to avoid substances that alter blood glucose levels (e.g., alcoholic beverages, cigarettes, any drug not prescribed by primary physician); role play peer pressure situations.
- Instruct to keep routine follow-up appointments and to notify physician with any problems.

☐ **EVALUATION CRITERIA/DESIRED OUTCOMES**

The child/parents
- Identify the type(s) of insulin prescribed

- Describe onset, peak actions, precautions for administration of insulin
- Store insulin correctly
- Administer prescribed dosages of insulin correctly
- Select and record injection sites correctly
- State the signs and symptoms of insulin reaction and identify measures to correct hypoglycemia

---

c. **Knowledge deficit** regarding glucose monitoring

Rationale: Insulin therapy is ordered and adjusted on the basis of direct/indirect monitoring of serum glucose levels. Urine testing was for many years the only home testing done to monitor diabetes and administer supplementary insulin. Recently, devices for blood glucose monitoring at home have become available and are more commonly prescribed/used as they provide direct rather than indirect measurement of serum glucose. In addition to glucose levels, the urinary acetone (ketone) level is monitored as well. Ketonuria may result when too little insulin is available for the body to metabolize glucose and the body instead begins to metabolize fats for energy.

☐ **GOAL**

The child/parents will assess blood glucose levels daily; will state when to call physician about glucose and acetone levels.

☐ **IMPLEMENTATION**

- Demonstrate how to test for serum glucose level using the device or method the child will be using after discharge; use the package insert or instruction manual so that the child/parents can follow along with you; follow the package insert/instructional manual precisely when timing, wiping, and interpreting test results.
- Instruct when to test blood sugars
  - to maintain strict control, test glucose levels 4 times a day (e.g., before meals and at bedtime); if the child is in school and under good control, only urine testing can be done at lunch
  - check blood sugar if illness/infection present or hypo/hyperglycemic episode suspected
  - call results into the physician's office as directed or bring to follow-up visits; *keep updated/ accurate records at home*
- Ensure child/parents have a written copy of the plan for the use of supplemental insulin if insulin coverage is ordered on the basis of serum glucose levels; instruct when to call physician.
- Demonstrate the test for glucose and acetone in the urine; use the product that will be used at

home; have the child/parents follow along with the package insert.
- Have child drink a glass of water and void again in 15–30 minutes if specimen is positive for sugar.
- Instruct to inform the physician of the presence of ketones in the urine, whether or not the serum and urinary glucose levels are elevated.

☐ **EVALUATION CRITERIA/DESIRED OUTCOMES**

The child/parents
- Perform serum/urinary glucose and acetone monitoring using the methods to be used in the home after discharge
- Interpret urine testing results correctly
- Demonstrate ability to administer supplemental insulin when indicated by elevated serum glucose levels as prescribed by physician
- List indications for informing physician of glucose or acetone levels

---

d. **Knowledge deficit** regarding appropriate exercise/activity regimen

Rationale: Exercise is important in the treatment of diabetes as it increases the body's sensitivity to insulin and decreases the blood sugar and percentage of fat in the body. Decreased anxiety and stress result from regular exercise, promoting a more positive self-image—a very important attitude to foster when confronting a chronic disease.

☐ **GOAL**

The child/parents will have sufficient information to understand, accept, and plan an age-appropriate exercise/activity regimen to be followed after discharge.

☐ **IMPLEMENTATION**

- Discuss with physician recommended exercise/activity regimen for the child.
- Explain that the exercise regimen has been planned with child's age, physical limitations, and present life-style in mind; specify the type of activity and how much exercise child needs to develop and maintain physical fitness.
- Suggest planning exercise/activity at the same time daily as the child may have to adjust insulin dose and diet.
- Advise to avoid strenuous exercise if the child has just resolved an insulin reaction, or is feeling symptomatic.
- Advise to return to normal physical education classes in school after hospitalization and to schedule gym as first class in morning or right after lunch.

- Stress that child should resume normal activities at home and not limit self because of diabetes.
- Tell to wear loose-fitting cotton clothes while exercising and to be sure to have properly fitting shoes.
- Encourage to choose an aerobic activity s/he enjoys to assure compliance.
- Remind that vigorous exercises (e.g., skiing, long hikes) need not be avoided but additional food should be eaten.

☐ **EVALUATION CRITERIA/DESIRED OUTCOMES**

The child/parents
- Describe an individualized plan for regular exercise/activity and state intention to follow it

---

e. **Knowledge deficit** regarding complications

Rationale: Because of the chronic nature of diabetes and because, at present, it can only be controlled, not cured, it is important that the child/parents be aware of common long-term complications associated with diabetes in order to promptly seek medical attention. They should also know that good control of diabetes may decrease the occurrence of complications, which include reduced vision and blindness, kidney problems leading to renal failure, foot problems leading to possible amputation, acute high blood sugar and diabetic ketoacidosis, and adverse outcomes of pregnancy.

☐ **GOAL**

The child/parents will recognize early warning signs of common complications of diabetes.

☐ **IMPLEMENTATION**
- Teach that complications are caused by arteriosclerosis, which is accelerated in diabetes by thickening of the capillary membranes and by the alterations in carbohydrate, fat, and protein metabolism due to the altered insulin levels; teach that complications can be minimized if child is in good control of diabetes from the beginning.
- Discuss with adolescents that weight, diet, and blood pressure control; stress reduction; avoidance

of smoking; and increased awareness of the signs of complications can decrease their incidence.
- Teach the importance of adhering to the prescribed treatment regimen and informing the physician promptly when changes (e.g., unplanned weight loss, changes in vision or urinary output, chronic infections, skin ulcers that do not respond to treatment) are noticed.
- Encourage to see an ophthalmologist and dentist yearly.

☐ **EVALUATION CRITERIA/DESIRED OUTCOMES**

The child/parents
- Comply with preventive health care
- Identify significant signs of complications
- Know when to seek appropriate attention for signs of problems

---

f. **Knowledge deficit** regarding community resources

Rationale: If diabetes is newly diagnosed or if the child/parents have not demonstrated compliance with the treatment regimen prescribed, it may be helpful to provide information about available community resources.

☐ **GOAL**

The child/parents will identify community resources helpful in adjusting to diabetes.

☐ **IMPLEMENTATION**
- Provide with address and phone number of the local chapter of the American Diabetes Association.
- Encourage participation in educational offerings and self-help groups.
- Discuss the importance of wearing a Medic-Alert bracelet.

☐ **EVALUATION CRITERIA/DESIRED OUTCOMES**

The child
- Wears Medic-Alert bracelet

The child/parents
- List community resources
- Express intent to use resources

Table 6
Differentiating Between Hypoglycemia and Hyperglycemia

	Symptoms	Signs	Treatment
Hypoglycemia Occurs when serum glucose level is below normal limits, usually less than 60 mg/dl.	Sweating; pale, cool, or clammy skin; headache; trembling or nervousness; hunger; dizziness or drowsiness; tingling of lips or fingertips; weakness or fatigue; blurred vision, behavioral changes: irrational, easily angered, aggressive, or appearing drunk; slurred speech; slow uncoordinated movement	Shallow, rapid respirations; tachycardia; dilated pupils	MUST BE INITIATED RAPIDLY OR CHILD MAY LOSE CONSCIOUSNESS • Give a simple fast-acting form of carbohydrate (e.g., 4 oz orange juice, 5–7 LifeSavers, or commercial preparations per hospital protocol). • Wait 10–15 min; repeat treatment if symptomatic; check blood sugar 1 hour later • If child unconscious, do not force food, rather administer IV Glucagon, IM Glucagon at home. • Draw stat serum glucose sample and send to lab, or use blood sugar monitoring device. • Notify physician of reaction. • Give juice again in 1 hr if blood sugar is still decreased even if child is asymptomatic; give juice sooner if no relief of symptoms.
Hyperglycemia Occurs when serum glucose level is elevated, usually greater than 250 mg/dl. Slower in onset than hypoglycemia; early recognition and treatment key in preventing ketoacidosis and coma.	*Early* • frequent urination/nocturia • dry mouth, thirst • fatigue, drowsiness • blurred vision • dry, itchy skin • polyphagia *Late* • nausea and vomiting • abdominal pain, constipation	*Late* • flushed, dry skin • fast, labored respirations • weak, rapid pulse • acetone (fruity) breath odor • hypotension • coma	• Keep child in bed and warm if symptomatic (especially late signs/ symptoms). • If conscious, have child drink sugar-free liquids (e.g., water, soda, coffee, tea, broth). • Record I&O. • Draw stat serum glucose; send to lab or use bedside blood sugar monitoring device. • Check/record vital signs, LOC. • Notify physician. • Administer insulin and parenteral fluids as ordered.

The Child with Diarrhea/Gastroenteritis

Definition/Discussion

Diarrhea is an increase in the volume, fluidity, or frequency of bowel movements relative to the usual habits of an individual. Diarrhea is a symptom of a pathophysiologic process within the intestinal tract, not a disease itself. Acute infectious gastroenteritis is an inflammation of the stomach and intestinal tract caused by pathogenic microorganisms. Diarrhea/gastroenteritis can be caused by recent travel or canned, perishable, possibly contaminated foods/formula. Antidiarrheals, adsorbents, and narcotics are rarely given in young children with diarrhea.

Nursing Assessment

☐ PERTINENT HISTORY

Course of illness (length, characteristics); others sick at home; home care regarding diet, fluids; normal weight of child; child/parent idea of possible causes; alteration in usual activities, normal bowel pattern/routine

☐ PHYSICAL FINDINGS

Vital signs, level of consciousness, level of hydration, stool characteristics and pattern (e.g., frequency, amount, color, presence of blood, reducing substances or sugar [test with Clintest tablets], protein, pH); stool specimens (e.g., culture, ova, parasites); abdominal distension/cramping, condition of the skin, behaviors/verbalizations indicating pain

☐ PSYCHOSOCIAL CONCERNS/ DEVELOPMENTAL FACTORS

Developmental level, coping mechanisms, habits (e.g., what comforts child, sleeping/eating routines, favored objects); impact of isolation

☐ PATIENT AND FAMILY KNOWLEDGE

Complications (e.g., dehydration, seizures, malnutrition), communicability, diet, level of knowledge, readiness and willingness to learn

Nursing Care

☐ LONG-TERM GOAL

The child will regain normal intestinal motility and function essential to continued growth and well-being; the child will return to a level of health associated with the reestablishment of fluid/electrolyte balance followed by a return to normal dietary intake.

NURSING DIAGNOSIS #1

Fluid volume deficit related to vomiting, diarrhea

Rationale: Diarrhea and vomiting cause imbalances since diarrheal stools and vomitus are fluid/electrolyte-rich substances. Excessive output without replacement leads to fluid deficit.

☐ GOAL

The child will be well hydrated; will be free from fluid/electrolyte deficit.

☐ IMPLEMENTATION

- Monitor vital signs at least every 4 hours or as needed; report abnormalities.
- Monitor for signs of increasing dehydration (e.g., less elastic skin turgor, depressed fontanels, sunken eyes, weight loss, rapid pulse, dry mucous membranes, decreasing urine output); chart and report to physician.
- Monitor IV every hour; regulate through microdrip chamber/mechanical regulator; restrain child as needed to maintain IV patency; check restraints every hour for pressure and position; protect venipuncture site with padded plastic cup; check every hour for infiltration; refer to *The Child with an Intravenous Catheter*, page 174.
- Record intake and output accurately, weigh diapers.
- Check urine specific gravity every 4 hours.
- Weigh child daily, or more frequently if neces-

sary, on same scale, in the same clothes, at the same time.
- Monitor lab reports (e.g., electrolytes, pH, hematocrit, serum albumin, urine specific gravity) daily; evaluate response to therapy.
- Reduce insensible fluid loss (via skin and lungs); dress lightly in minimal clothing, administer medications, and give tepid sponge baths if fever present.
- Maintain NPO until/unless otherwise ordered.

☐ EVALUATION CRITERIA/DESIRED OUTCOMES

The child
- Shows improving skin turgor with no tenting present
- Has moist mucous membranes
- Demonstrates lab values and urine output within normal limits for age
- Returns to preillness weight

NURSING DIAGNOSIS #2

Alteration in nutrition: less than body requirements related to inadequate absorption of nutrients

Rationale: With vomiting and diarrhea the body cannot absorb enough nutrients to meet metabolic demands. The child loses weight and growth and development may suffer.

☐ GOAL

The child will experience a cessation of vomiting and loose, watery stools; will maintain/regain weight.

☐ IMPLEMENTATION

- Keep NPO; provide oral hygiene.
- Monitor total parenteral nutrition infusion if ordered; see *The Child Receiving Total Parenteral Nutrition*, page 276.
- Resume oral fluids gradually when permitted using an electrolyte solution or clear liquids; progress from half-strength to full-strength formulas.
- Reintroduce solid foods with a bland BRAT (i.e., *b*ananas, *r*ice, *a*pplesauce, *t*oast) diet.
- Change previous diet/food preparation depending on causative agent; place infants on a soy formula until any lactose intolerance has resolved (4–6 weeks).
- Report tolerance of new diet, reappearance of vomiting or diarrhea.

☐ EVALUATION CRITERIA/DESIRED OUTCOMES

The child
- Retains food and fluids
- Resumes normal bowel elimination patterns
- Demonstrates appropriate growth pattern for age

NURSING DIAGNOSIS #3

Impairment of skin integrity related to frequent loose stools

Rationale: Diarrheal stools are alkaline and contain enzymes that readily cause excoriation when in contact with skin.

☐ GOAL

The child will experience no diaper rash, impaired perianal skin integrity.

☐ IMPLEMENTATION

- Clean diaper area with water and mild soap after each bowel movement (commercial cleaning wipes contain alcohol and may cause further irritation/pain).
- Apply medicated powder to area (preparations such as Desitin may be used but are difficult to wash off); do not apply hydrocortisone cream if using plastic pants as plastic can increase absorption of the hydrocortisone with resulting side effects.
- Teach parents that baby powder is not necessary but if used it should be sprinkled in their hands and then applied to baby; keep powder away from infant's face to avoid inhalation; never give powder container to infant to hold.
- Use cloth diapers when available; line disposable diapers with disposable wash cloths if irritation is increased by diapers.
- Leave diaper area open to air as much as possible; expose diaper area at least 5–10 minutes with each diaper change.
- Use heat lamp (60-watt bulb, 15–18 inches from child and objects) on area for 5–10 minutes every 2–4 hours; wipe any ointment off before treatment to prevent burns.

☐ EVALUATION CRITERIA/DESIRED OUTCOMES

The child
- Shows no excoriation of diaper area
- Is free from secondary infection

NURSING DIAGNOSIS #4

Alteration in comfort: pain related to abdominal cramps/distension

Rationale: Increased bowel transit time and a hyperosmotic load cause stretching and spasms in the intestines. When diarrhea or vomiting are present, abdominal cramping and distension are often accompanying symptoms that cause discomfort/pain.

GOAL

The child will be comfortable; will experience relief from cramping.

IMPLEMENTATION

- Give medications sparingly; monitor effects carefully.
- Change position at least every 2 hours.
- Hold young children.
- Minimize crying to reduce amount of swallowed air that adds to distension; burp as necessary to expel swallowed air.
- Place warm cloth on abdomen for cramping; do not apply heat if acute abdomen or inflammation such as appendicitis or peritonitis is suspected.

EVALUATION CRITERIA/DESIRED OUTCOMES

The child
- Has soft, nondistended abdomen
- Demonstrates no verbal/nonverbal indications of pain
- Sleeps comfortably
- Plays happily

NURSING DIAGNOSIS #6

Diversional activity deficit related to illness/hospitalization

Rationale: Illness/hospitalization is a disturbance to normal individual/family functioning, restrictions are often imposed that stress new/previous coping mechanisms and methods of meeting developmental milestones.

GOAL

The child will be free from boredom/emotional disturbances related to illness/hospitalization.

IMPLEMENTATION

- Schedule time every hour for verbal and physical contact; speak soothingly, stroke and comfort, especially when parents are unable to stay with child.
- Reposition every 1–2 hours; remove restraints.
- Do range-of-motion exercises; refer to *The Child Requiring Range-of-Motion Exercises*, page 237.
- Encourage parents to visit and interact with child.

- Provide the young infant and child with sucking stimulation (e.g., pacifier, teething toy).
- Use brightly colored washable/disposable toys, pictures, and mobiles to stimulate and vary environment.
- Provide musical background when parents or nurse not in room.
- Encourage age-appropriate developmental tasks/therapeutic play as condition permits.
- Explain all procedures to child/parents; provide explanation that is appropriate for developmental level.

EVALUATION CRITERIA/DESIRED OUTCOMES

The child
- Performs appropriate age-related tasks

NURSING DIAGNOSIS #7

Knowledge deficit regarding signs of complications, dietary restrictions, communicability

Rationale: If knowledge deficit exists, child/parents cannot appropriately manage treatment or detect complications of diarrhea/gastroenteritis before the child becomes more seriously ill. If appropriate infection-control and isolation techniques are not maintained, disease may spread to family and community.

GOAL

The child/parents will verbalize an understanding of dietary restrictions, potential complications, methods of treating diarrhea/gastroenteritis.

IMPLEMENTATION

- Instruct parents in the proper method of making, storing, and giving formula/meals.
- Obtain consultation with dietician if appropriate.
- Teach parents dietary management of vomiting and diarrhea.
- Use facts and examples to teach good handwashing technique and sanitation habits; observe return demonstration.
- Teach danger signs of diarrhea/vomiting (e.g., more than 3 episodes within a 4-hour period, loss of appetite, inability to retain fluids or food, fever, change in breathing/sensorium, diminished urination).
- Explain need for isolation if appropriate; teach isolation techniques.
- Explain reason for reporting communicable disease to local health department for epidemiologic follow-up if appropriate.
- Teach parents to notify pediatric clinic or public health nurse if symptoms are not gone in 1 week or if there are repeated episodes of diarrhea over a period of weeks or months.

☐ EVALUATION CRITERIA/DESIRED OUTCOMES

The child/parents

- State how to prevent a recurrence
- Demonstrate proper handwashing and sanitation techniques
- Isolate child from possible sources of infection
- State the importance of keeping the child well hydrated
- List danger signs of diarrhea and the need for prompt medical care

The Child who is Dying/Terminal

Definition/Discussion

Societal and cultural values influence both children and adults in their acceptance of death. Understanding those values influences the perceptions of/reactions to the knowledge that a child is dying. Previous experiences with death (e.g., pet, family member, friend, peer) will influence the child's perception of/reaction to death. Children convey their feelings and understanding of impending death through symbols and behaviors.

The age of the child must be considered in relation to his/her level of understanding regarding death and dying. Young children may equate death with separation, going into a grave, or sleep. The apparent lack of understanding on the child's part about what is happening does not mean the child has no anxiety about death and dying. Children perceive alterations in staff and family behavior around them and may adjust their own reaction to death based on adult behavior.

The development of a concept of death takes place in stages related to the child's maturing cognitive abilities, rather than the child's chronologic age. Factors such as cultural background, religious socialization, and real-life experiences with death and dying processes influence the concept formation. Children learn to cope with death mainly through observing parents, other family members, and friends. Emotional support and teaching of the family promote adaptive coping with death in both children and parents. Exposure to death in a matter-of-fact, non-frightening manner and at a developmentally appropriate level tends to be less fearful. This results in more adaptive coping compared to those who have not had this developmentally appropriate presentation.

Nursing Assessment

☐ PERTINENT HISTORY

Course of illness (e.g., length, characteristics), social and cultural values of family, previous experiences with death (e.g., relative, friend, pet), home measures to maintain child's comfort and to relieve anxiety

☐ PHYSICAL FINDINGS

Level of consciousness, vital signs, level of hydration, amount of pain/discomfort, energy available for self-care and diversional activities

☐ PSYCHOSOCIAL CONCERNS/ DEVELOPMENTAL FACTORS

Age and developmental level, coping mechanisms of child/family, support systems and resources available, behavior of parents and siblings around the child, expectations of child/family, habits/rituals of child at home

☐ PATIENT AND FAMILY KNOWLEDGE

Causes, options, level of knowledge, readiness and willingness to learn

Nursing Care

☐ LONG-TERM GOAL

The child will maintain physiologic/emotional functioning with comfort and reduced anxiety during the terminal process; the family will move toward acceptance and resolution of the terminal process so they can assist in providing comfort and support to the dying child.

NURSING DIAGNOSIS #1

Alteration in comfort: pain related to disease process

Rationale: *Throughout the course of the illness and in particular close to the time of death, the pain the child experiences becomes the parent's pain, and the apprehension that the parents have is transferred to the child, increasing discomfort.*

☐ GOAL

The child will experience minimal pain and discomfort, thus easing the parent's pain as well

☐ IMPLEMENTATION

- Refer to *The Child Experiencing Pain*, page 216.
- Prepare the parents in advance for the pain the child may be experiencing.
- Assure the family that care givers are monitoring the child, and prepared to help.

116

- Make sure the family knows how often the pain medication can be given and the time that it is due.
- Assess pain and provide medication PRN; use oral medications whenever possible; attempt to reserve heavy doses of any narcotics/shots until late in illness.
- Position the child to relieve pain.
- Give analgesic 30 minutes before painful procedures.
- Use gentle touch, soothing voice, distraction techniques (e.g., imagery, music) as appropriate.

☐ **EVALUATION CRITERIA/DESIRED OUTCOMES**

The child
- Exhibits behaviors indicating comfort
- Denies pain verbally
- Sleeps comfortably

NURSING DIAGNOSIS #2

Anticipatory grieving related to probability of death

Rationale: As the child's illness progresses, emotional changes take place in the child and family reflecting stages of awareness and understanding of the terminal process. This grieving also occurs in care givers.

☐ **GOAL**

The child/family will express feelings, fears, anxieties and guilt; will verbalize their understanding of the child's physical health status and the terminal process.

☐ **IMPLEMENTATION**
- See Table 7—The Child's Conception of Death.
- Assess acceptance of the physical-health status; tell child/family that others in the same situation experience many kinds of feelings; ask what it is like for them.
- Allow and encourage parents to express feelings without the child being present.
- Provide opportunities for the child to share feelings without the parents.
- Accept feelings and expressions in a nonjudgmental manner.
- Permit expressions of anger and hostility, but do not allow unacceptable behavior; the child may perceive this as hopelessness and abandonment.
- Provide age-appropriate tools (e.g., toys, pens, pencils) that will enable the child to have normal experiences and symbolically express level of understanding about death; refer to *The Child Requiring Play Therapy*, page 226.

- Avoid false cheerfulness and evasiveness that may prevent the child from trusting/expressing true feelings.
- Allow discussion of the physical manifestations of the illness, the diagnosis, and possible outcomes; use language that can be understood by all.
- Give information to the child and family about changes that are occurring in the body.
- Encourage family members, friends, peers, to continue interaction with the child; be available to them if the child withdraws from their attempt to comfort.
- Allow the child to make decisions regarding physical care (e.g., setting the time for procedures and participating in daily activities whenever possible).
- Allow the family to assist with care, or if that is not feasible, to assist with the care of other children on the unit (if the child/family desire and accept this).
- Keep the family informed on the daily medical and nursing regimen so they can be kept abreast of the child's physical and emotional functioning.
- Assess the parents' coping behavior so that when they need support, or are unable to be with the child and need to be alone, feelings of guilt will be avoided; seek consultation from a psychiatric/mental health nurse if necessary.
- Assess the strengths of the parents; utilize those strengths in planning the management of the child.
- Provide opportunities for staff discussion of home care options.
- Explain the decision for home care is not irreversible if the family cannot cope.

☐ **EVALUATION CRITERIA/DESIRED OUTCOMES**

The child/parents
- Identify feelings
- Express understanding of prognosis
- List resources available for support

NURSING DIAGNOSIS #3

Self-care deficit: feeding, bathing/hygiene, dressing/grooming, toileting related to debilitated state

Rationale: As the terminal illness progresses, the child becomes weaker and less able to meet physical needs, and physiologic demands of illness manifest in fever, bleeding, drainage, and incontinence that increase physical care demands.

☐ **GOAL**

The child will maintain as much independence as possible in activities of daily living (ADL); will maintain physiologic functioning with comfort for as long as possible; the family will participate in the child's physical care.

☐ IMPLEMENTATION

- Encourage the child's participation in ADL as long as the child's energy levels are not depleted.
- Use passive/active range-of-motion exercises as tolerated; refer to *The Child Requiring Range-of-Motion Exercise*, page 237; encourage as much ambulation as possible.
- Ensure adequate intake of fluid and food; use supplements when necessary; allow child choice of food when possible.
- Preserve skin integrity (e.g., massage, bathe, use lotions, sheepskins, water mattress); reposition every 2 hours and as necessary.
- Maintain a pleasing physical environment (e.g., allowing adequate ventilation of the room, use of room deodorants when necessary, permitting toys/material objects of importance to the child to be present).
- Allow the child to wear own clothing when possible.

☐ EVALUATION CRITERIA/DESIRED OUTCOMES

The child
- Remains clean and dry
- Is positioned comfortably every 2 hours

The parents
- Demonstrate moving and hygiene techniques

NURSING DIAGNOSIS #4

a. **Diversional activity deficit** related to immobility, lack of energy, isolation from friends
b. **Social isolation** related to separation from family, friends

Rationale: A child with a terminal illness may lack the physical stamina to engage in previous accustomed play activities. The child may withdraw from friends in preparing for death, friends may stay away because they are uncomfortable, friends/parents may prohibit visiting ill child so as to protect healthy child (physically/emotionally).

☐ GOAL

The child will not be bored; will accomplish age-appropriate activities as stamina permits.

☐ IMPLEMENTATION

- Talk with child to assess wants/desires regarding play, favorite activities.
- Provide age-appropriate play activities (e.g., play-

ing jacks, baking cookies, making paper dolls, coloring, finger painting, clay modeling, reading, watching favorite movies/TV, listening to music, caring for pets, walking outside, riding in wagon).
- Include child in family activities as much as possible; if at home, suggest child be placed in central area where family gathers.

☐ EVALUATION CRITERIA/DESIRED OUTCOMES

The child
- Shows no listlessness/irritability from lack of activity
- Does not complain, demonstrate behaviors of boredom

NURSING DIAGNOSIS #5

Knowledge deficit regarding preparation for transfer of child to home or nonacute setting

Rationale: Given the right set of circumstances and supportive help for the family, a death at home (or in a more home-like setting) can be more comfortable and more personal for both the child and the family. Training the parents to become the primary care givers can often help the family to overcome the feelings of helplessness and loss of control that accompany a death in the hospital setting.

☐ GOAL

The child will maintain current level of functioning in new setting; the child/family will perceive that home/nonacute hospital care is a viable alternative; the family will demonstrate understanding of the child's care; will state potential complications, and list community resources.

☐ IMPLEMENTATION

- Assist family members to learn the skills necessary to care for the child's physical needs at home (e.g., administration of medications, positioning, range-of-motion exercises, bathing, skin care, use of equipment, bedside commodes, suctioning devices).
- Assist to recognize need for pain medications and the amount necessary to maintain comfort.
- Make home visit to assist family in setting up the home for the child prior to discharge.
- Refer to appropriate agencies (e.g., VNA, health department, home health agency, hospice) for additional professional assistance.
- Assist the family in anticipating funeral arrangements; arrange for social service agencies and resource persons (e.g., clergy) to be available.
- Refer to self-help groups in their community; keep a list available at your nursing unit for convenient

use; refer to the American Cancer Society or Community Mental Health Center for additional resources.
- Give family list of names/phone numbers to call in case of questions/emergency.

The child/family
- Demonstrates technical skills needed to care for self/child at home
- Acknowledges the decision for home care is not irreversible if the family cannot cope
- Understands arrangements for the use of community resources including support/self-help group and clergy

Table 7
The Child's Conception of Death

Concepts	Nursing Implications
Infant (0–14 months) • Elementary sense of the meaning of separation. • Until about 5 months, the loss means the deprivation of the basic needs for food, comfort, and security. • Separation anxiety develops beginning with stranger anxiety about 7–8 months and then the concept of object permanence around 9 months. • Child is sensitive to parental reactions (e.g., anxiety, anger, sadness, crying).	• Note behaviors indicative of response to separation (e.g., excessive crying, irritability, apathy, listlessness, feeding disorders, weight loss, developmental delays). • Assist parents to deal with feelings about loss and death, which will allow the build-up of emotional reserves to meet the needs of the infant. • Provide visual, auditory, and tactile stimulation (e.g., talk to, play with, hold infant). • Provide age-appropriate play activities (e.g., peek-a-boo, "all-gone").
Toddler (15 months–2½ years) • Comprehension of loss remains limited in scope, but child can extend concept beyond the maternal figure to people and objects in the world around him. • Separation anxiety reaches its peak around 2 years. • Learns through repeated separations that reunions are an inevitable outcome; therefore, death is temporary.	• Note behaviors indicative of response to separation (e.g., anger, tantrums, depression, withdrawal, inappropriate attachment). • Listen attentively and be matter of fact and honest: "Grandpa can't come to dinner because he's dead and in (heaven, cemetery, or other explanation)." Use correct terms "death," "died," "buried," to prevent confusion; do not use "sleep" to describe death as toddler will be afraid to sleep. • Know that toddlers are adept at sensing inconsistencies between verbal and nonverbal messages; withholding real feelings will make toddler anxious. Say, "Crying makes me feel better when I'm sad," or "Grownups need to cry and be sad, too." • Provide appropriate play activities (e.g., hide and seek, peek-a-boo, jack-in-the-box).
Preschooler (2½–6 years) • Death does not imply cessation of life but an altered state of living (e.g., sleep, immobility). • Attributes life and consciousness to the dead. • Egocentric thinking results in the notion that dead people can be fed or given medicine to bring them back to life, because these kinds of things make the child feel better. Television and cartoons reinforce that death is not final. • Does not understand intent or reasons behind events; attributes magical or supernatural causes to what is seen and cannot be understood; may perceive death as a punishment or retribution for wrongdoing.	• Note behaviors that indicate a response to the death: ritualistic or superstitious behaviors (e.g., continuing to set a place at the table; may lie awake at night to ward off monsters; has repeated questions, may continue to ask when the deceased is coming home, or when will be the next time to see the person, why did the person die). • Utilize familiar situations to talk about death (e.g., talk about dead birds, bugs, autumn leaves, or dead flowers; read age-appropriate books and let child draw pictures). • Allow child to have funeral ritual for deceased pets (curious child may dig up the remains to see if still in ground). • Give concise and frequent explanations as requested by child regarding the death. • Explain death in terms child can understand (e.g., "Dead people [animals] cannot eat or run or play or be sad or happy"). • Explain that people cannot be "wished away"; inform child that everyone has these wishes sometimes and that thoughts and wishes cannot hurt others.

Table 7
The Child's Conception of Death, Cont.

Concepts	Nursing Implications
	• Know that preschoolers accept literal meaning of words; listen to thoughts and feelings and clarify understanding of death; familiarize yourself with words or phrases that connote death to the preschooler, and use them when referring to the deceased. Do not use them in association with the preschooler. For example, if child says pet is "sleeping," do not put child to bed stating "It is time to go to sleep." Use child's terms of "nite-nite," "bedtime," "tuck me in time." • Accept expressed feelings; give support until child feels safe enough and has enough self-control to grieve and begin to resolve loss. • Hold and comfort the child. Say "It's OK to cry or be angry"; let child know that s/he was not at fault or responsible for death.
School-age (6–12 years) • By 9 years, equates death with the cessation of life; is more reality oriented and logical in thought. • Increased cognitive abilities facilitate an understanding of time and transformation of states. • Considers death as something that happens to someone else until about 9 years old, then death becomes universal. • May feel varying degrees of responsibility; can still interpret death as punishment. • Has pronounced fears of mutilation.	• Note behaviors that indicate a response to death: anxiety about changes in routine; creation of rituals or setting routines as magical or protective; nailbiting, thumbsucking; hyperactivity; mood swings; inappropriate gaiety. • Assess understanding and clarify meanings of statements and questions; ask "What do you think makes people (animals) die?" This age group responds well to logical explanation. • Listen to religious orientation and beliefs; allow child to talk about feelings; provide aggressive outlets through play, as well as opportunities to draw, write, read and tell stories. Use physical contact and bedtime rituals to encourage conversation about the happenings of the day, joys, fears, concerns, questions. • Allow child to attend or discuss funeral and burial services; tell what to expect in matter-of-fact way; arrange for friend or family member to sit with child and take child out of service if child wants to leave. Take child to burial site to visit grave if child desires. Answer questions about postdeath activities (e.g., mortuary, autopsy, or funerals). • Know that support given to parents about their concerns and feelings about death will help child. Allow child to laugh and play during periods of bereavement; play is the work of child and will facilitate grief work. • Acknowledge child's concerns and fears about parents' possible death; let child know that they are not dying and who would care for the child if they did. • Provide appropriate play activities; reassure that child is not responsible for the death, that child did nothing wrong to cause the death. Reinforce that no physical harm will come to child because of the death.

Table 7
The Child's Conception of Death, Cont.

Concepts	Nursing Implications
Adolescent (13–18 years) • Understands death is universal, including self, but still does not accept it as believed reality (practices denial); anxiously avoids thought of death; directs energies at obtaining a sense of self and one's place in the world.	• Note behaviors that may indicate a response to the death: defiance, drug/ETOH abuse, reckless driving; tachycardia, tachypnea, flushed skin tone, diaphoresis; restlessness, pacing; mood swings; may ask many questions; will fear and resent any intrusion on independence; may regress in behavior and become demanding of help with the simplest tasks. • Listen to thoughts and feelings about death; answer questions honestly; discuss movies, television, and books with theme of death. • Treat with respect and as an individual who needs guidance and support and needs to retain independence, control, and decision-making power; facilitate peer-group contact. • Accept expressed feelings of anger or resentment; assist family to regard unpredictable outburst or projection of anger toward staff or parents as normal response to grief and mourning; observe for misconceptions and leftover "magical thinking" or responsibility/guilt for death. Focus on normalcy of experimentation with independence, sexuality, and aggression so that adolescent will release inappropriate guilt. Listen and give support to parents so they can support adolescent and believe in his/her growing process as mature person. • Discuss plans for future. Reinforce the need to be responsible for personal safety and have adolescent problem solve way to provide this.

The Child with Epilepsy

Definition/Discussion _____

Epilepsy is a symptom of a disorder of the central nervous system characterized by seizures (i.e., sudden and periodic lapses of consciousness caused by abnormal electrical discharges in the brain). Seizures may be local or general, accompanied or not accompanied by clonic movements, and may be followed by periods of confusion or drowsiness. Children may also display incoherent speech/extreme restlessness following a seizure persisting for minutes or hours. The child may also be incontinent. Diagnosis is made by electroencephalogram (EEG) recordings.

Status epilepticus (SE) refers to seizures that are repetitive without periods of consciousness, or seizures lasting longer than 30 minutes. Precipitants of SE include withdrawal from alcohol, sedatives, or antiepileptic drugs, fever, trauma, intoxication, and sleep deprivation. EEG monitoring may be needed to differentiate SE-related from nonconvulsive (stuporous) seizures so that appropriate effective antiepileptic drugs can be selected.

Nursing Assessment _____

☐ PERTINENT HISTORY

Course of child's epilepsy: length of time since onset of seizure, date of last seizure and persons present; cause (if known), characteristics of seizures; home care for seizures; names and dosages of medications; normal weight; known precipitating factors

☐ PHYSICAL FINDINGS

Seizures (e.g., onset, duration, characteristics), level of consciousness (LOC), vital signs, side effects of medications (e.g., phenytoin-induced gingival hyperplasia, hirsutism)

☐ PSYCHOSOCIAL CONCERNS/ DEVELOPMENTAL FACTORS

Developmental level, coping mechanisms, habits of child/family; impact of hospitalization/diagnostic testing; educational history; peer relations; school activities

☐ PATIENT AND FAMILY KNOWLEDGE

Acceptance of limitations imposed by disease, medication regimen; level of knowledge, readiness and willingness to learn

Nursing Care _____

☐ LONG-TERM GOAL

The child will lead a relatively normal/healthy life, participating in social and athletic activities; the child will be seizure free; the child will cope effectively, demonstrating positive feelings of self-worth and self-confidence consistent with realistic education/career goals. The child/family will accept the reality of a lifelong condition.

NURSING DIAGNOSIS #1
a. **Potential for injury** related to falling, aspiration during or after seizure
b. **Ineffective airway clearance** related to aspiration of mucus, foreign objects, or obstruction by tongue

Rationale: *During the seizure (i.e., ictal phase) or after (i.e., postictal phase), the child may be injured by falling, hitting a sharp object, or aspirating (e.g., mucus, foreign objects). First aid measures for lay people specifically indicate that tongue blades or other objects should not be placed in a child's mouth during a seizure.*

☐ GOAL

The child will sustain no injuries; will maintain patent airway.

☐ IMPLEMENTATION

- Tape plastic oral airway (for possible use by physician or qualified nurse) in a clearly designated, easily accessible place (e.g., head of bed) and have an alternate available when the child leaves room.

- Keep bed rails up and padded when in bed; explain to child and obtain cooperation.
- Take only rectal or axillary temperatures.
- Have readily accessible for immediate use: oxygen and suction equipment, IV supplies, parenteral antiepileptic drugs (e.g., diazepam, phenobarbital, phenytoin, valproic acid), cardiac and respiratory stimulants, and IV bicarbonate.
- Remain calm, reassuring, matter-of-fact during seizure activity, as attitudes influence behavior of onlookers.
- Urge onlookers to leave scene once a seizure begins; assure them that you will cope with situation.
- Remain with child once a seizure begins
  - place in a side-lying position if possible
  - loosen clothing at neck and waist
  - remove glasses
  - protect head with your arms, lap, cushion, or safe substitute; protect from environmental dangers (e.g., furniture, walls, equipment)
  - maintain an open airway by extending neck, turning face to side if possible
  - intubate with oral airway if available and indicated
  - use padded tongue blade if able to insert prior to seizure; *do not* force anything between clenched teeth
  - suction secretions as necessary
  - prepare IV fluids with antiepileptic drugs (usually quick-acting diazepam to start) and monitor frequently to ensure a slow infusion rate
  - observe closely for respiratory and cardiac depression
  - monitor vital signs at least every 15 minutes
  - arrange for transfer to intensive care unit or provide one-to-one nursing observation and care
- Record observations without interpretations or judgments in chronologic sequence
Preictal phase
  - time
  - onset of unusual behavior
  - environmental stimulants or other possible pre-seizure factors (e.g., photosensitivity, chill, fatigue, stressors)
Ictal phase
  - location and type of tonic/clonic contractions
  - incontinence
  - skin color and condition
  - automatisms (e.g., eye fluttering, lip smacking)/ eye movements and pupillary changes
  - duration of seizure
  - medications given and effectiveness
Postictal phase
  - progress of child's condition, sensorium
  - level of awareness
  - speech difficulty, weakness, pain
  - length of time it takes for child to be reoriented and stabilized

- Check vital signs and LOC immediately after seizure and every 2 hours.
- Observe and report unusual behavior.
- Do not try to stop purposeless behavior; do not touch, annoy, or argue with a child who is not in control.

☐ EVALUATION CRITERIA/DESIRED OUTCOMES

The child
- Sustains no injury during/after seizures
- Maintains normal respiratory pattern

NURSING DIAGNOSIS #2

Alteration in thought processes related to seizure activity, loss of consciousness

Rationale: *A seizure involves a sudden, brief loss of contact with the environment; afterwards, the child may be sleepy, confused, exhausted, complain of a headache, but will not remember the seizure.*

☐ GOAL

The child will be oriented after seizure.

☐ IMPLEMENTATION

- Check vital signs and level of consciousness every 2 hours; observe and report unusual behavior.
- Reorient child to name, time, place, and surroundings; speak slowly.
- Remain with child until fully conscious and oriented or until child is stable although asleep.
- Allow child to eat or sleep after seizure when possible.

☐ EVALUATION CRITERIA/DESIRED OUTCOMES

The child
- Is oriented after seizure
- Has normal vital signs after seizure

NURSING DIAGNOSIS #3

Disturbance in self-concept: body image/self-esteem related to loss of control over body, reactions of others to child

Rationale: *Children with epilepsy and their families must cope with social stigma/rejection because of the public's misconceptions and prejudices about seizure disorders. The child is often confused/embarrassed following a seizure and under such circumstances may feel insecure and resentful, and develop behavioral/emotional difficulties.*

GOAL

The child will maintain positive self-esteem; will cope effectively with the seizures and reactions of others.

IMPLEMENTATION

- Explain child's behavior during/after a seizure to child, parents, witnesses; do not allow child to be subjected to embarrassment because of behavior.
- Encourage open expression of feelings; indicate that feelings of resentment, frustration, and scepticism are normal.
- Encourage discussion concerning misconceptions, fears, the reality of public discrimination and the social stigma of epilepsy.
- Inform parents of the importance of treating their child as any other child.
- Assist the parents to plan age-appropriate developmental activities for the child.
- Do not discipline because of or immediately following a seizure.
- Prepare child to assume self-care activities.
- Assist the child/parents to utilize community support resources, as appropriate

EVALUATION CRITERIA/DESIRED OUTCOMES

The child
- Achieves age-appropriate developmental tasks
- Has balanced, active childhood

NURSING DIAGNOSIS #4

Knowledge deficit regarding use of medication in preventing seizures, realities of epilepsy

Rationale: Child/parents cannot manage treatment of epilepsy or detect symptoms of drug side/toxic effects if a knowledge deficit exists. Misconceptions are fostered when there is a lack of understanding/ knowledge.

GOAL

The child/parents will comply willingly with drug regimen; will identify/report symptoms of side and toxic effects; will list factors that alter seizure threshold; the parents will manage seizures safely; will describe seizures accurately.

IMPLEMENTATION

- Teach/counsel regarding reality of epilepsy, need for compliance with continuing medical regimen.
- Explain necessary information about each medication: name, action, dosage, time of administration, side and toxic effects to report.
- Emphasize the necessity of maintaining a therapeutic blood level by not missing or postponing doses; explain protocol for a missed dose; explain that it may take several months to find the best combination of drugs or the most effective dosage levels.
- Teach actions to minimize side effects of drugs (e.g., proper oral hygiene, gum stimulation to decrease gingival hyperplasia; taking some medications with meals to decrease gastric irritation).
- Teach that seizure threshold can be lowered by fatigue, sleep deprivation, infection, fever, injury, psychologic stress; help plan life-style that minimizes the occurrence of these factors, especially stress.
- Promote and facilitate an open discussion among child, parents, teachers, and physician.
- Provide auxiliary medical personnel, parents, child's friends with information regarding child's particular type of seizure.
- Teach parents how to observe and describe seizures accurately.
- Teach safe, appropriate first aid measures to be provided during and after a seizure.
- Tell parents of the need to provide this information to child's teacher, school nurse/officials; provide written materials to take to school officials.

EVALUATION CRITERIA/DESIRED OUTCOMES

The child
- Takes drugs as prescribed

The child/parents
- Explain the importance of medication in preventing seizures
- State name, action, dosage, time of administration, and side/toxic effects of medications to be reported
- Identify and report symptoms of side effects and toxic reactions

The parents
- Identify support services to be utilized as needed
- Describe first aid measures to be provided during and after a seizure

The Child with Failure to Thrive (Nonorganic)

Definition/Discussion

Failure to thrive (FTT) is the deviation of an infant's or child's growth rate below a normal standard. The weight may persist below the third percentile for age or may decrease to become less than 80% of ideal weight for age. The deceleration or persistence at a low weight may be the result of organic or nonorganic (psychosocial) etiologies.

- *organic:* physiologic cause is known to contribute to growth failure such as defects in digestion (e.g., cystic fibrosis) or absorption (e.g., gastroenteritis), failure to metabolize (e.g., inborn errors), disruption in utilization (e.g., infection, malignancy, cardiac disease), neurologic disorders (e.g., diencephalic syndrome)
- *nonorganic:* dysfunctional patterns of interaction between primary caretaker (usually mother) and infant/child; caretaker appears to be "out of touch" with the child

Nursing Assessment

☐ PERTINENT HISTORY

Prenatal history; birth and neonatal course (e.g., birth weight, discharge weight); past medical problems; height and weight of other family members; illnesses; nutritional intake; method and type of feeding; food preparation; behaviors during feeding; developmental milestones

☐ PHYSICAL FINDINGS

Weight, height, head circumference, vital signs, hydration status, presence of vomiting, characteristics of stool, cardiac/respiratory/gastrointestinal/genitourinary/neurologic status; observed behavior of child and parents during feeding

☐ PSYCHOSOCIAL CONCERNS/ DEVELOPMENTAL FACTORS

Family social history (e.g., father/mother employment, availability at home, relationship between parents, known/suspected child abuse, ability of family income to meet basic needs), age when major developmental milestones were achieved, comparison of child's development with any siblings or parental expectations, availability of support systems

☐ PATIENT AND FAMILY KNOWLEDGE

Appropriate interactional patterns, willingness to change and to accept support from outside the family, level of knowledge, readiness and willingness to learn

Nursing Care

☐ LONG-TERM GOAL

The infant/child will attain normal growth rate and establish functional patterns of interaction with caretaker.

NURSING DIAGNOSIS #1

Alteration in nutrition: less than body requirements related to insufficient caloric intake, difficulties in feeding

Rationale: The growing body has specific caloric intake requirements related to stages of growth and development. Insufficient intake of calories results in a growth deficit. Protein is necessary for tissue healing and fluid balance. Hypoproteinemia may lead to edema, which interferes with cellular nutrition. Anemia reduces oxygen-carrying capacity of the blood and may result in tissue hypoxia. Vitamins and minerals are necessary for many aspects of cell membrane formation and stability. Dehydration leads to decreased tissue perfusion. Infants and children with FTT can be frustrating to feed; they may turn away, refuse the nipple, fall asleep, vomit, spit, or fight feeding. Prior feeding experiences may have been unpleasant.

GOAL

The child will ingest an adequate diet for age; will eat without resistance.

IMPLEMENTATION

- Monitor and record intake and output accurately.
- Provide adequate caloric intake (may need 150–200 cal/kg/day); focus on protein intake.
- Offer small amounts of high-protein food and fluids at frequent intervals; consult dietician as needed.
- Weigh child daily on same scale, in same clothes, at same time.
- Include primary caretaker as much as possible in feeding care; observe interaction patterns.
- Demonstrate nurturing by holding, cuddling, and talking to child during feeding; teach parents to nurture during feeding.
- Provide feeding times that are conflict free.
- Encourage and praise child/parents for any behaviors that are conducive to successful feeding.
- Teach parents regarding the current developmental level of child; explain that child is not purposefully refusing to eat in order to frustrate them.

EVALUATION CRITERIA/DESIRED OUTCOMES

The child
- Gains weight
- Resumes normal growth pattern for developmental level
- Eats without resistance

The parents
- Participate in feeding
- Describe child's current developmental level
- State realistic expectations for child's feeding behavior

The child/parents
- Interact appropriately with each other

NURSING DIAGNOSIS #2

Alteration in parenting related to low self-esteem

Rationale: Parents who have low self-esteem are not confident in their roles and may be depressed. These feelings disrupt healthy parent-child interaction and reduce chances for effective parenting.

GOAL

The parents will express positive feelings and demonstrate adequacy in the parenting role.

IMPLEMENTATION

- Provide time for parents to express feelings/concerns/doubts about parenting roles.

- Encourage parents to participate as much as possible in all aspects of child care.
- Praise even the smallest parental attempts to participate in care giving and nurturing.
- Show parents developmentally appropriate child care techniques.
- Role model positive parenting behaviors (e.g., talk soothingly to child, praise child for appropriate behavior, use distraction as appropriate to stop undesirable behavior in child instead of verbally belittling or physically handling child).
- Identify parental support groups (e.g., Parents Anonymous) available in the community.

EVALUATION CRITERIA/DESIRED OUTCOMES

The parents
- Care for child appropriately
- Verbalize positive feelings about parenting
- Demonstrate realistic, developmentally appropriate expectations for their child

---

NURSING DIAGNOSIS #3

Impairment of skin integrity related to decreased nutritional intake

Rationale: Children who fail to thrive often are emaciated and dehydrated as a result of insufficient nutritional intake. Any interference with cellular nutrition will disrupt skin integrity.

GOAL

The patient will maintain intact skin surfaces while undergoing nutritional therapy.

IMPLEMENTATION

- Bathe daily with mild soap and rinse completely; leave no residue on skin to contribute to breakdown.
- Clean diaper area quickly and gently after soiling.
- Use lubricating cream on entire body to prevent drying of surface.
- Reposition child every 1–2 hours.

EVALUATION CRITERIA/DESIRED OUTCOMES

The child
- Has no drying, cracking, peeling skin
- Maintains perineal skin integrity

NURSING DIAGNOSIS #4

Alteration in health maintenance related to impaired family dynamics, lack of resources

Rationale: Families of children who fail to thrive characteristically are isolated from the mainstream of society. They often have no extended family in the vicinity or a dysfunctional extended family. Mothers may withdraw from the family; fathers may be unable/unwilling to help or are not present. These families may demonstrate ineffective or non-existent use of medical and community resources. They may either not know about available resources or reject outside help.

☐ GOAL

The family will identify existing medical and community services; will accept assistance.

☐ IMPLEMENTATION

- Establish a trusting relationship with the family; use nonjudgmental listening techniques; acknowledge their concerns.
- Give family a list of community services available.
- Alert interdisciplinary team of need for social work involvement.
- Use relationship with the family to introduce the outside support; introduce social worker to family.
- Assist with scheduling of appointments for follow-up care prior to discharge (this will let family know they are not alone).

☐ EVALUATION CRITERIA/DESIRED OUTCOMES

The family
- Allows nurse to interact with them
- Accepts outside assistance/support
- Establishes and keeps follow-up appointments

NURSING DIAGNOSIS #5

Knowledge deficit regarding normal child growth and development

Rationale: Parents who lack knowledge of normal growth and development will have unrealistic expectations for child behavior as each new developmental stage approaches. Expecting behavior beyond the child's capabilities, or labeling a child's normal behavior as spiteful, reduces the effectiveness of parenting.

☐ GOAL

Parents will understand normal behaviors in the next stage of child's development.

☐ IMPLEMENTATION

- Refer to *Normal Growth and Development*, pages 300–314, and *Guidelines for Teaching Parents and Children*, page 316.
- Teach parents about normal childhood growth and development; give them written material or suggest references to reinforce teaching.
- Praise parents for increased knowledge about their child.
- Identify resources available to assist with continued learning.

☐ EVALUATION CRITERIA/DESIRED OUTCOMES

The parents
- Participate in teaching sessions
- List normal behaviors in the next stage of child's development
- Verbalize positive feelings regarding new knowledge

The Child with a Fever

Definition/Discussion

Fever itself is not an illness, but a sign that accompanies many different illnesses. Most fevers in children are caused by an alteration in the thermoregulating center of the hypothalamus. The febrile state results from a higher-than-normal setting for this "thermostat" as opposed to a dysfunction in the heat loss/heat production mechanism. "Normal" body temperature is 37°C (98.6°F). A child with a rectal temperature exceeding 38°C (101°F) or an oral temperature of 37.9°C (100.2°F) is considered febrile. Skin temperature is unreliable as an indicator of body temperature, which must be elicited with a thermometer.

Low-grade temperatures (37°C [98.6°F] to 37.9°C [100.2°F] orally or 38°C [101°F]) are usually not important in asymptomatic children except newborns. "Brain damage" caused by fever alone is not a possibility unless temperature exceeds 41.1°C (106°F).

Antipyretics are the treatment of choice for fevers but they only reduce the temperature and may not affect the underlying cause. Bathing or sponging with cold water or alcohol to reduce a fever makes a child uncomfortable; alcohol is irritating to the respiratory tract and can cause a rapid change in body temperature that may elicit shivering, thus increasing body temperature.

Nursing Assessment

☐ **PERTINENT HISTORY**

Previous exposure to illness, progression of illness; rashes (persistent or recurrent), headache or neck stiffness, crying when picked up, vomiting or diarrhea, localized pain, respiratory status (runny nose, cough), unusual or persistent irritability, appetite, pattern of behavior/sleep/feeding/playing; parents' perception of progression (better, same, worse); fluid intake and urine output (number of ounces/ 24 hours); pattern of temperature elevations; recent immunization (past 7–10 days); exposure to communicable disease in past 3 weeks; use of medications (antipyretics, antibiotics, herbal remedies, folk remedies); sponge bathing

☐ **PHYSICAL FINDINGS**

Vital signs; hydration status; amount of spontaneous activity; interest in visual surroundings (looking at examiner or spontaneously looking about room); motor activity (sitting still or lying down compared to moving arms or legs voluntarily)

☐ **PSYCHOSOCIAL CONCERNS/ DEVELOPMENTAL FACTORS**

Usual pattern of behavior for developmental level, usual pattern of behavior in medical settings (if known), previous experiences with health care

☐ **PATIENT AND FAMILY KNOWLEDGE**

Recognition of "fever" as symptom, ability to assess temperature and report other signs and symptoms accurately, measures for fever control; level of knowledge, readiness and willingness to learn

Nursing Care

☐ **LONG-TERM GOAL**

The child will return to and maintain normal body temperature.

NURSING DIAGNOSIS #1
a. **Hyperthermia** related to increased metabolic rate, illness, dehydration
b. **Alteration in comfort** related to the febrile state

Rationale: Hyperthermia is a state in which body temperature is elevated above normal range. Children experience subjective feelings of discomfort when febrile, regardless of the cause of the temperature elevation.

☐ **GOAL**

The child will have a normal temperature; will express comfort verbally or through behavior.

☐ **IMPLEMENTATION**

• Monitor temperature and other vital signs every 4 hours and as necessary.
• Administer antipyretic (acetaminophen) as or-

dered; monitor effectiveness 30–60 minutes post-administration.
- Dress child in light-weight clothing; cover lightly when in bed; avoid shivering as this produces and conserves heat.
- Give tepid (not cool) sponge baths as ordered only for temperatures at or above 104°F (40°C).

☐ EVALUATION CRITERIA/DESIRED OUTCOMES

The child
- Maintains a normal temperature
- Verbalizes/demonstrates feeling comfortable
- Resumes some normal play activity, rests quietly, or sleeps as appropriate

---

NURSING DIAGNOSIS #2

Fluid volume deficit related to the febrile state

Rationale: As body temperature increases so does the body's metabolism. Without replenishment of fluid lost through diaphoresis, evaporation, respiration, and usual body excretions the child will experience dehydration.

☐ GOAL

The child will maintain normal hydration status.

☐ IMPLEMENTATION

- Monitor for signs of dehydration (e.g., lack of tear formation, dry mucous membranes, poor skin turgor, sunken eyes, sunken fontanel, increased pulse rate, decreased urination) at least every 4 hours.
- Maintain accurate intake and output.
- Weigh daily on the same scale, at the same time, in the same clothing.
- Calculate amount of fluid required (e.g., maintenance replacement).
- Monitor IV replacement carefully; refer to *The Child with an Intravenous Catheter*, page 174.
- Provide favorite fluids if possible; play games, use funny straws/cups to increase willingness to drink.
- *Do not* administer tepid bath if signs of dehydration are present (will increase vasoconstriction and heat retention, thereby increasing child's temperature and furthering dehydration).

☐ EVALUATION CRITERIA/DESIRED OUTCOMES

The child
- Has good skin turgor, moist mucous membranes, tearing, flat fontanel, and normal pulse rate
- Has balanced intake and output

NURSING DIAGNOSIS #3

Sensory-perceptual alteration related to elevation of body temperature

Rationale: Elevated body temperature may result in confusion or delirium. The cause of this phenomenon is poorly understood but may be related to alterations in certain neuromodulators in fever or to interferon levels that increase with viral infections. Parental anxiety may increase child's anxiety, thus increasing child's mental confusion.

☐ GOAL

The child will maintain sensory-perceptual orientation.

☐ IMPLEMENTATION

- Monitor level of consciousness every 4 hours and as necessary.
- Report changes in behavior.
- Explain child's confusion to parents; elicit their feelings about seeing child in this state.
- Maintain safe environment for child: use side rails, restraints as necessary, provide appropriate toys (soft, no sharp edges), monitor child closely.
- Orient child to person, place, time as developmentally appropriate.

☐ EVALUATION CRITERIA/DESIRED OUTCOMES

The child
- Returns to afebrile state of consciousness (or orientation)
- Recognizes parents
- Responds appropriately to questions
- Arouses easily

NURSING DIAGNOSIS #4

Knowledge deficit regarding cause of fever, care of child with fever, prevention and detection of a fever

Rationale: Many parents do not understand the cause of fever, do not know how to take a temperature, and have misconceptions about fever management and potential changes in body function.

☐ GOAL

The parents will demonstrate increased understanding of causes of fever, taking temperatures, and resolving misconceptions about fevers.

☐ IMPLEMENTATION

- Teach to take an accurate temperature (e.g., methods, timing, reading).
- Educate parents about normal diurnal variation of body temperature, what temperatures are considered to be "fever."
- Explain the importance of administering antipyretic at correct dose and appropriate time intervals.
- Teach parents regarding the use of aspirin and its relationship to Reye's syndrome; tell them not to use with children under age 16 years for varicella, flu (or flulike symptoms), viral illness.
- Correct misconceptions about fevers.
- Provide a factsheet regarding fever, treatment of fever, and misconceptions about fever to reinforce teaching.

☐ EVALUATION CRITERIA/DESIRED OUTCOMES

The parents

- Take temperature correctly
- State association of Reye's syndrome with aspirin use
- State accurate information about fevers

The Child with Gastroesophageal Reflux

Definition/Discussion

Gastroesophageal reflux (GER) occurs when stomach contents reflux up into the esophagus as a result of a relaxed or incompetent lower esophageal sphincter. GER occurs more frequently in infants with cerebral palsy, Down's syndrome or other developmental disabilities, and following tracheoesophageal fistula or esophageal atresia repair. Treatment varies depending on the severity of reflux present, but usually includes specific positioning (depending on severity and physician preference) to prevent vomiting. Surgical repair (fundoplication) may be performed for severe problems.

Nursing Assessment

☐ PERTINENT HISTORY

Presence of congenital defects, feeding patterns, characteristics of vomiting (e.g., duration, occurrence, appearance, presence of blood/bile, effect of change in position), complaints of discomfort/heartburn (in nonverbal infant presence of irritability, especially after eating), respiratory symptoms (e.g., coughing, pneumonia, bronchitis), weight gain/loss patterns

☐ PHYSICAL FINDINGS

Weight, length, head circumference (in infants); skin turgor, respiratory status (e.g., rales, rhonchi, wheezes, retractions), abdomen (e.g., pain, tenderness, masses, bowel sounds)

☐ PSYCHOSOCIAL CONCERNS/ DEVELOPMENTAL FACTORS

Feeding environment at home, parents' feelings about feeding child, developmental level of child, habits (e.g., bedtime/eating routines, favored objects, what comforts child)

☐ PATIENT AND FAMILY KNOWLEDGE

Implication of defect, acceptance of treatment modalities; level of knowledge, readiness and willingness to learn

Nursing Care

☐ LONG-TERM GOAL

The child will retain feedings; the child will gain weight.

NURSING DIAGNOSIS #1

Alteration in nutrition: less than body requirements related to reduced nutrient intake, vomiting

Rationale: *Frequent vomiting results in loss of nutrients and inadequate intake. Infants and young children need to maintain sufficient nutritional intake to permit optimal growth.*

☐ GOAL

The child will maintain normal growth pattern; will not be malnourished.

☐ IMPLEMENTATION

- Keep accurate intake and output.
- Record amount, characteristics of vomiting, time since last feeding.
- Encourage feeding child in a relaxed manner since child responds to parental anxiety/frustration.
- Thicken formula with rice cereal to consistency at which spoon remains upright in bottle.
- Feed slowly in small amounts (depending on age of child) every 2–3 hours with child in an upright position.
- Handle child gently and burp after every 1–2 ounces.
- Position appropriately after feeding (refer to Nursing Diagnosis #2).
- Refeed amount vomited, if ordered.
- Observe parent-child interaction during feeding.
- Refer to *The Child with a Gastrostomy*, page 135, as necessary.

EVALUATION CRITERIA/DESIRED OUTCOMES

The child
- Maintains weight, height, head circumference measurements along growth curve
- Has no signs of protein, carbohydrate, fat, vitamin deficiencies

---

NURSING DIAGNOSIS #2
a. **Impaired physical mobility** related to positioning
b. **Diversional activity deficit** related to positioning

Rationale: The prone position is recommended to prevent GER. It is used when minimal symptoms are present and is used for 4–6 months until the child outgrows the reflux. Maintaining this position limits the child's opportunity to explore the environment or to develop gross motor skills. If child is not stimulated to move, contractures can develop.

GOAL

The child will be free from contractures; will perform gross motor tasks within age-appropriate range; will resume normal tasks shortly after positioning is discontinued (if positioning is for 24 hours/day).

IMPLEMENTATION

- Maintain upright position as much as possible when changing, bathing infant; carry child in upright position (slouching may increase intraperitoneal pressure thus promoting reflux).
- Position on abdomen for 2–3 hours after feeding.
- Prop young infant's head with towels/blankets to ensure proper head and neck position.
- Promote normal growth and development; refer to *Normal Growth and Development: Infant*, page 300.
- Make environment stimulating (e.g., place mobile/bright pictures in line of vision, cradle gym in front of infant, toys in reach); play music, sing, talk frequently to infant; use direct eye contact; put in room with others, touch frequently, spend time playing with infant when awake.
- Schedule active play prior to meals.
- Encourage parents to have others learn child's routine (gives parents a break and may provide different stimulation).
- Prevent torticollis/contractures by changing direction child is facing (e.g., face crib in different directions, move slant board around room, walk around) so child must turn neck to follow you.

If upright on slant board
- Position infant correctly; check neurovascular status on lower extremities every 2 hours.

- Explain to parents that usual length of treatment on board is 24 hours/day for 6–8 months.
- Restrain infant at all times while on board.
- Elevate legs for several minutes just prior to feeding if lower leg edema develops.

EVALUATION CRITERIA/DESIRED OUTCOMES

The child
- Is free from contractures
- Has good muscle tone and movement present in all muscle groups
- Performs age-appropriate developmental tasks
- Is alert, interested in environment
- Meets language and fine motor milestones
- Interacts with environment and other people

NURSING DIAGNOSIS #3

Impaired gas exchange related to immobility, aspiration, postsurgical atelectasis

Rationale: When one position is maintained for long periods secretions pool in the lungs and hypostatic pneumonia may occur. Refluxed material may easily be aspirated into the lungs. Surgery may further compromise the child's respiratory status.

GOAL

The child will experience no respiratory difficulty.

IMPLEMENTATION

- Monitor respiratory status at least every hour.
- Maintain prescribed position, encourage holding/exercising as feeding schedule/condition permits.
- Encourage deep breathing (e.g., blowing bubbles, have child imitate deep breathing), occasional crying (if does not worsen reflux).
- Perform chest physical therapy postoperatively every 2–4 hours as tolerated.

EVALUATION CRITERIA/DESIRED OUTCOMES

The child
- Has normal breath sounds
- Is free from coughing, fever

NURSING DIAGNOSIS #4

Alteration in comfort: pain related to reflux of stomach contents, gas/incisional pain following surgery

Rationale: Esophagitis may be caused by frequent contact between the esophagus and acidic stomach contents. If a fundoplication is performed the child cannot burp or vomit immediately after surgery and *gas accumulates causing distension/pain. Skin, muscles, and nerves are cut during surgery with resultant pain.*

☐ GOAL

The child will be free from pain, abdominal distension.

☐ IMPLEMENTATION

- Refer to *The Child Experiencing Pain,* page 216.
Preoperatively
- Administer drugs (e.g., antacids, cimetidine) as ordered; monitor effectiveness.
- Decrease chance for reflux (e.g., position carefully, handle gently, allow minimal movement for 1–2 hours after feedings).
- Obtain baseline abdominal circumference.
Postoperatively
- Monitor abdominal circumference every 4 hours or as necessary.
- Carefully maintain nasogastric/gastrostomy tube; use free drain or low suction as ordered; position tube(s) securely and restrain child to prevent pulling tube(s) out.
- Unclamp gastrostomy if abdomen becomes tense and distended.

☐ EVALUATION CRITERIA/DESIRED OUTCOMES

The child
- Sleeps comfortably
- Has no abdominal distension
- Is free from apparent physical distress, does not cry excessively, is not irritable

---

NURSING DIAGNOSIS #5
a. **Potential for infection** related to surgical incision
b. **Impairment of skin integrity** related to leakage of gastric contents

Rationale: Surgery interrupts normal skin integrity. A gastrostomy may be inserted at this time with the potential for leakage of gastric contents.

☐ GOAL

The child will be free from infection; the child's incision will heal with no excoriation around gastrostomy tube.

☐ IMPLEMENTATION

- Inspect incision/gastrostomy sites for erythema, edema, warmth, excoriation every 2 hours and report to physician as necessary.

- Position gastrostomy securely; monitor for leakage of stomach contents; notify physician of problems.
- Clean incision and around gastrostomy tube with sterile swabs soaked in a 1:1 solution of sterile water and hydrogen peroxide; rinse with sterile normal saline.
- Consult enterostomal therapist if skin around gastrostomy becomes excoriated; use Karaya ring or Karaya powder to protect skin.

☐ EVALUATION CRITERIA/DESIRED OUTCOMES

The child
- Is afebrile
- Has clean incision and gastrostomy site
- Has no excoriation around gastrostomy

NURSING DIAGNOSIS #6
a. **Alteration in parenting** related to feelings of inadequacy, hospitalization
b. **Grieving** related to loss of a perfect baby

Rationale: Parents anticipate the birth of a perfect baby. When the child has medical problems, parental expectations are altered and they must work through the subsequent grief feelings. Frequent vomiting and the child's resulting weight loss often make parents feel inadequate in their parenting skills. These feelings may be further reinforced by well-meaning relatives who may tell parents they are not feeding or burping the infant correctly.

☐ GOAL

The parents will feel adequate in their parenting skills; will accept and nurture their baby appropriately.

☐ IMPLEMENTATION

- Explain that reflux is not uncommon in neonates and frequently resolves when child begins eating thicker foods.
- Observe parent-child interactions, teach skills/behaviors (e.g., gastrostomy care, proper positioning, feeding, talking to infant, making eye contact) as necessary; observe return demonstrations.
- Involve parents in feeding and physical care, provide reinforcement for positive behavior.
- Encourage parents to ventilate feelings; discuss how others react to child.
- Point out and help parents to focus on child's positive characteristics/behaviors.
- Support parents in all aspects of care, especially when introducing oral feedings after surgery, which may be particularly stressful if negative feeding behaviors developed before surgery.

- Support positive parenting activities/skills.

☐ **EVALUATION CRITERIA/DESIRED OUTCOMES**

The parents
- Hold, feed, and interact with child
- State they feel comfortable when caring for child
- Discuss feelings of loss of the healthy child they expected

The child
- Smiles, responds to parental presence within capabilities
- Develops age-appropriate social, language, fine and gross motor skills

---

NURSING DIAGNOSIS #7

Knowledge deficit regarding condition, positioning, feeding, incision/gastrostomy care

Rationale: Parents need information to provide optimal care for child and prevent complications.

☐ **GOAL**

The parents will care for child appropriately.

☐ **IMPLEMENTATION**
- Explain anatomy of the esophagus/stomach, causes of GER, and why the ordered position is beneficial.
- Teach proper positioning/feeding techniques; observe return demonstrations.
- Demonstrate incision and gastrostomy care; observe parents delivering care.
- Discuss potential complications and methods to prevent them.
- Teach infant-stimulation exercises and explain developmental milestones; refer to *Normal Growth and Development: Infant,* page 300.
- Teach to provide short periods of exercise just before meals.

☐ **EVALUATION CRITERIA/DESIRED OUTCOMES**

The parents
- State cause of GER
- Demonstrate proper positioning, feeding, incision and gastrostomy care

The Child with a Gastrostomy

Definition/Discussion

A gastrostomy is a temporary or permanent opening directly into the stomach through the abdominal wall. Gastrostomies are performed for feeding and stomach decompression following gastric or esophageal surgery.

Nursing Assessment

☐ **PERTINENT HISTORY**

Medical/surgical history; disease or condition necessitating procedure, including primary GI surgery, congenital defects (e.g., tracheoesophageal fistula, esophageal atresia), caustic burns, trauma, oral-motor dysfunction, gastroesophageal reflux, organic disease causing profound anorexia and malnutrition

☐ **PHYSICAL FINDINGS**

Pre-op: nutritional status, findings related to condition requiring gastrostomy placement
Post-op: vital signs, gastrostomy and nasogastric (NG) tube drainage, skin condition of gastrostomy site

☐ **PSYCHOSOCIAL CONCERNS/ DEVELOPMENTAL FACTORS**

Age, developmental level, available coping mechanisms, support systems, strengths and limitations, routines/habits (e.g., eating, sleeping, playing), body image

☐ **PATIENT AND FAMILY KNOWLEDGE**

Surgical procedure including potential complications, administration of gastrostomy feeding, care of gastrostomy; level of knowledge, readiness and willingness to learn

Nursing Care

☐ **LONG-TERM GOAL**

The child will recover from a gastrostomy placement free from preventable complications; the child will maintain adequate nutrition via a gastrostomy feeding tube; the child/ parents will cope adaptively with body-image change and will assume responsibility for enteral therapy, when appropriate.

NURSING DIAGNOSIS #1
Anxiety/fear related to impending surgery

Rationale: *The child/parents usually have inadequate knowledge of surgical procedure, indications for it, and post-op expectations causing fear and anxiety. Adequate preparation helps to decrease fear and anxiety while increasing understanding and ability to cope.*

☐ **GOAL**

The child/parents will have adequate knowledge of the surgical intervention and perioperative care; will express feelings and concerns.

☐ **IMPLEMENTATION**

- Refer to *Normal Growth and Development*, pages 300–314, and *The Child Requiring Play Therapy*, page 226.
- Use developmentally appropriate teaching techniques (e.g., drawings, dolls) to explain procedure and post-op appearance; let child handle tube similar to one that will be inserted; refer to clinical nurse specialist if available.
- Provide opportunity for child/parents to express fears/concerns; clarify misconceptions.
- Review post-op routine (e.g., frequent vital signs); demonstrate cough and deep-breathing exercises and have child practice.
- Follow specific physician orders or hospital protocol for pre-op preparation.

☐ **EVALUATION CRITERIA/DESIRED OUTCOMES**

The child/parents
- Verbalize knowledge of surgical procedure
- Demonstrate intellectual/emotional acceptance of need for surgery

NURSING DIAGNOSIS #2

a. **Fluid volume deficit** related to vomiting, losses from nasogastric (NG)/gastrostomy tube
b. **Alteration in nutrition: less than body requirements** related to pre-op condition, intake dependent on gastrostomy feedings

Rationale: Fluid loss can occur via NG and gastrostomy tube drainage. The child who was dehydrated from pre-op emesis, diarrhea, diaphoresis, or NPO status is at increased risk for these diagnoses. The child may be malnourished preoperatively due to the medical condition. A temporary gastrostomy is occasionally performed to supply food in the pre-op or early post-op period of some major surgeries, although it will be several days before gastrostomy feedings will be initiated postoperatively. Long-term gastrostomy feedings may be required for some conditions.

☐ GOAL

The child will maintain adequate hydration; will be well nourished.

☐ IMPLEMENTATION

- Monitor blood pressure, pulse every 4 hours.
- Keep accurate intake and output; measure urine specific gravity on each voided specimen.
- Weigh child daily at the same time on the same scale in the same clothes.
- Monitor for signs of dehydration (e.g., dry mucous membranes, thirst, decreased skin turgor).
- Administer IV fluid and electrolyte replacement as ordered; monitor effectiveness; refer to *The Child with an Intravenous Catheter*, page 174.
- Report vomiting and excessive bleeding immediately.
- Administer antiemetics if ordered; evaluate effectiveness.
- Measure abdominal girth every 4 hours and as necessary; palpate for tenseness.
- Provide oral hygiene frequently to keep mucous membranes moist and prevent discomfort.
- Maintain placement, patency of NG tube and secure connection to low, intermittent suction as ordered; refer to *The Child Requiring Nasogastric Intubation*, page 194.
- Irrigate NG tube with prescribed amount of normal saline, record amount used and returned.
- Note color and amount of drainage.
- Monitor return of bowel sounds every 8 hours and as necessary.
- Attach gastrostomy tube to gravity drainage, initially, as ordered to prevent buildup of gas and gastric juices in stomach; irrigate as ordered.
- Clamp gastrostomy tube when bowel sounds become active and gastric drainage starts to decrease.
- Vent stomach after each feeding and as necessary.
- Administer initial clear liquid feeding in small amounts; increase amount of fluids as tolerated; monitor tolerance of continuous drip or bolus feedings; refer to *The Child Requiring Tube Feedings*, page 288.
- Progress feeding (e.g., special formula, elemental diet formula [e.g., Vivonex], or regular blended food) if there is no leakage of fluid around the tube and if child tolerates the clear liquids.
- Unclamp tube before each feeding and check for residual; return residual of less than 50% of previous feeding; delay feeding if a residual is 50% or more of previous feeding; report finding to physician.
- Place child on right side or prone with head elevated to enhance gastric emptying.
- Warm feeding to room temperature.
- Let prescribed feeding flow in by gravity or with the use of a feeding pump over a 15- to 20-minute period; flush with 5–15 cc of water depending on child's size and clinical status.
- Allow child to suck on a pacifier during feeding if age is appropriate.
- Monitor bowel elimination; report diarrhea or constipation; take corrective measures.

☐ EVALUATION CRITERIA/DESIRED OUTCOMES

The child
- Has normal skin turgor, moist mucous membranes, urine output of at least 1 cc/kg/hour
- Maintains lab values within normal limits
- Has active bowel sounds
- Has gastric residual less than 50% of prior feeding
- Stabilizes and demonstrates consistent weight gain

NURSING DIAGNOSIS #3

a. **Impairment of skin integrity** related to enzymatic action of gastric juices on skin
b. **Potential for infection** related to microbial contamination of gastrostomy incision

Rationale: Contact of the skin surrounding the gastrostomy with the drainage, containing digestive enzymes, can lead to erythema and excoriation. Any break in the skin's integrity is a risk factor for microbial contamination.

☐ GOAL

The child will maintain skin integrity.

IMPLEMENTATION

- Inspect skin around gastrostomy for leakage, erythema, induration, warmth, and tenderness at least every 4 hours.
- Cover skin around tube with a sterile dressing if indicated; inspect dressing and change as needed; note color, amount, consistency, and odor of drainage.
- Clean gastrostomy site with half-strength hydrogen peroxide and water/saline every 8 hours; after immediate post-op period and when site is well healed, clean gastrostomy site with soap and water, pat dry.
- Expose site to air as much as possible.
- Apply a protective ointment/Karaya powder around stoma if irritation or leakage is present.
- Monitor temperature every 4 hours and as necessary.

EVALUATION CRITERIA/DESIRED OUTCOMES

The child

- Is free from wound and skin erythema, induration, drainage
- Is afebrile

NURSING DIAGNOSIS #4

Alteration in comfort: pain related to incision, tension on gastrostomy tube

Rationale: Incisional discomfort is expected to be most evident during the first 48 hours after surgery, gradually subsiding by 3–4 days postoperatively. An added source of discomfort is the tension of the gastrostomy tube sutured in place.

GOAL

The child will be comfortable.

IMPLEMENTATION

- Monitor the level of discomfort using age developmentally appropriate self-rating scale (e.g., 0–10 point, color scale).
- Monitor nonverbal behaviors indicating pain (e.g., crying, withdrawing, moaning, changing behaviors).
- Identify location, type, duration, intensity, and pattern of pain.
- Reposition child and use proper support; assure that position change will not injure gastrostomy.
- Administer analgesics and determine effectiveness.
- Utilize nonmedicinal pain-relief techniques (e.g., distraction, relaxation, guided imagery, cutaneous stimulation); refer to *The Child Experiencing Pain*, page 216.

EVALUATION CRITERIA/DESIRED OUTCOMES

The child

- Is free from crying, moaning, grimacing, restlessness
- Verbalizes pain less than 4 on a scale of 0–10 if appropriate

---

NURSING DIAGNOSIS #5

a. **Disturbance in self-concept: body image** related to perceptions of change in body integrity, function
b. **Grieving** related to perceptions of loss of body function
c. **Ineffective individual coping** related to inability to taste or swallow food/liquids
d. **Altered growth and development** related to lack of stimulation during feeding

Rationale: The psychologic trauma of not being able to eat normally is usually severe. The child may become depressed and need a great deal of encouragement. Normal oral stimulation, an important avenue of development in infants, may be reduced. The child/parents must also deal with an unnatural opening into the stomach, which may create body-image concerns.

GOAL

The child/parents will adapt realistically to an altered body image; will cope effectively with the loss of normal eating patterns, accepting the gastrostomy and the care involved.

IMPLEMENTATION

- Refer to *The Parent Experiencing Grief and Loss*, page 139, and *The Child Experiencing a Body-Image Disturbance*, page 30.
- Help to express feelings regarding not being able to eat normally; use drawings, puppets, favorite doll with gastrostomy tube and dressing to communicate with younger child; refer to *The Child Requiring Play Therapy*, page 226.
- Encourage child/parents to administer feedings and care for gastrostomy to promote independence and increase self-esteem.
- Provide pacifier for infant when administering feeding to promote associating sucking with a feeling of satiety; hold/cuddle/talk during feeding.
- Initiate appropriate referrals if available (e.g., enterostomal therapist, gastrostomate visitor, clinical nurse specialist) to assist child in coping with gastrostomy.
- Encourage child to sit at table during mealtimes to promote normalizing behaviors.
- Encourage adolescent to verbalize feelings (e.g.,

body image, sexuality) regarding the gastrostomy, to discuss concerns with significant other; inform that counseling is available.

☐ EVALUATION CRITERIA/DESIRED OUTCOMES

The child
- Achieves expected developmental milestones

The child/parents
- Verbalize/play out beginning adaptation to altered body image and loss of normal eating patterns
- Administer feedings and care for gastrostomy correctly

NURSING DIAGNOSIS #6

Knowledge deficit regarding management of gastrostomy

Rationale: The child/parents must learn care of the gastrostomy in order to leave the hospital and reintegrate into family and society.

☐ GOAL

The child/parents will manage care of the gastrostomy.

☐ IMPLEMENTATION

- Teach how to anchor tube securely at insertion site (e.g., using feeding nipple, gauze roll, tape).
- Discuss necessary food preparation (e.g., blenderized, special formula).

- Demonstrate proper position for eating/feeding.
- Demonstrate correct method of giving the feeding; provide opportunity for return demonstration.
- Provide information regarding cleaning and storing equipment.
- Stress the importance of maintaining peristomal skin integrity.
- Discuss trouble-shooting and safety measures (e.g., maintaining tube patency; anchoring tube and securing under clothing to prevent dislodgment).
- Assist to make plans for returning to usual activities.
- Review symptoms requiring immediate medical attention (e.g., tube dislodgment, occlusion, bleeding, infection, nausea and vomiting, excessive diarrhea, polyuria or excessive thirst, leakage of fluid around opening).
- Stress the need for medical follow-up.
- Refer to community resources as necessary (e.g., home health agency, social services, occupational therapy).

☐ EVALUATION CRITERIA/DESIRED OUTCOMES

The child/parents
- Demonstrate competent administration of feeding
- Care for gastrostomy safely
- Identify appropriate trouble-shooting techniques, corrective actions
- Verbalize symptoms requiring immediate medical attention
- List appropriate community agencies

The Parent Experiencing Grief & Loss

Definition/Discussion

Grief is the set of normal responses a person goes through following the death of a loved one, or the loss of an idealized perfect child because of birth defects or prematurity. Mourning is the psychologic process that results from a loss. The grief and mourning process is the process of coping with and adapting to the loss. According to Engel (1965), the grief and mourning process involves three states: 1) shock and disbelief, 2) developing awareness of the loss, and 3) restitution. Full restitution may take a year or more and some people never completely recover. Each stage has its own adaptive responses and time frame.

Nursing Assessment

☐ **PERTINENT HISTORY**

Medical history of child, length/type of illness, nature/cause of condition (e.g., hereditary, accidental, self-destructive)

☐ **PHYSICAL FINDINGS**

General level of wellness/illness, ability to sleep, appetite

☐ **PSYCHOSOCIAL CONCERNS/ DEVELOPMENTAL FACTORS**

Developmental stage and tasks; expectations for the outcome of the illness; meaning of the loss; past experiences with loss: what previous losses have occurred, rate of progression through the grief process, what helped them cope; support system; normal expression of emotions, communication patterns; degree of success in completing previous stages of development; habits/rituals (e.g., sleeping, eating, playing)

☐ **PATIENT AND FAMILY KNOWLEDGE**

Stages of grief, what to expect in each stage; community resources; level of knowledge, readiness and willingness to learn

Nursing Care

☐ **LONG-TERM GOAL**

The parents will cope with the loss by completing each stage of the grief and mourning process.

NURSING DIAGNOSIS #1

Grieving related to the death of a child, birth of an infant with major defects

Rationale: Grief is the expected and normal response to the death of a child or loss of the idealized perfect infant.

☐ **GOAL**

The parents will go through the stages of grief in their own manner and reach resolution.

☐ **IMPLEMENTATION**

- Help parents to talk about their feelings (e.g., "Would you like to talk about what has happened?" "What is it like for you just now?").
- Expect a variety of grief reactions; know that all are adaptive and should be supported except suicidal ideation, destructive reactions; anger and hostility may be projected; know that it is not meant for you personally; do not reject the parents but rather give support (e.g., "You must be feeling very angry right now," or "I feel that you are really hurting inside"); continue to spend time with them.
- Provide empathic listening (probably the most helpful intervention); do not challenge statements, but encourage more expressions of feelings.
- Recognize individual responses to grief, which are determined by ego strengths, perception and meaning of loss, previous experience, and present support systems.
- Avoid platitudes (e.g., "You're healthy, you'll be able to have another child").
- Ask the parents if they wish to see the baby/child;

ask if they have seen a dead person before if the child is dead and they wish to view the body; assess expectations and provide information accordingly; wrap/cover the body in a blanket; handle it tenderly and carefully.

- Discuss the positive and negative aspects about seeing the body if parents are ambivalent; know that some view this as helpful to shorten the period of shock and disbelief.
- Adjust visiting hours if necessary to allow family/friends to visit and provide needed support.
- Be prepared to discuss such things as signing of autopsy or death certificate, disposing of child's clothes, possible future surgery and hospitalization for living baby.
- Have the same nurse each shift sit and talk with parents twice/shift if possible; allow family or friend to remain at bedside.
- Explain to the parents that the next stage of adaptive resolution involves behaviors of: asking questions (e.g., about the cause of death or deformity, what can be done for the living child); making outbursts (e.g., crying, anger, hostility); and feeling overwhelmed, interspersed with reality.
- Continue to support the grieving process; reinforce positive, adaptive grieving.
- Share the importance of allowing self to grieve openly rather than suppressing it; stress that both parents need to grieve and may not be able to support each other.
- Discuss with parents/family how they expect to cope at home; assess the need for ongoing support (e.g., public health or home health nurse, referral to a mental health clinic or a private mental health worker).
- Provide referrals and follow-up as needed; work with family so they can continue to give the parents support after discharge.

☐ **EVALUATION CRITERIA/DESIRED OUTCOMES**

The parents
- Talk about the child and about feelings of loss
- Move through the stage of shock, disbelief, anger,

and progress to developing an awareness of the reality of the loss
- Verbalize an understanding of the time span needed to complete the grief process

---

NURSING DIAGNOSIS #2

Knowledge deficit regarding the process of grief

Rationale: The experience of grief makes it difficult for the parents to take in and retain information. The parents may be experiencing a major loss for the first time.

☐ **GOAL**

The parents will verbalize where to obtain information and support for grieving.

☐ **IMPLEMENTATION**

- Discuss responses to grief, point out how responses are common and necessary, that others experiencing a loss have many of the same responses.
- Tell what to expect next in the grieving process.
- Explain that restitution will eventually occur and that frightening feelings/responses will diminish over time.
- Provide follow-up as necessary and when possible; tell parents they can call hospital staff for further support.
- Provide a written list of books on grief and community support services.

☐ **EVALUATION CRITERIA/DESIRED OUTCOMES**

The parents
- State expectations for the future
- Explain that responses to grief are limited in time
- Identify resources available for information, support, and referral

The Child with a Head Injury

Definition/Discussion

Head injuries are either direct (e.g., a blow to the head) or indirect (e.g., acceleration or deceleration of the head due to sudden jolt). Injuries to the head include skull fractures, concussion, cerebral contusions, lacerations, cerebral edema, and hemorrhage. Refer also to *The Child with Increased Intracranial Pressure*, page 160.

Nursing Assessment

☐ PERTINENT HISTORY

Cause and site of injury, direction and force of blow, secondary injury resulting from fall after blow; loss of consciousness (duration, method of arousal), seizures (description); length of time since injury; behavior since injury (e.g., level of alertness or responsiveness); treatment administered after injury; other history of falls, seizures, head injuries, or illnesses; current medications

☐ PHYSICAL FINDINGS

Vital signs, neurologic status (e.g., level of consciousness [LOC], muscular strength, pupillary response, response to stimuli, reflexes), inspection of head and scalp, scalp wounds, skull lumps, or tenderness, bruising behind ear (Battle's sign), periorbital ecchymosis ("raccoon eyes"), otorrhea, or rhinorrhea (blood or cerebrospinal fluid [CSF]); bleeding or discharge from ears, eyes, nose, mouth; headache, vomiting, weakness; emotional irritability; amnesia (retrograde: events prior to injury; antegrade: events during or following injury); aphasia or dysphasia

☐ PSYCHOSOCIAL CONCERNS/DEVELOPMENTAL FACTORS

Developmental level/coping mechanisms, usual routines of child/family, perceptions of responsibility for the injury, rituals/habits (e.g., sleeping, eating, playing)

☐ PATIENT AND FAMILY KNOWLEDGE

Anticipated treatment plan, safety measures to prevent injuries; level of knowledge, readiness and willingness to learn

Nursing Care

☐ LONG-TERM GOAL

The child will return to home as fully recovered as possible; the parents will prevent future injuries through implementation of safety measures (if accidental injury occurred) or through counseling (if injury was nonaccidental); the parents will care for the child to maximize return to more normal functioning, OR to sustain with compassion and dignity until life-support systems are disconnected; the parents will cope with loss and grief.

NURSING DIAGNOSIS #1
a. **Potential for injury** related to history of head trauma, sequelae of head injury
b. **Alteration in tissue perfusion: cerebral** related to head trauma

Rationale: Depending on the severity of the head injury, the child's LOC may range from alert and oriented to comatose. Assessment and early nursing intervention can reduce the risk of further injury should the child have a sudden change in LOC (e.g., become combative, have seizure activity). Head trauma may cause increased intracranial pressure (ICP) leading to alterations in cerebral perfusion. Increased intrathoracic and intra-abdominal pressure (e.g., Valsalva maneuver, hip flexion), sudden movement/startle, restlessness, and fear will further increase ICP.

☐ GOAL

The child will not sustain further injury.

☐ IMPLEMENTATION

- Refer to *The Child with Increased Intracranial Pressure*, page 160.
- Describe behavior clearly, carefully, and comprehensively or use standardized, neurologic observation record (e.g., Glasgow coma scale); check LOC every 15 minutes.
- Assess for presence of mind/behavior-altering sub-

stances (e.g., alcohol, marijuana, street drugs); know that neurologic findings may be due to injury, mind-altering substances, or a combination of both.

- Check gag, swallow, and deep tendon reflexes; note presence or absence of Babinkski's sign; review and assess function of cranial nerves.
- Check ability to speak without hoarseness or dysphasia.
- Accompany child for tests (e.g., CT scan) to provide constant, consistent nursing care and monitoring, especially if child is in critical condition; assist lab and x-ray personnel with necessary tests to minimize disturbances and movement.
- Do not elevate child's head or flex neck until spinal injury has been ruled out; apply cervical collar until cervical spine films are taken and diagnosis is clear.
- Elevate head of bed 15°-30° to promote cerebral venous drainage if there is no spinal injury.
- Monitor intake and output carefully; record urine output and specific gravity every hour.
- Restrict fluid intake except for cases of hypovolemic shock; use microdrip IV tubing sets and monitor rate of parenteral therapy closely; refer to *The Child with an Intravenous Catheter*, page 174.
- Protect child from injuries due to restless movements, disorientation, and seizures; avoid physical restraints unless absolutely necessary and ordered.
- Refer to *The Child with Epilepsy*, page 122.
- Maintain functional body alignment; avoid hip flexion; turn child slowly and gently, logrolling to keep body straight; have child exhale while turning to prevent Valsalva maneuver.
- Assess, report, and attempt to correct causes of restlessness (e.g., pain, distended bladder due to a kinked or clamped catheter, tight casts or bandages, respiratory distress, bleeding).
- Have family member or close friend present if child is regaining consciousness; encourage them to hold child's hand, stroke or talk to calm child and reduce ICP.
- Avoid unnecessary sedation that may cause respiratory depression and mask neurologic symptoms.
- Monitor effect of medications, physical movements, or conditions that may affect, mask, or potentiate signs of ICP or make interpretation and accurate assessment more difficult.

☐ **EVALUATION CRITERIA/DESIRED OUTCOMES**

The child
- Is oriented
- Has no neurologic deterioration
- Does not injure self

NURSING DIAGNOSES #2 through #6
Refer to *The Child with Increased Intracranial Pressure*, page 160.

NURSING DIAGNOSIS #7
Knowledge deficit regarding follow-up care for the child

Rationale: For the child who is discharged home following observation in the ER or after an overnight stay in the hospital, parents will need to know how to care for the child and how to observe for signs of complications. For the child who is being released home following a moderate-to-severe head injury, the parents must know the care regimens as well as the signs of complications.

☐ **GOAL**

The family will provide adequate, competent care for their child at home; will recognize signs of complications that need to be reported to the physician.

☐ **IMPLEMENTATION**

- Tell parents to awaken child every 2 hours for the first 24 hours to answer age appropriate questions.
- Give only aspirin or acetaminophen for headaches, nothing stronger; do not give sedatives, tranquilizers, antihistamines, or other medications.
- Give bland diet as tolerated for first 24 hours after head injury.
- Instruct to return to hospital if child cannot be awakened, is disoriented or has a severe headache, persistent vomiting, unequal pupils or vacant, staring look; is weak, limp, or loses feeling in arms or legs; has any kind of seizure or stiffness; or shows any increased drowsiness, change in behavior, drainage from nose or ears.
- Explain that the normal aftereffects of an acute, minor head injury (e.g., headache; dizziness; some drowsiness and fatigue; emotional irritability and periodic euphoria or depression; difficulty speaking, remembering, computing sums, writing paragraphs) may last from a few days to a month or longer.
- Teach daily care regimen (e.g., treatments, range-of-motion exercises [ROM], diet, bowel/bladder care).
- Instruct about actions, doses, side effects of medications.

- Support realistic hopes; prepare family for prolonged recovery and rehabilitation usually needed for children with serious head injuries; help family to think through the decisions regarding practical arrangements and adjustments that are necessary for each member of the nuclear family (e.g., siblings, nearby grandparents, step-parents, close friends).
- Make referrals for assistance from community agencies as necessary (e.g., community health nurse, social services, physical therapy, speech therapy, occupational therapy, board of education for home-bound teachers, or special education classes).

☐ **EVALUATION CRITERIA/DESIRED OUTCOMES**

The parents
- Describe care of child, including medications
- Verbalize signs of complications
- Seek out appropriate help when necessary

The Child Requiring Hemodialysis

Definition/Discussion

Hemodialysis removes toxic waste products and fluids from the systemic circulation to maintain the body in homeostasis when the kidneys are not functioning adequately.

Time involved for hemodialysis is approximately 3-4 hours, depending on the child's condition and the type of dialyzer used. It is usually done 3 times a week.

The artificial kidney machine contains a semipermeable membrane that separates the child's blood from the dialyzing solution. Hemodialysis is based upon three principles of fluid and particle movement, diffusion, osmosis, and ultrafiltration. Through diffusion and osmosis, molecules and ions of waste products pass from the area of higher concentration (the child's blood) to the area of lower concentration (the dialyzing solution) until a degree of equilibrium between the two is achieved. Molecules may also pass from the dialyzing solution into the blood, thus the electrolyte content of the dialysate can be manipulated to meet the child's needs based on blood chemistries and clinical evaluation. Ultrafiltration involves movement of fluid across a semipermeable membrane as a result of an artificially created pressure gradient.

Types of access to the child's circulation include

- *external arteriovenous shunting (cannulization):* a Silastic-Teflon cannula is surgically inserted and fixed in an artery (usually the radial artery of the nondominant arm or the posterior tibial artery of either leg); another cannula is fixed in a nearby vein. Arterial blood is shunted through the artificial kidney and returned to the child via the venous cannula. After dialysis is completed, both cannulae are connected so that the flow of blood from artery to vein through the "shunt" is continuous.
- *arteriovenous graft:* permanent access created by suturing an artificial device to the child's own vessels. Two needles are inserted: one to carry the blood to the artificial kidney, and one to return the blood to the child. The needles are removed and reinserted for each treatment. This is the most commonly used internal access for children because of the small size of their blood vessels.
- *internal arteriovenous fistulization:* a tiny opening is surgically created between an artery and a nearby

vein; this enables the arterial blood to enter into and engorge the vein, which is then easily punctured at time of dialysis. No external or artificial device is used and problems of clotting and infection are minimized. Patency of the fistula is achieved by the rapid flow of blood.

- *femoral or vein catheterization:* a temporary access site that is used for emergency (acute) hemodialysis
- *subclavian vein catheterization:* a temporary access using a double lumen catheter; this is being utilized more in the pediatric population instead of the external arteriovenous shunt to preserve the peripheral vessels for future access.

Nursing Assessment

☐ **PERTINENT HISTORY**

High and rising serum potassium level, acute renal failure, end-stage renal disease, severe fluid/electrolyte imbalance, severe pulmonary edema or congestive heart failure (CHF), chemical or drug toxicity

☐ **PHYSICAL FINDINGS**

Lethargy, restlessness, confusion, pallor, anorexia, oliguria or anuria, general edema, possible cardiac dysrhythmias, elevated BUN, creatinine, serum proteins, decreased hematocrit, hemoglobin

☐ **PSYCHOSOCIAL CONCERNS/ DEVELOPMENTAL FACTORS**

Anxiety/fear regarding treatment/disease, especially if acute dialysis or initial session; body-image disturbances; depression/powerlessness with long-term condition; hopelessness/fear of dying (with end-stage renal disease); habits/rituals (e.g., sleeping, eating, playing)

☐ **PATIENT AND FAMILY KNOWLEDGE**

Purpose/expected effects of procedure; postdischarge regimen (e.g., diet, medications, scheduled dialysis sessions); evaluation procedure for renal transplant; community resources; level of knowledge, readiness and willingness to learn

Nursing Care

☐ **LONG-TERM GOAL**

The child/parents will adhere to prescribed regimen to aid recovery from the acute renal failure and to return to usual roles; OR the child/parents will adapt to the reality of long-term dialysis and will live within its accompanying limitations.

NURSING DIAGNOSIS #1

a. **Anxiety** related to limited understanding of hemodialysis procedure, expected course of renal dysfunction
b. **Powerlessness** related to perceived lack of control over disease, treatment
c. **Disturbance in self-concept: body image** related to loss of renal function, use of artificial device to achieve bodily function
d. **Altered growth and development** related to dependency on family members and hospital personnel, frequent hospitalizations, and social isolation from peers

Rationale: Lack of knowledge and fear of the unknown cause high anxiety and stress levels. Depending upon the precipitating indication for hemodialysis, the child/parents may have had little time to prepare for the procedure.

Children undergoing dialysis usually have many conflicts regarding being dependent on a machine and health team for life, and these may be expressed by a variety of feelings and emotions. During the first few weeks, the child often feels increasingly better physically. Next, s/he may become discouraged and easily depressed. Finally, most children achieve some degree of acceptance of medical condition and imposed limitations, display fewer negative feelings, and, along with their parents, plan for changes in life-style. Acceptance of the child's feelings by the nurse in a nonjudgmental way will facilitate the adjustment to dialysis.

Changes in physical appearance may result in a lessened sense of self; this is often increased by changes in usual role functioning. Intervention may need to be directed at family members to decrease the child's feelings of dependency and promote a sense of control over at least some aspects of the prescribed regimen. Some children may grieve for the loss of their kidneys and may require assistance in accepting the necessity for dialysis. Other dialysis children can become very attached to "their" machine and incorporate it into their body image.

☐ **GOAL**

The child will identify those aspects of the disease process/treatment regimen s/he can control; will in-corporate new body image into self-concept; the child/parents will indicate decreased level of anxiety.

☐ **IMPLEMENTATION**

- Assess level of anxiety before each dialysis treatment; validate your observations by using input from family members along with verbal and nonverbal cues; provide empathic listening.
- Encourage to ask questions regarding the disease process and treatment.
- Accept and acknowledge all verbalizations; indicate that these are usual and expected feelings.
- Initiate measures to prevent communication breakdown (e.g., setting up family, child, and staff conferences with psychiatric clinical specialist, psychiatrists, social worker, or other mental health person); ensure that all care givers are aware of health team decisions.
- Help to adjust to body-image changes by giving recognition for any involvement, by eliciting feelings and listening carefully to what child says, and by reminding child of previously successful coping mechanisms for stressful situations.
- Provide opportunities for child/parents to exert some degree of control over planning and managing care (e.g., scheduling of medications, fluids, foods); reassure that increasing independence from the health team is a sign of progress, and not rejection by staff.
- Encourage increased independence in the adolescent with procedures during dialysis treatment (e.g., cleaning sites).
- Explain the importance of allowing child to perform own self-care tasks as much as possible.
- Encourage parents and siblings to attend support group, if available, in hospital or community.

☐ **EVALUATION CRITERIA/DESIRED OUTCOMES**

The child
- Expresses acceptance of dialysis by verbal and nonverbal cues during treatment
- Reaffirms self-worth by participating in age-appropriate activities (e.g., play, school, dating)

The child/parents
- Participate in decision making regarding plan of care
- Verbalize decreased anxiety regarding dialysis

NURSING DIAGNOSIS #2

a. **Fluid volume deficit** related to rapid volume depletion
b. **Alteration in cardiac output: decreased** related to dysrhythmias, fluid removal
c. **Impaired gas exchange** related to decreased cardiac output, anemia, dialysis procedure

Rationale: With excessive ultrafiltration, there is a risk of rapid volume depletion because too much fluid is removed in too short a time. Rapid fluid reduction may cause hypotension with resultant hypoxia.

Even when the fluid volume remains stable, the child may show signs of a decreased cardiac output if there are electrolyte imbalances that cause cardiac dysrhythmias. Hyperkalemia causes changes in cardiac conduction that may result in cardiac standstill while a too-rapid reduction in potassium can also cause dysrhythmias secondary to hypokalemia.

Fluid congestion within the pulmonary circulation causes an alteration of the ventilation/perfusion ratio and results in impaired gas exchange. The child should demonstrate improved exchange after dialysis as the excess fluid removed from the systemic circulation will decrease the workload and increase the efficiency of the heart as a pump, improving pulmonary as well as the systemic circulation.

Anemia may be present because decreased red blood cell production results from decreased erythropoietin production in the diseased kidneys, even when blood loss in dialyzer and from blood sampling is kept to a minimum. Anemia reduces the oxygen-carrying capacity of the child's blood and the child develops symptoms reflecting impaired gas exchange.

☐ GOAL

The child will maintain fluid and electrolyte balance; will maintain cardiac output sufficient to promote normal gas exchange.

☐ IMPLEMENTATION

- Review vital signs before initiating dialysis to establish baseline data; monitor EKG for dysrhythmias if indicated.
- Inform physician of predialysis laboratory results (e.g., serum electrolytes, BUN, hematocrit/hemoglobin).
- Monitor blood pressure, pulse, and respirations every 5-10 minutes during the first half hour of dialysis and every 15-30 minutes throughout the procedure; watch for signs of fluid volume deficit (e.g., decreased blood pressure, increased pulse, nausea, vomiting, dizziness); inform physician of deficit and decrease rate of dialysis, adjust concentration of dialysate, or administer blood components as ordered or per hospital protocol; refer to *The Child Receiving Blood and Blood-Product Transfusions*, page 24.
- Administer volume expanders or vasopressors as ordered; note effectiveness; monitor for signs of fluid overload (with volume expanders) or hyper-

tension; discontinue infusion and contact physician if untoward effects noted.
- Position with feet elevated if signs of shock (e.g., decreased BP, increased pulse, decreased peripheral perfusion) appear; give normal saline/hypertonic solutions (e.g., 5% saline, 50% dextrose) into venous blood line.
- Elevate head 15°-30° if dyspneic, and administer oxygen as ordered.
- Assess throughout dialysis for symptoms of decreased cardiac output and related hypoxia (e.g., irregular or weak pulse, dizziness, labored respirations, mental confusion).
- Monitor cardiac rhythm as ordered; report/record presence of dysrhythmias and related symptoms; administer medications as ordered; watch for expected effectiveness and toxicity.
- Auscultate lungs at least every hour.
- Monitor arterial blood gases as ordered; watch for decreased pO_2 and acidosis; assess for symptoms of respiratory insufficiency (e.g., increased respiratory rate, shallow or labored respirations, irritability/agitation, loss of consciousness) and inform physician; prepare for possible intubation and mechanical ventilation.

☐ EVALUATION CRITERIA/DESIRED OUTCOMES

The child
- Has stable blood pressure, pulse and acceptable lab values (e.g., serum electrolyes, hematocrit, hemoglobin)
- Has normal respirations and breath sounds

NURSING DIAGNOSIS #3
a. **Potential for injury** (hemorrhage) related to heparinization, vulnerability for dislodgment of vascular access
b. **Potential for injury** (air embolism) related to air entering hemodialysis tubing
c. **Potential for infection** related to impaired skin integrity at vascular access site, increased susceptibility for hepatitis and AIDS through frequent blood transfusions
d. **Potential for injury** related to seizures, electrolyte imbalances

Rationale: Hemorrhage may occur by accidental needle dislodgment, disconnection of the shunt, or rupture of a dialyzer during the procedure. Heparin, which requires about 4 hours to metabolize, is used to prevent clotting of the blood as it is cycled through the dialysis machine. The risk for bleeding continues until the heparin has been metabolized.

Any opening in the hemodialysis system can become a port of entry for air. When an air bolus greater than 3 cc (rapidly delivered) enters the child's vascular space, there is the risk of air embolism developing. Given the large vessels used for cannulization and the active pumping action of the machine, it can be expected that air entering through the dialysis system would reach the heart and lungs faster than air entering through an ordinary peripheral or central IV line.

Infection at the access site is a potential problem. Local infection may lead to systemic infection, especially for children with CRF whose immune system is compromised. When frequent transfusions are required to treat anemia secondary to renal failure and hypovolemia during dialysis, the child is at increased risk for developing hepatitis and AIDS as the viruses causing these conditions can be transmitted through blood from an infected donor. Hospital staff are also at risk when administering transfusions and should exercise caution when performing venipunctures and handling blood.

BUN levels become elevated in the interdialytic period often in excess of 100 mg/100 cc. Once dialysis is initiated, excess urea is removed from the systemic circulation, causing an osmotic gradient between the blood and the cells in the surrounding tissues. The fluid will shift from the blood into the cells, resulting in symptoms of cerebral edema.

Cerebral edema requires additional time to resolve; therefore, the child continues to be at risk for seizures during and after dialysis.

☐ GOAL

The child will remain free from injury and infection.

☐ IMPLEMENTATION

- Inspect access site every 15-30 minutes during dialysis for patency and signs of bleeding or infection; notify physician of significant findings; have protamine sulfate available to counteract effects of heparin as needed.
- Check patency of shunt or fistula every 4 hours when child not being dialyzed: observe blood flow through external shunt (e.g., color, temperature); auscultate for bruit and palpate for thrill in internal fistula; if decreased or if patency not verified, notify physician.
- Initiate measures to prevent introduction of air into dialysis system
  - tape all connections securely
  - avoid kinks in the tubing and negative pressures between the pump and the child
  - avoid infusing solutions in vented containers
  - keep air detector functioning at all times
- Monitor coagulation and hematology studies according to orders or unit protocol; inform physician of significantly prolonged times or decreased hematocrit and hemoglobin.
- Ensure that no punctures are made in external

shunt; do not take blood pressure nor withdraw blood from access extremity; post a sign (at bedside or door to child's room) to remind all members of the health team to observe these precautions; explain reasons to child.
- Watch for signs of air embolism (e.g., chest pain, cyanosis, decreased blood pressure, weak, rapid pulse, coughing, loss of consciousness); if present, turn child onto left side and elevate upper body, notify physician immediately, discontinue dialysis, administer oxygen/IV fluids as ordered, and prepare for possible intracardiac aspiration by physician.
- Monitor for signs of systemic infection (e.g., increased temperature, pulse, and respirations; decreased blood pressure; changes in skin color or mental status).
- Administer antibiotics as prescribed; watch for toxicity.
- Monitor liver function studies (e.g., SGOT, SGPT, LDH) for elevations indicative of hepatitis; monitor serology reports for positive hepatitis B surface antigen; assess for signs of hepatitis (e.g., fatigue, jaundice, fever); institute isolation precautions as ordered; explain purpose.
- Monitor hematology studies for indications of immunosuppression (decreased white blood cell count and lymphocytes) and serology studies for positive AIDS antigen (HTLV/III); confer with physician in interpreting test results; initiate protective isolation precautions as ordered; explain purpose.
- Monitor BUN; know that if greater than 100 mg/dl, mannitol may be ordered prophylactically.
- Monitor for signs of increased intracranial pressure (e.g., hypo/hypertension, bounding pulse, nausea, vomiting, headache, restlessness, respiratory pattern changes) during and after dialysis; administer mannitol as ordered if signs occur, titrating according to orders or hospital protocol; monitor for effectiveness and toxicity.
- Maintain seizure precautions; refer to *The Child with Epilepsy*, page 122; administer antiseizure medications as ordered; monitor for effectiveness and toxicity; record/report seizure activity.

☐ EVALUATION CRITERIA/DESIRED OUTCOMES

The child
- Has stable vital signs, is afebrile
- Is free from seizure activity

NURSING DIAGNOSIS #4

Alteration in comfort: pain related to fluid volume excess, hypertension, electrolyte imbalances

Rationale: *Fluid overload experienced between dialysis sessions may cause hypertension which may in turn cause headache. This is related to the increased total blood volume in the small vessels of the brain causing increased dilitation in a closed space. Electrolyte imbalances (e.g., rapid shifts in sodium, potassium, and calcium ion concentrations) can cause muscle cramping, abdominal pain, and nausea and vomiting.*

☐ GOAL

The child will be comfortable; will be free from headache, muscle cramping, abdominal pain, nausea and vomiting.

☐ IMPLEMENTATION

- Assess regularly for signs of discomfort; implement measures to promote relief.
- Administer prescribed analgesic for headache.
- Apply heat or pressure to cramping areas of the upper and lower extremities, massage.
- Explain reasons for discomfort.
- Assist child in using distraction/imagery to control discomfort; refer to *The Child Experiencing Pain*, page 216.

☐ EVALUATION CRITERIA/DESIRED OUTCOMES

The child
- Is free from headache, muscle cramping, abdominal pain

NURSING DIAGNOSIS #5

Knowledge deficit regarding care of shunt, fistula, or subclavian catheter

Rationale: *To promote compliance with the hemodialysis schedule, the child/parents require information about care of the shunt, fistula, or subclavian catheter, and schedule for hemodialysis sessions. Predischarge teaching should also cover the prescribed diet, medication and community resources; refer to The Child with Chronic Renal Failure, page 66 for discussion of these knowledge deficits. All teaching must be individualized depending on the child's age and development, as well as the parents' level of understanding, motivation, and support.*

☐ GOAL

The child/parents will demonstrate proper shunt, fistula, or subclavian care; will describe dialysis schedule.

☐ IMPLEMENTATION

- Demonstrate skin-cleansing technique at shunt site using aseptic technique and following hospital protocol; provide opportunity for return demonstration.
- Instruct to check for patency by palpating the thrill and listening for the bruit in the internal fistula.
- Teach to check external shunt site for swelling, coolness, redness, or other discoloration of skin, and to report these to dialysis team.
- Instruct to check subclavian dressing and catheter for drainage or leaking and report these to dialysis team.
- Teach necessary restrictions for bathing, swimming when external shunt or subclavian catheter is used; ensure child has 2 clamps at all times in case of accidental separation of cannulae; ensure child/parents know how to use them.
- Teach to protect shunt from injury; instruct to avoid constrictions/pressures on arm (e.g., blood pressure cuff, tourniquet, tight clothing); stress not to carry purse or packages on affected arm; teach to avoid sleeping on arm or using weights.
- Teach to keep the subclavian catheter protected by the use of a cotton T-shirt underneath child's clothing.
- Reinforce what physician has told child/parents concerning anticipated dialysis sessions after discharge; ensure that child has a written schedule for outpatient dialysis appointments.
- Give daytime, nighttime, and weekend phone numbers of dialysis unit and nephrologist on call if problems arise.
- Answer questions and refer to local chapter of National Kidney Foundation for additional information as needed.

☐ EVALUATION CRITERIA/DESIRED OUTCOMES

The child/parents
- Demonstrate proper shunt or fistula care
- State indications for notifying physician
- Describe schedule for dialysis sessions

The Child with Hydrocephalus

Definition/Discussion

Hydrocephalus is an excessive accumulation of cerebrospinal fluid (CSF) in the cerebral ventricles, subarachnoid space, or subdural space. This accumulation may be caused by an increase in the production of CSF, an obstruction of the flow of CSF through the ventricles (noncommunicating), or an inability to reabsorb the fluid (communicating). Noncommunicating hydrocephalus is the most common form of the condition in children under the age of 2 and is generally associated with a developmental defect.

The symptoms of hydrocephalus are dependent upon the rate at which the fluid accumulates, the child's age, and the causes (e.g., meningitis, tumor). Clinical manifestations are primarily the signs/symptoms of increased intracranial pressure (ICP). Children less than 2 years old have an enlarged head in association with the increased pressure because the cranial sutures have not yet closed. As the fluid accumulates, the skin/skull covering the brain becomes thin/stretched, and the scalp veins become engorged.

The treatment of hydrocephalus is aimed at decreasing the pressure either by eliminating the cause or shunting the fluid to other parts of the body (e.g., peritoneal cavity). The prognosis is good for children who are treated early (approximately 1/3 being physically/developmentally normal). Without treatment, the child is likely to be severely retarded or die at a very young age.

The information contained in this guide reflects the care of the child with uncomplicated hydrocephalus. For information regarding the care of a child with one of the many frequently associated conditions (e.g., myelomeningocele, meningitis, developmental disabilities), refer to the appropriate guide.

Nursing Assessment

☐ **PERTINENT HISTORY**

Symptoms leading to diagnosis, when was diagnosis made, recent signs of increased intracranial pressure or infection

☐ **PHYSICAL FINDINGS**

General appearance, signs of increased ICP (e.g., elevated blood pressure with decreased pulse, decreased responsiveness, headache, nausea and vomiting, seizure activity, bulging fontanels in infants), signs of infection (e.g., elevated temperature, poor feeding, vomiting), head circumference

☐ **PSYCHOSOCIAL CONCERNS/ DEVELOPMENTAL FACTORS**

Developmental level, coping mechanisms, usual routines of child and family, previous hospital experiences

☐ **PATIENT AND FAMILY KNOWLEDGE**

Hydrocephalus and treatment regimens, level of knowledge, readiness and willingness to learn

Nursing Care

☐ **LONG-TERM GOAL**

The child will recover from surgical correction of hydrocephalus free from preventable complications and will resume growth and development; the child/parents will participate in treatment plan and will cope effectively with long-term management.

NURSING DIAGNOSIS #1

a. **Alteration in tissue perfusion: cerebral** related to increased CSF volume
b. **Potential for injury** related to shunt malfunction
c. **Sensory-perceptual alteration** related to measures taken to reduce ICP, increased ICP
d. **Impairment of skin integrity** related to difficulty in moving enlarged cranium

Rationale: *Shunt malfunctions may cause an increase in ICP that can result in decreased level of consciousness, brain damage, or death. Increased size of head may cause stretching of skin and possible development of pressure areas or breakdown. The head may also be large enough so the child has difficulty moving.*

☐ GOAL

The child will be free from preventable complications; will have a properly functioning shunt; will be free from skin breakdown of the scalp.

☐ IMPLEMENTATION

- Measure head circumference every 8 hours using paper tape measure.
- Monitor fontanel fullness every 4 hours and as necessary.
- Position on unoperated side; keep head flat to avoid sudden reduction of ICP.
- Check neurologic status every 15 minutes until vital signs are stable, then as ordered; refer to *The Child with Increased Intracranial Pressure*, page 160.
- Report immediately any change in behavior (e.g., irritability, decreased level of consciousness) or vital signs (e.g., increased blood pressure, decreased pulse).
- Check dressing for bleeding and area around operative site for redness and swelling every 15 minutes until vital signs are stable, then every 2 hours.
- Change position every 2 hours and as necessary; use sheepskin or water mattress and position head to prevent development of pressure areas.

☐ EVALUATION CRITERIA/DESIRED OUTCOMES

The child
- Has stable neurologic signs
- Is free from bleeding
- Is free from skin breakdown of scalp

NURSING DIAGNOSIS #2

Potential for infection related to surgical placement of shunt

Rationale: Surgical placement/revision of a shunt results in a break in skin integrity. The shunt is a foreign object and therefore a possible source for infection. Compressing the reservoir chamber of shunt may be ordered immediately post-op to prevent occlusion by cells or tissue. The more frequent the infection/revision, the poorer the long-term prognosis for child.

☐ GOAL

The child will be free from infection.

☐ IMPLEMENTATION

- Report any change in vital signs (e.g., increase in temperature) or behavior (e.g., irritability, decrease in levels of consciousness) immediately.
- Monitor operative site for signs of redness/swelling.

- Maintain shunt; compress reservoir as ordered.
- Know that infection of the shunt usually requires removal and replacement.

☐ EVALUATION CRITERIA/DESIRED OUTCOMES

The child
- Has stable vital signs
- Has no visible signs of infection

NURSING DIAGNOSIS #3
a. **Alteration in family processes** related to diagnosis of child with potentially life-threatening condition
b. **Fear** related to inability of parents to control child's health
c. **Anticipatory grieving** related to possible death of child.
d. **Alteration in parenting** related to stressors of having a physically/mentally disabled child, hospitalization

Rationale: When a child is diagnosed with a potentially life-threatening condition, parents and other family members will begin the grief process. Parents may be drawn to the ill child, leaving siblings feeling ignored; or parents may reject the ill child because of physical appearance. The enlarged head of the child with hydrocephalus can be very disconcerting to parents/family members.

☐ GOAL

The parents will accept the child into the family; will seek support systems to assist with grief resolution; will identify behaviors that indicate high risk for child abuse.

☐ IMPLEMENTATION

- Provide opportunity for parents/family members to discuss feelings/concerns; do not condemn negative statements.
- Role model behaviors that indicate acceptance of the child (e.g., hold child, talk to child, comfort child).
- Encourage parents to assist with child's care; allow them to do as much as possible.
- Explain all procedures, treatments.
- Support positive parenting behaviors; be alert to negative behaviors (e.g., not picking the child up, avoiding/yelling at the child).
- Discuss behaviors indicating a high level of frustration; role play new coping strategies.
- Discuss resources available within the community (e.g., clergy, parental support groups).
- Refer for counseling as necessary.

☐ EVALUATION CRITERIA/DESIRED OUTCOMES

The parents
- Participate in care
- Hold, comfort, and talk to child
- List community resources available
- Identify negative behaviors requiring outside intervention

NURSING DIAGNOSIS #4

Knowledge deficit regarding expected care, development of child, signs of complications, follow-up care requirements

Rationale: If knowledge deficits exist, parents may not understand their child's care or their role during hospitalization. Parents may not have realistic expectations regarding growth and development of the child, cannot appropriately manage post-op treatment, or detect signs of complications early.

☐ GOAL

Parents will verbalize treatment plans for child; will discuss realistic developmental expectations, potential complications; will demonstrate follow-up care.

☐ IMPLEMENTATION

- Explain all treatments and procedures; be present when information is given by other health-team members; reinforce and clarify this information.
- Encourage parents to express feelings/concerns and to participate in care of child as they feel comfortable.
- Assist parents to individualize growth and development expectations for child; help develop methods to promote achievement of milestones; refer to *Normal Growth and Development*, pages 300–314.
- Reinforce child's needs for touch, love, security.
- Teach signs of infection and increased ICP; discuss indications for seeking medical care.
- Demonstrate required care (e.g., how to check shunt functioning, how to position child); provide opportunity for return demonstration.
- Instruct parents about medications (e.g., names, actions, dosages, and side effects).
- Provide a list of telephone numbers to use when problems occur.

☐ EVALUATION CRITERIA/DESIRED OUTCOMES

The child/parents
- Verbalize an understanding of the treatment plan
- State realistic expectations of child
- List signs of infection and increased ICP
- Demonstrate required care
- Explain medications the child is to receive including schedule, side effects, and importance of maintaining drug levels

The Neonate with Hyperbilirubinemia

Definition/Discussion

Hyperbilirubinemia, an elevation of serum bilirubin, is a condition characterized by jaundice of the skin, the sclera of the eyes, the mucous membranes, and body fluids. It is caused by the deposition of bilirubin pigment, released when the red blood cells undergo hemolysis. Phototherapy is the most widely used treatment of hyperbilirubinemia; it accelerates bilirubin turnover and excretion by photo-oxidation. Indications for an exchange transfusion include length of gestation, age, weight condition, and diagnosis. In a two-volume exchange, 86% of circulating blood will be replaced by alternating withdrawal of a small amount of blood with replacment of an equal amount of donor blood in order to remove accumulated bilirubin.

Nursing Assessment

☐ **PERTINENT HISTORY**

Hemolytic disorder (e.g., Rh or ABO incompatibility), polycythemia, infection, hematomas, bruising, liver or metabolic disease, bowel obstruction, diabetic mother, breast-feeding

☐ **PHYSICAL FINDINGS**

Jaundice, pallor; dark, concentrated urine; lethargy, hypotonia; poor sucking reflex; irritability, tremors, convulsions; high-pitched cry

☐ **PSYCHOSOCIAL CONCERNS/ DEVELOPMENTAL FACTORS**

Effect of having a "sick" baby (e.g., guilt, bonding problems), separation

☐ **PATIENT AND FAMILY KNOWLEDGE**

Causes and treatment, follow-up care, familiarity with other neonates with jaundice, level of knowledge, readiness and willingness to learn

Nursing Care

☐ **LONG-TERM GOAL**

The neonate's serum bilirubin will decrease; the neonate will not suffer long-term sequelae; the neonate will grow to full potential.

NURSING DIAGNOSIS #1

Impairment of skin integrity related to jaundice, diarrhea

Rationale: Bilirubin and enzymes excreted in the stool of neonates with hyperbilirubinemia can be very irritating to the skin.

☐ **GOAL**

The neonate will maintain intact skin.

☐ **IMPLEMENTATION**

- Document the color and condition of the skin on admission, every 8 hours, and as necessary.
- Monitor direct and indirect bilirubin levels; notify physician of results.
- Position on sides or prone; change position every 2 hours; monitor skin condition and massage bony prominences with each position change.
- Keep clean and dry.

☐ **EVALUATION CRITERIA/DESIRED OUTCOMES**

The neonate's
- Skin remains intact

NURSING DIAGNOSIS #2
a. **Potential for injury** related to phototherapy
b. **Sensory-perceptual alteration: visual** related to eye shields

Rationale: Phototherapy may be a technically simple procedure but it requires very careful application and monitoring to ensure the neonate does not experience complications. Eye shields are necessary to protect the neonate's eyes from the bili lights yet they restrict the visual observation/interaction capabilities of the neonate.

GOAL

The neonate will develop no signs of visual/sensory deprivation.

IMPLEMENTATION

- Place neonate approximately 18 inches from light sources.
- Do not diaper or clothe neonate.
- Cover closed eyes with eye shields, eye pads, or stockinette cap to protect eyes from light source.
- Ensure patches do not slip down and block the nose.
- Turn off lights and uncover eyes every 8 hours to inspect scleral color.
- Remove eye pads for feedings or any time neonate is removed from phototherapy.
- Talk to, touch neonate gently during nursing care.
- Encourage parents to visit and participate in care.

EVALUATION CRITERIA/DESIRED OUTCOMES

The neonate
- Is free from preventable complications
- Makes eye contact when eyeshields are removed
- Responds to voice/touch by quieting

NURSING DIAGNOSIS #3

a. **Alteration in body temperature** related to age, phototherapy
b. **Ineffective thermoregulation** related to immaturity, environmental temperature

Rationale: Exposure of neonate's skin to air during phototherapy may compromise thermoregulation

---

GOAL

The neonate will maintain a stable body temperature.

IMPLEMENTATION

- Provide a neutral thermal environment (i.e., an environmental temperature that maintains the neonate's temperature at a stable level); use a radiant warmer or Isolette as needed.
- Maintain axillary temperature of 36.5°-37°C (97.7°-98.6°F) to avoid cold/heat stress.
- Check other vital signs every 2-4 hours and as necessary.

EVALUATION CRITERIA/DESIRED OUTCOMES

The neonate's
- Temperature remains stable within acceptable range

NURSING DIAGNOSIS #4

Fluid volume deficit related to inadequate fluid intake, phototherapy-induced diarrhea

Rationale: Phototherapy increases bowel motility, a potential side effect of which is loose stools. Phototherapy also increases insensible water loss.

GOAL

The neonate will be adequately hydrated.

IMPLEMENTATION

- Record number and quality of stools.
- Monitor skin turgor and mucous membranes.
- Monitor intake and output.
- Administer feedings as soon as possible after birth, as ordered.
- Offer feedings at specific times; do not skip feedings.
- Offer water between breast- or bottle-feeding.

EVALUATION CRITERIA/DESIRED OUTCOMES

The neonate
- Maintains good skin tugor
- Voids at least 10 cc/hour with urine specific gravity of less than 1.010
- Has moist mucous membranes and flat fontanels

NURSING DIAGNOSIS #5

Alteration in parenting related to enforced separation

Rationale: The need for phototherapy restricts the amount of time the neonate can be in contact with the parents.

GOAL

The neonate and parents will display attachment behaviors; the parents will express an understanding of the bonding process.

IMPLEMENTATION

- Have parents come to nursery or take neonate to mother's room for feedings.
- Ensure the neonate is held during feedings.
- Encourage parents to talk to neonate, use *en face* positioning.
- Involve parents in as much of care as possible.
- Keep parents informed of neonate's treatment and progress to allay fears.
- Allow parents to express feelings.

The neonate/parents
- Show attachment behaviors

The parents
- Attempt to engage in eye contact with neonate
- Hold neonate close to trunk
- Speak positively to neonate

NURSING DIAGNOSIS #6

Alteration in tissue perfusion related to hypo-/hypervolemia during exchange transfusion

Rationale: As blood is removed from the neonate and replaced, fluid volume and electrolytes (especially calcium and sodium bicarbonate) remain in delicate balance.

□ **GOAL**

The neonate will undergo successful exchange transfusion free from preventable complications; will decrease the bilirubin level.

□ **IMPLEMENTATION**

Preprocedure Care
- Prepare radiant warmer, cardiac and respiratory monitoring equipment, and pacifier (if needed).
- Maintain NPO status 3-4 hours prior to exchange.
- Check blood date, type, and crossmatch information according to hospital protocol.
- Warm blood as ordered.
- Restrain all 4 extremities.
- Assist physician with insertion of umbilical arterial or venous catheter as necessary.
- Ensure that all preprocedure lab work (e.g., complete blood count; total and direct bilirubin; platelet count; serum nitrogen, potassium, glucose, calcium; blood cultures) has been drawn.
- Ensure parental consent has been obtained.

Procedural Care
- Save first and last 10 cc removed from infant for lab work as ordered (e.g., fractionated bilirubin, electrolytes, calcium, hemoglobin, hematocrit, and total protein; a CBC and type and crossmatch may be included in the final specimen).
- Note respiratory and cardiac rates every 15 minutes.
- Check axillary temperature every 15-30 minutes (unless a temperature probe is utilized).
- Suction as necessary.
- Observe for any abnormal behavior (e.g., lethargy or seizure activity, abnormal or changed cry).
- Check all tubing connections periodically during procedure.
- Record amounts of blood withdrawn and re-

placed, time of each exchange, and cumulative records of the total volume exchanged.
- Observe for signs of exchange transfusion reaction; refer to *The Child Receiving Blood and Blood-Product Transfusions*, page 24.
- Notify physician when 100 cc blood have been exchanged (depending on the preservative used for the blood, calcium may be given).
- Offer pacifier as necessary.

Postprocedure Care
- Handle neonate minimally and gently for 2-4 hours.
- Monitor cardiac and respiratory rate every 15 minutes for 1 hour; then if stable, every 30 minutes for 2 hours; and if stable, every 4 hours.
- Check axillary temperature every 1-3 hours for 48 hours.
- Measure intake and output accurately.
- Obtain a blood glucose immediately following and 1 and 2 hours following completion of procedure.
- Maintain IV infusion as necessary.
- Continue to monitor serum bilirubin levels as ordered.
- Observe for cord bleeding every 5-15 minutes for 1-2 hours, then periodically after umbilical line is withdrawn.
- Resume oral feedings 4-6 hours after transfusion; feed slowly or gavage feed as ordered.
- Reinforce physician's explanation as needed.
- Encourage parents to visit neonate after procedure and involve them in care as much as possible.

□ **EVALUATION CRITERIA/DESIRED OUTCOMES**

The neonate
- Has reduced serum bilirubin level
- Is free from preventable complications
- Maintains electrolytes, vital signs, and blood glucose in normal range

---

NURSING DIAGNOSIS #7

Knowledge deficit regarding jaundice, treatments, care of neonate

Rationale: If parents do not understand causes, reasons for treatments, and potential complications of hyperbilirubinemia they may not be able to emotionally support neonate or deliver appropriate care.

□ **GOAL**

The parents will verbalize understanding of care; will identify symptoms to report to health team.

□ IMPLEMENTATION

- Be present during physician's explanations to parents, reinforce concepts and clarify misconceptions.
- Encourage parents to visit and care for neonate as they are able, evaluate care they deliver and offer positive reinforcement or be a role model for appropriate behaviors as indicated.
- Teach parents signs of jaundice (e.g., yellow tinge to skin, sclera) and to report them to health team.
- Give parents phone numbers and names to call in case of questions, illness of neonate, recurrence of jaundice.

□ EVALUATION CRITERIA/DESIRED OUTCOMES

The parents

- State causes of hyperbilirubinemia
- List complications
- State importance of ongoing care, including follow-up lab tests
- Receive counseling if pathologic hyperbilirubinemia is diagnosed

The Child at Risk for Hazards of Immobility

Definition/Discussion

Immobility is the temporary or permanent state of not being able to move. Physical complications from immobility can occur after only 2 days of immobilization. Children who are confined to bed/immobilized are usually sufficiently active to minimize the physical consequences of immobility, and the nursing challenge may be to minimize activity. The physical effects of immobility result from complete immobility (e.g., coma, paralysis from trauma or CNS infection) or partial immobility or weakness (e.g., myelomeningocele, trauma, infection, degenerative disease).

Nursing Assessment

☐ **PERTINENT HISTORY**

Medical/surgical history, previous periods of immobility and any complications related to them, mechanism of injury (if appropriate), medication history, allergies

☐ **PHYSICAL FINDINGS**

Pulmonary, cardiovascular, gastrointestinal (GI), genitourinary (GU) functions; joint mobility, muscle strength; nutritional status, general physical condition

☐ **PSYCHOSOCIAL CONCERNS/ DEVELOPMENTAL FACTORS**

Age, sex, developmental level, usual coping mechanisms, family/living situation, available social support, routines/habits (e.g., sleeping, eating, playing)

☐ **PATIENT AND FAMILY KNOWLEDGE**

Complications associated with immobility and preventive measures to avoid them; level of knowledge, readiness and willingness to learn

Nursing Care

☐ **LONG-TERM GOAL**

The child will be free from pulmonary, cardiovascular, skin, musculoskeletal, GI, and GU complications resulting from immobility; the child/parents will demonstrate adap-

tive coping responses in dealing with the temporary or permanent loss of mobility.

NURSING DIAGNOSIS #1

Impaired gas exchange related to immobility

Rationale: When children are bedbound, the lungs do not fully expand because of the pressure created by the bed. Activity and movement allow the lungs to expand fully, to blow off excess carbon dioxide, and to stimulate the movement of secretions and respiratory waste products out of the lungs via the cilia. When children are immobile, atelectasis, congestion, and hypostatic pneumonia can occur. These conditions will impair the efficient exchange of gases between the alveoli and the vascular system.

☐ **GOAL**

The child will be free from pulmonary complications; will demonstrate effective gas exchange.

☐ **IMPLEMENTATION**

• Have child change position, cough, and take 5 deep breaths (holding on inspiration for 3 seconds if possible) every 1-2 hours; encourage alternative methods of deep breathing, short periods of crying, and games (e.g., blowing bubbles, pinwheels).

• Instruct in use of incentive spirometer; provide reward system (e.g., stickers, stars, special activity) to encourage use.

• Monitor for signs and symptoms of respiratory infection/other complications (e.g., elevated temperature and pulse, pain upon inspiration, rales, rhonchi, productive cough with green or yellow sputum).

• Monitor arterial blood glases for indications of hypoxia.

• Consider the use of respiratory therapy to assist child in respiratory function.

EVALUATION CRITERIA/DESIRED OUTCOMES

The child

- Coughs, turns, takes deep breaths at least every 2 hours
- Uses incentive spirometer and consistently increases inspired tidal volume
- Is free from signs or symptoms of respiratory complications
- Exhibits no indications of acid-base imbalance

NURSING DIAGNOSIS #2

Alteration in tissue perfusion: peripheral related to immobility

Rationale: When children are immobile, there is often excessive pressure on the vessels and the peripheral nerves. This pressure compromises circulation to the affected area and causes decreased perfusion of the surrounding tissues. Immobility may also cause thrombophlebitis from venous stasis.

GOAL

The child will be free from peripheral nerve damage and thrombophlebitis.

IMPLEMENTATION

- Assess daily for signs of phlebitis and stasis (e.g., pain, swelling in lower extremities); elevate all extremities to promote venous return.
- Check toes for temperature, color, sensation, and mobility every hour.
- Check peripheral pulses at least once a shift.
- Apply antiembolic stockings or elastic wraps to facilitate venous return from lower extremities; remove them for 10 minutes twice a day to inspect for tightness and bunching; do same procedure for splints.
- Encourage to flex toes, ankles, and feet every hour.
- Avoid pillows and pads under the knees or calves.

EVALUATION CRITERIA/DESIRED OUTCOMES

The child

- Wears antiembolic stockings/elastic wrap/splints
- Performs ankle, toe, and feet exercises on a regular basis
- Is free from signs/symptoms of thrombophlebitis or stasis
- Has normal peripheral pulses

NURSING DIAGNOSIS #3

a. **Impairment of skin integrity** related to immobility
b. **Potential for injury** related to improper alignment

Rationale: When the blood supply to an area falls below that required for survival, the skin and the underlying tissues are destroyed. With immobility, there is excessive pressure placed on the peripheral vessels, compromising circulation to the area and causing decreased perfusion of the surrounding tissues, which can result in a pressure sore or decubitus ulcer. Permanent misalignment and decreased range of motion (ROM) of the extremities may result if the body is not properly aligned while the child is immobile.

GOAL

The child will be free from decubitus ulcers; the child will maintain joint mobility; will be free from musculoskeletal complications.

IMPLEMENTATION

- Monitor for signs of impaired circulation (e.g., reddened areas of the skin, skin blanching) and massage back and other bony prominences every 2 hours and as necessary.
- Turn at least every 2 hours; use caution to avoid mechanical irritation (e.g., friction from sheets; pressure from traction, ropes, braces, casts).
- Use available resources (e.g., sheepskin, egg-crate, rotating-pressure beds) to minimize pressure.
- Provide a padded foot board to keep the feet at right angles; use a bed cradle to keep the weight of the bed linens off the feet; remind/help child to maintain appropriate alignment (e.g., place sticker on overhead bar/trapeze in correct position and tell child to keep nose right under sticker).
- Instruct in active or passive ROM exercises for all joints; perform exercises 4 times a day; refer to *The Child Requiring Range-of-Motion Exercises*, page 237.
- Remind child to perform gluteal and quadricep exercises.
- Provide weight bearing on lower extremities via tilt table or standup exercises.
- Position properly
  - *supine:* head in line with the spine; trunk positioned so that flexion of the hip is minimized; legs extended; heels suspended in a space between the mattress and the footboard; toes pointed straight up; small trochanter rolls under the hip joint area; small folded towel in the lumbar region for support
  - *side-lying:* head in line with the spine; trunk in

alignment and not twisted; uppermost hip joint slightly forward and supported by a pillow in a position of slight abduction; upper arm flexed at the elbow and shoulder and supported by a pillow; upper leg slightly flexed at the hip and knee and supported by a pillow

- *prone:* head turned to the side and in alignment with the rest of the body; arms abducted and externally rotated at the shoulder joint; toes suspended over the edge of the mattress; a small, flat support under the area from the umbilicus to the upper thigh to support the pelvis

• Refer to physical therapist to assist with progressive exercise and to instruct regarding transfer techniques as appropriate.

☐ EVALUATION CRITERIA/DESIRED OUTCOMES

The child

• Is free from decubiti
• Is free from foot drop, wrist drop, muscle atrophy/spasm/contracture, and external rotation of the hip
• Performs active/passive ROM to all joints
• Changes positions at least once every 2 hours; maintains proper alignment in all positions

---

NURSING DIAGNOSIS #4

a. **Alteration in nutrition: less than body requirements** related to condition
b. **Alteration in fluid volume: deficit** related to condition, immobility
c. **Alteration in bowel elimination: constipation** related to decreased physical activity

Rationale: Children who are immobile are often physically debilitated and unable or unwilling to consume an adequate amount of fluids and nutrients to meet their metabolic needs. All children who have physical illness have increased nutritional requirements to promote healing. Immobility slows the digestive process and contributes to problems of constipation.

☐ GOAL

The child will maintain weight within the normal growth curve; will maintain prehospital elimination pattern.

☐ IMPLEMENTATION

• Serve favorite foods in an attractive manner; encourage parents to bring food from home.
• Record intake and output; maintain fluid intake above normal for age/weight (unless there are fluid restrictions).

• Maintain a diary to monitor actual intake of fluids and nutrients; enlist child's help in keeping diary.
• Record baseline weight; weigh daily on same scale, at same time, in same clothes.
• Encourage to eat small, frequent (5-7) meals rather than a few, large ones; consider the use of high-protein liquid nutritional supplements.
• Encourage family and friends to visit during mealtime; move child to hallway and encourage having other children/staff eat with child.
• Establish a bowel program to ensure adequate bowel function
  - provide foods high in fiber (e.g., bran, raw fruits, vegetables)
  - encourage to be as physically active as permitted
  - administer stool softener prophylactically, laxatives and enemas as ordered to facilitate elimination
• Allow to use a bedside commode if possible.

☐ EVALUATION CRITERIA/DESIRED OUTCOMES

The child

• Drinks more than maintenance fluid requirement daily
• Maintains or increases weight as appropriate
• Verbalizes no feelings of distension in the stomach
• Consumes foods high in fiber and bulk daily
• Has a bowel movement of normal consistency and color at least every other day

---

NURSING DIAGNOSIS #5

a. **Potential for infection** related to urinary retention, placement of an indwelling urinary catheter
b. **Functional incontinence** related to immobility, cognitive deficit

Rationale: Children who are immobile are at increased risk for urinary retention, infection, and formation of calculi. Immobile children often become incontinent of urine requiring the placement of an indwelling urinary catheter and are, therefore, unable to practice their usual pattern of urinary elimination.

☐ GOAL

The child will maintain an adequate urinary output; will be free from calculi formation, urinary retention, and urinary tract infection.

☐ IMPLEMENTATION

• Assess for signs and symptoms of urinary retention (e.g., decreased urinary output, bladder dis-

tension) every shift; if severe retention continues, insert an indwelling catheter as ordered; refer to *The Child with a Urethral Catheter*, page 294.
- Monitor for signs and symptoms of urinary infection (e.g., dark, foul-smelling, concentrated urine; frequency; urgency; dysuria; elevated temperature) with each voiding.
- Monitor urinary function every shift (e.g., urine color, amount, frequency, turbidity, specific gravity, and pH).
- Allow to stand/use a bedside commode if at all possible.
- Be alert to indications of renal calculi (e.g., low abdominal distension or pressure, flank pain).

☐ EVALUATION CRITERIA/DESIRED OUTCOMES

The child
- Empties bladder completely
- Is free from urinary infection or calculi

NURSING DIAGNOSIS #6
a. **Diversional activity deficit** related to inability to participate in recreational activities
fb. **Altered growth and development** related to lack of control over environment, restriction on usual outlets for feelings

Rationale: *Mobility affects all aspects of growth and development and is an important avenue for expression of feelings, learning about the environment, and dealing with stress, anxiety, and frustration. Restriction of activities may decrease environmental stimuli and give the child an altered perception of self and environment. The child who is immobilized may demonstrate anger and acting-out behaviors (e.g., aggression, withdrawal, regression). These children need as much diversion and attention as possible.*

☐ GOAL

The child will participate in developmentally age-appropriate activities; will not be bored; will comply with mobilization restrictions.

☐ IMPLEMENTATION

- Include child in planning the daily routine; allow as many choices/decisions as possible.
- Maintain consistent daily routine when possible.
- Provide age-appropriate diversions (e.g., radio, tapes, games, mobiles, television, visitors, a roommate, a clock, a calendar); move bed to hallway, playroom if possible; encourage family to bring in personal possessions; refer to *The Child Requiring Play Therapy*, page 226; arrange for child life workers/volunteers to play with child.
- Plan your daily schedule to allow time to sit with the child.

☐ EVALUATION CRITERIA/DESIRED OUTCOMES

The child
- Participates in developmentally appropriate activities
- Verbalizes decreased boredom
- Complies with immobilization restrictions
- Participates in planning the daily schedule

NURSING DIAGNOSIS #7
Knowledge deficit regarding the hazards of immobility

Rationale: *Children who will be going home with continued mobilization restrictions and their parents require much instruction about the hazards of immobility to avoid the associated complications.*

☐ GOAL

The child/parents will understand the potential complications of immobility; will demonstrate measures to avoid complications.

☐ IMPLEMENTATION

- Discuss potential complications of immobility; teach methods of prevention.
- Instruct in proper positioning of the child; have family position child; give feedback.
- Discuss methods that can be used at home to avoid boredom and depression.
- Determine the need for a home physical therapy consult to assist with organizing a safe home environment; make appropriate referral.
- Assess the need for a referral to social services for supportive counseling in the home and assistance with community resources.

☐ EVALUATION CRITERIA/DESIRED OUTCOMES

The child/parents
- List at least 3 complications from each of the pulmonary, cardiovascular, skin, musculoskeletal, GI, and GU systems
- List at least 10 measures to prevent the complications of immobility
- Demonstrate proper positioning on a consistent basis
- Describe at least 4 techniques to provide diversion and avoid boredom and depression

The Child with Increased Intracranial Pressure

Definition/Discussion

Increased intracranial pressure is a rise above normal of the pressure of the cerebrospinal fluid (CSF) in the subarachnoid space. Normal intracranial pressure (ICP) ranges between 0 and 15 mm Hg.

Conditions that cause an *increase in brain size* include tumors, surgical manipulation, infarction, anoxic event (e.g., drowning, asphyxia, smoke inhalation, accidents, cardiac or respiratory arrest), head injury, brain abscess, metabolic disorder (e.g., chemical toxicity, diabetic acidosis), and Reye's syndrome. Conditions that *increase intracranial blood volume* include hypercapnia, hypoxemia, or hyperthermia causing cerebral vasodilation; tumor; cerebral hematoma; an aneurysm or arteriovenous malformation; and subarachnoid hemorrhage causing intracerebral bleeding. Conditions that *increase CSF volume* include tumors of the choroid plexus; subarachnoid hemorrhage meningitis, or cerebripseudotumor causing decreased CSF absorption; hydrocephalus, tumor, or trauma causing a blockage of CSF flow.

Nursing Assessment

☐ PERTINENT HISTORY

Presence of congenital defects, medical and surgical history, onset of symptoms (e.g., duration, location, description), mechanism of injury/insult, medications, allergies

☐ PHYSICAL FINDINGS

Altered level of consciousness (LOC)/responsiveness, irritability, pupillary changes, motor/sensory changes in extremities; vital sign changes (e.g., Cushing's triad: increased blood pressure, decreased heart rate, and widening pulse pressure), changes in depth, rate, and pattern of respirations; papilledema, enlarging head circumference, bulging fontanels, high-pitched cry, seizures; complaints of blurred/double vision, headache, vomiting; increased ICP on ICP monitor (i.e., epidural, intraventricular, or subarachnoid); presence/absence of gag reflex, deep tendon reflexes, Babinski's sign (normal under 1 year of age)

☐ PSYCHOSOCIAL CONCERNS/ DEVELOPMENTAL FACTORS

Age, developmental level, coping strategies; personal/family interaction patterns; habits/routines (e.g., what comforts child, bedtime routine, favored objects) acceptance of condition

☐ PATIENT AND FAMILY KNOWLEDGE

Etiology, treatment, outcomes, signs/symptoms of increased ICP; level of knowledge, readiness, willingness and ability to learn

Nursing Care

☐ LONG-TERM GOAL

The child will maintain stable vital functions with minimal complications through the period of actual or potential increased intracranial pressure; the child will experience reduction of increased intracranial pressure with no residual neurologic deficits.

NURSING DIAGNOSIS #1

Alteration in tissue perfusion: cerebral related to an increase in brain tissue, intracranial blood volume, CSF volume

Rationale: ICP is indicative of the balance in the intracranial volume (i.e., brain tissue, blood, and CSF). An alteration in either the arterial pressure or ICP alters cerebral perfusion. Cerebral perfusion pressure (CPP) is the amount of pressure needed in the cerebral vasculature to supply oxygen and nutrients to the brain. CPP can be calculated by subtracting the mean ICP from the mean arterial blood pressure. Normal CPP is 60-90 mm Hg (50 mm Hg is minimum for adequate cerebral perfusion).

☐ GOAL

The child will maintain/regain adequate cerebral perfusion.

☐ IMPLEMENTATION

- Monitor child's neurologic status every 1-2 hours and as necessary
  - LOC
  - behavior
  - reflexes
  - motor/sensory function (symmetry; movement: spontaneous, to command, to painful stimuli)
  - pupil symmetry, size, reactivity, deviation
- Monitor vital signs every 15 minutes to 1 hour and as necessary.
- Monitor intake and output, electrolytes, and urine specific gravity to determine potential fluid imbalance contributing to cerebral edema.
- Monitor ICP every 15 minutes to 1 hour and as necessary if ICP monitoring device is in place; maintain proper functioning of ICP monitoring device (e.g., check for closed system, position of transducer, calibration, air in system).
- Elevate head of bed and align head/neck to maintain venous outflow from the brain.
- Describe and record behavior carefully.
- Administer fluids within fluid restriction to prevent cerebral edema.
- Instruct older child to refrain from activities that increase intrathoracic or intra-abdominal pressure (e.g., straining for bowel movement, isometric exercises, holding breath when turning in bed, hip flexion, coughing, blowing nose).
- Prevent unnecessary crying.
- Utilize restraints only when absolutely necessary (agitation will increase ICP).
- Observe for increased ICP (e.g., irritability, high-pitched cry, headache, nausea, vomiting).
- Organize nursing care to allow child optimal rest periods.
- Employ strict aseptic technique and infection control measures regarding tubing and dressing changes (infection increases metabolic rate, cerebral blood flow, and cerebral edema).
- Administer steroids, diuretics (e.g., mannitol, furosemide), barbiturates, or short-acting narcotics, antiemetics, analgesics, stool softeners as ordered; monitor effectiveness.
- Drain CSF via intraventricular drain if appropriate.

☐ EVALUATION CRITERIA/DESIRED OUTCOMES

The child
- Has ICP of 0-15 mm Hg, CPP greater than 50 mm Hg
- Maintains/improves neurologic status

NURSING DIAGNOSIS #2
a. **Ineffective breathing pattern** related to increased ICP, alteration in LOC
b. **Ineffective airway clearance** related to increased ICP, alteration in LOC
c. **Impaired gas exchange** related to increased ICP, alteration in LOC

Rationale: There are a number of abnormal respiratory patterns associated with increased ICP. As pressure increases, vital centers located in the brainstem are affected. Cheyne-Stokes breathing consists of waxing and waning of respirations with periodic apnea. Central neurogenic hyperventilation, associated with lesions in the lower midbrain and upper pons, is characterized by continuous, regular, rapid, deep respirations. Pressure in the mid to lower pons region causes prolonged inspiration followed by prolonged expiration and a pause (apneustic breathing). Cluster breathing or irregular spurts of breathing interspersed with apnea is associated with lesions in the lower pons and upper medulla. Finally, a completely irregular pattern of breathing that may progress to apnea (ataxic or Biot's breathing) is indicative of pressure on the medulla.

A change in consciousness or responsiveness may impair the child's ability to clear pulmonary secretions or aerate adequately, causing acid-base disturbances. Acid-base imbalances and altered oxygenation will further increase the intracranial pressure.

☐ GOAL

The child will demonstrate effective air exchange; will be free from respiratory complications.

☐ IMPLEMENTATION

- Maintain a patent airway; utilize airway adjuncts as needed.
- Place child in side-lying position when comatose; place a small linen roll under shoulders to extend airway when supine.
- Suction the oropharynx as necessary; if intubated, hyperventilate by giving 6-8 breaths with Ambu-bag before and after suctioning; limit suctioning to 10-15 seconds.
- Monitor respiratory rate, rhythm, and depth every 15 minutes to 1 hours; auscultate breath sounds every 2-4 hours.
- Assess circulatory status (e.g., pulse, blood pressure, skin color) every hour; monitor ABGs and report findings.
- Administer oxygen as ordered; monitor effectiveness.
- Encourage deep breathing and limited coughing

every 1-2 hours; avoid percussion and postural drainage.
- Assess color, amount, consistency of pulmonary secretions.
- Initiate aerosol/nebulized treatments to break up secretions if appropriate.

☐ EVALUATION CRITERIA/DESIRED OUTCOMES

The child
- Has ABGs within normal limits
- Maintains regular respiratory rate within normal limits for age
- Has clear breath sounds
- Has no retractions, nasal flaring

NURSING DIAGNOSIS #3
a. **Alteration in fluid volume: excess** related to steroid therapy, syndrome of inappropriate antidiuretic hormone (SIADH)
b. **Fluid volume deficit** related to diuretic therapy, fluid restriction, diabetes insipidus

Rationale: Management of cerebral edema or increased ICP with drug therapy/fluid restriction can result in fluid and electrolyte imbalances. Syndrome of inappropriate secretion of antidiuretic hormone (SIADH) can occur with a variety of brain disorders, the stress of surgery, anesthesia, and certain medications.

☐ GOAL

The child will demonstrate adequate fluid balance.

☐ IMPLEMENTATION

- Monitor intake and output every hour; notify physician of urinary output of less than 0.5/greater than 2 cc/kg/hour; check specific gravity every 1-4 hours.
- Monitor laboratory findings (e.g., electrolytes, BUN, creatinine).
- Weigh daily on same scale, at same time, in same clothing.
- Monitor central venous, pulmonary artery, and pulmonary capillary wedge pressures; skin turgor; and mucous membranes at least every 1-2 hours.
- Administer fluids and medications as ordered; monitor effectiveness.

☐ EVALUATION CRITERIA/DESIRED OUTCOMES

The child
- Excretes at least 1 cc urine/kg/hour
- Maintains electrolytes, urine specific gravity within normal limits

- Has good skin turgor, moist mucous membranes
- Is free from edema

NURSING DIAGNOSIS #4
a. **Self-care deficit: total** related to decreased responsiveness
b. **Potential for injury** related to unresponsiveness, seizure activity
c. **Impaired physical mobility** related to neurologic insult
d. **Impairment of skin integrity** related to immobility, hypothermia therapy

Rationale: The child with an altered LOC caused by increased ICP or a therapeutically induced barbiturate coma will not be able to care for or move self, requiring either total or partial assistance.

Physical injury may occur during periods of seizure activity; or the child may experience gastrointestinal (GI) bleeding because of the corticosteroids used to treat/prevent increased ICP. The child in a coma is at risk for corneal abrasion because of an absent corneal reflex.

Hypothermia may be utilized to reduce metabolism, body's oxygen requirements, and cerebral blood flow. This places the child at risk for skin breakdown.

☐ GOAL

The child will maintain/regain motor function; will have all care needs met; will be free from injury, skin breakdown.

☐ IMPLEMENTATION

- Refer to *The Child at Risk for Hazards of Immobility*, page 156.
- Give mouth care every 2-4 hours with saline or half-strength peroxide swabs (glycerine may increase crusting); clean tongue and teeth; apply cream to nostrils and lips.
- Check eyes for corneal irritation or conjunctivitis; irrigate eyes with artificial tears, normal saline, or other suitable solution every 2 hours; place eyepads over eyes, tape lids closed if necessary.
- Monitor for seizure activity; refer to *The Child with Epilepsy*, page 122; take seizure precautions.
- Provide Foley catheter care every 8 hours if in place to assure patency and prevent infections.
- Inspect skin every 8 hours for hydration and turgor, rashes, abrasions, contusions, infection, or phlebitis at puncture sites; bathe daily.
- Review hospital protocol prior to instituting hypothermia; ensure that all personnel use hypothermia equipment safely; refer to product manual for instruction regarding recommendations for skin care and temperature settings.

- Reposition/turn every 2 hours and as necessary; check for redness/pressure areas with each turn.
- Use an alternating pressure pad or flotation mattress, massage, and protection for heels, elbows, bony prominences to prevent skin breakdown.
- Prevent contractures with bed board, foot board, trochanter rolls, and devices to prevent hand deformities; give passive range-of-motion exercises; cooperate with physical therapy aims and program.
- Evaluate oral structures, gag and swallow reflexes, and motor ability prior to oral feeding attempts; position as appropriate for child; use symmetric midline orientation with flexed extremities; know that choice of foodstuffs may influence success of feeding (e.g., pureed foods are difficult to keep in mouth if motor function is impaired); calculate daily caloric intake.
- Insert a nasogastric (NG) tube as appropriate; refer to *The Child Requiring Nasogastric Intubation*, page 194; if NG tube in place, keep patent; check for gastrointestinal bleeding (e.g., observe and hematest gastric secretions) from stress or from glucocorticosteroids.
- Refer to *The Child Requiring Tube Feedings*, page 288 and *The Child Receiving Total Parenteral Nutrition*, page 276 as needed.
- Monitor elimination status; check for diarrhea (from tube feedings, medications) or constipation (from immobility, medications).

☐ EVALUATION CRITERIA/DESIRED OUTCOMES

The child
- Maintains or improves level of motor function
- Has no contractures
- Has intact skin and mucous membranes
- Gains weight at a slow, steady pace
- Is free from injury

NURSING DIAGNOSIS #5
a. **Altered growth and development** related to imposed hospitalization, sensory deficits, altered LOC
b. **Sensory-perceptual alteration** related to sensory overload/deprivation, sensory deficits, altered LOC

Rationale: The child in a coma is not able to interpret the environment. The ability to see, hear, and feel may be altered as a result of the condition contributing to the increased ICP (e.g., a tumor pressing on the auditory nerve, meningitis). The child with actual or potential increased ICP will often be hospitalized in a critical care setting where constant monitoring, extensive equipment, and numerous personnel contribute to sensory overload/deprivation.

☐ GOAL

The child will interpret incoming stimuli in an age-appropriate way; will attain developmental milestones within limits of functional capabilities.

☐ IMPLEMENTATION

- Refer to *Normal Growth and Development*, pages 300–314.
- Reorient to environment frequently; place familiar objects (e.g., blanket, stuffed animal, pictures) in bed.
- Explain all tests, procedures, and routines even if you think child cannot hear or is too young to understand.
- Allow for uninterrupted rest periods to prevent sleep deprivation; allow child to assume favored sleeping position within restrictions of equipment; follow home bedtime routine if possible.
- Talk with child and play child's favorite music for stimulation; remind parents that child can often hear and understand, that unresponsive children may be soothed by familiar voices and sounds.
- Modify approach to child based on present deficits (e.g., approach from unaffected side, utilize touch, talk to child).
- Increase/decrease stimuli as appropriate to correct sensory deprivation/overload.
- Avoid talking about the child in his/her presence as if child did not exist.

☐ EVALUATION CRITERIA/DESIRED OUTCOMES

The child
- Is oriented to environment
- Responds appropriately to stimuli
- Obtains adequate rest
- Attains age-appropriate developmental milestones as able

NURSING DIAGNOSIS #6
a. **Fear** related to perceptions of uncertain future, unfamiliar environment
b. **Ineffective individual/family coping** related to actual or perceived loss of well-being, unfamiliar environment, separation from parents
c. **Alteration in family process** related to actual or perceived loss of well-being of child

Rationale: Increased ICP causes an alteration in the child's neurologic status, either temporary or permanent. This uncertainty and stress, in addition to the stress of hospitalization, can inhibit the coping abilities of the child/family.

GOAL

The child/family will effectively adapt to actual or potential altered abilities.

IMPLEMENTATION

- Keep family informed of child's progress, prognosis, and current plan of treatment; encourage them to assist with care whenever possible and to spend as much time as possible with child.
- Note family's emotional reaction to child's condition; determine effectiveness of coping strategies.
- Encourage family to express fears, feelings of helplessness, guilt, anger, and despair outside the child's hearing range; arrange for spiritual and emotional counseling as needed.
- Encourage child's expression of fears (e.g., about environment, procedures, prognosis) and feelings as condition warrants; refer to *Normal Growth and Development*, pages 300–314, and *The Child Requiring Play Therapy*, page 226.
- Explain tests, procedures, need for frequent assessments, treatments; use short, simple explanations; use pictures to augment comprehension.
- Utilize other personnel (e.g., child life worker, social worker, pastor, clinical nurse specialist, support group members) to assist child/family in coping with child's condition.

EVALUATION CRITERIA/DESIRED OUTCOMES

The child/family
- Verbalizes/plays out feelings related to fears
- Discusses ways to adapt to child's changed status

NURSING DIAGNOSIS #7

Knowledge deficit regarding disease process, treatment, prognosis

Rationale: The child and parents are usually inadequately prepared because of the unexpected and sudden hospitalization related to a head injury, cardiac arrest, or similar traumatic event. They will need specific instruction regarding the home care, depending on the cause of the problem.

GOAL

The child/parents will demonstrate adequate knowledge of ICP (potential and actual), prognosis, home care needs.

IMPLEMENTATION

- Correct any misinformation, fill in gaps of needed information.
- Ask child/parents to repeat information to ensure understanding.
- Keep informed about child's progress, prognosis, and plan of care.
- Identify resources and support groups available.
- Encourage verbalization and questions about current situation.
- Refer to appropriate other guides for details regarding discharge plans.

EVALUATION CRITERIA/DESIRED OUTCOMES

The child/parents
- Verbalize cause of present condition
- State treatment procedures and rationale
- Describe home care needs accurately

The Child with Infectious Mononucleosis

Definition/Discussion

Infectious mononucleosis is an acute infection caused by the Epstein-Barr Virus (EBV). It most commonly effects the oropharynx and causes lymphadenopathy. Most children who develop infectious mononucleosis are cared for at home unless complications develop.

Nursing Assessment

☐ **PERTINENT HISTORY**

Medications, treatments at home; exposure to mononucleosis

☐ **PHYSICAL FINDINGS**

Low-grade fever, fatigue, malaise, sore throat, muscle soreness, abdominal discomfort; enlarged, mildly tender cervical, submandibular, posterior auricular, axillary, inguinal nodes; splenomegaly; petechiae on the palate; positive Monospot test; positive herterophil-antibody titer; atypical lymphocytes; decreased neutrophil count; abnormal liver function tests

☐ **PSYCHOSOCIAL CONCERNS/ DEVELOPMENTAL FACTORS**

Age (the younger the child, the less severe the symptoms); daily routine, usual environment (school/day care/employment)

☐ **PATIENT AND FAMILY KNOWLEDGE**

Causes of signs and symptoms, expected course, outcome of disease; understanding of short-term changes in life-style and ability to develop plan to adapt to these changes during illness

Nursing Care

☐ **LONG-TERM GOAL**

The child will recover from the acute phase free from preventable complications.

NURSING DIAGNOSIS #1

Alteration in comfort related to oropharyngitis, fever, muscle soreness, abdominal tenderness

Rationale: The Epstein-Barr virus causes enlargement of lymph nodes and organs (e.g., liver and spleen), and inflammation of the oropharynx. Muscle soreness and headache are systemic effects of the illness.

☐ **GOAL**

The child will report minimal discomfort; will sleep and rest comfortably.

☐ **IMPLEMENTATION**

- Offer antipyretic/analgesic medication every 4 hours; document findings and response to medications.
- Avoid aspirin.
- Report increase in abdominal tenderness/shoulder pain; do not palpate abdomen (one of the complications of infectious mononucleosis is splenic rupture).
- Assist to assume position that provides greatest comfort; offer backrub at least twice daily.
- Encourage to rest/sleep as often as possible.
- Create environment conducive to relaxation (e.g., quiet music, dim lights, plants, moving bed to window).
- Provide active range-of-motion exercises 3 times a day while child is on bedrest.

☐ **EVALUATION CRITERIA/DESIRED OUTCOMES**

The child
- Maintains temperature of 36.5°-37.5°C (97.7°F-99.5°F)
- Rests quietly/sleeps soundly
- Reports relief from sore throat, headache, and muscle soreness

NURSING DIAGNOSIS #2

a. **Fluid volume deficit** related to fever, decreased intake
b. **Hyperthermia** related to condition

Rationale: Fever increases metabolism, thus utilizing increased amounts of body water; the discomfort of oropharyngitis may discourage adequate oral fluid intake.

☐ GOAL

The child will maintain adequate hydration.

☐ IMPLEMENTATION

- Check vital signs at least every 4 hours, more frequently if temperature elevated; give antipyretic as ordered and monitor effectiveness.
- Calculate maintenance fluid requirement for weight; include additional fluids if febrile.
- Ascertain favorite fluids and offer frequently; try novel ways of offering fluids (e.g., Popsicles, frozen juices, having a tea party).
- Record intake and output every shift.
- Monitor for clinical signs of dehydration every 4 hours (e.g., poor skin turgor, dry mucous membranes, decreased urine output, elevated urine specific gravity).

☐ EVALUATION CRITERIA/DESIRED OUTCOMES

The child
- Maintains adequate intake and output for weight
- Has moist mucous membranes, good skin turgor
- Maintains urine specific gravity of 1.003-1.020

NURSING DIAGNOSIS #3

Alteration in nutrition: less than body requirements related to anorexia, malaise, sore throat

Rationale: Pharyngitis and the generalized feeling of fatigue and malaise associated with infectious mononucleosis will inhibit adequate intake of nutrients. Adequate nutrition, especially protein intake, will enhance the body's immune system.

☐ GOAL

The child will ingest adequate nutrients for age and metabolic needs.

☐ IMPLEMENTATION

- Calculate nutritional requirements for age/weight.
- Ascertain particular food likes and dislikes; offer

small meals frequently; utilize novel ways of serving food (e.g., cut into shapes, use colorful plates and napkins); if child is hospitalized, encourage family members to take meals with child.
- Allow child to help plan meals for the day; encourage to maintain a food diary.
- Weigh child every other day at same time, in same clothing, using same scale.
- Monitor child's elimination pattern; give laxatives if constipation occurs (foods containing fiber may be difficult to swallow because of sore throat).

☐ EVALUATION CRITERIA/DESIRED OUTCOMES

The child
- Maintains stable weight
- Ingests high-protein diet

NURSING DIAGNOSIS #4

Diversional activity deficit related to imposed activity restriction

Rationale: Rest is the primary treatment for infectious mononucleosis. Inadequate rest will prolong recovery and delay the return to typical activities. Inactivity, however, is difficult to enforce and requires creativity and patience on the part of the caretaker.

☐ GOAL

The child/parents will verbalize understanding of the need for decreased activity during recovery; will describe a plan for incorporating quiet activities and adequate rest into the daily routine.

☐ IMPLEMENTATION

- Ask to identify favorite quiet activities; encourage to identify additional quiet activities s/he is interested in learning.
- Assist to develop a plan for alternating quiet activities (e.g., listening to music, playing word games, doing artwork or stitchery) with periods of rest.
- Encourage parents to allow child's friends to visit for short periods; remind parents to caution friends to maintain a quiet environment.
- Allow child to participate in planning care; know that unless the child is involved in planning care, rebellion and noncompliance may be a problem.
- Assist parents to explore options regarding homebound teaching so that delayed school progress does not add to child's frustration.
- Encourage parents to bring family activities into the child's bedroom so that the child does not feel isolated.

EVALUATION CRITERIA/DESIRED OUTCOMES

The child/parents

- Describe a plan for quiet activities
- Recognize that fatigue and low energy may persist for months after acute symptoms subside
- Verbalize importance of adequate rest for recovery

NURSING DIAGNOSIS #5
Knowledge deficit regarding home care

Rationale: The presence of an ill child in the home will alter the typical living patterns of all family members. Well-planned home care will enhance the child's recovery and minimize the disruption of established living patterns.

GOAL

The child/parents will verbalize understanding of the disease and treatment plan.

IMPLEMENTATION

- Teach appropriate hygiene techniques (e.g., hand-washing, use of disposable plates and eating utensils, washing of tableware in hot soap and water).
- Reinforce need to maintain a restful environment.
- Discuss the need to avoid activities that may cause the spleen to rupture; instruct regarding the symptoms of splenic rupture and emphasize need to contact physician if symptoms occur.
- Instruct to avoid immunizations until physician confirms that cellular-immune reactivity has returned to normal.
- Initiate public health nursing referral if appropriate; discuss role of public health nurse as a resource person.

EVALUATION CRITERIA/DESIRED OUTCOMES

The child/parents

- Describe home care routine/hygiene practices correctly
- List signs and symptoms to be reported to physician
- Have phone numbers of resources to contact for assistance

The Child Undergoing Intracranial Surgery: Craniotomy, Craniectomy, or Cranioplasty

Definition/Discussion

Craniotomy is an opening in the skull to form a bone flap. *Craniectomy* is the removal of part of the skull to form a hole or holes of varying size. *Cranioplasty* is the placement of a bone graft or synthetic plate to repair a defect or opening in the skull. Intracranial surgery relieves intracranial pressure (ICP) by removing hematomas, fluid, tissue, or an arteriovenous malformation (AVM); clipping an AVM; redirecting fluid via a shunt; or repairing fracture injuries.

Nursing Assessment

☐ PERTINENT HISTORY

Past medical and surgical history; condition mandating surgery (e.g., hematoma following head injury, tumor, AVM, hydrocephalus; pre-op neurologic deficits; seizures); history of coagulation disorder; respiratory or cardiac problems; diagnostic tests and findings (e.g., CT scan, angiography, skull films); medications; allergies

☐ PHYSICAL FINDINGS

Level of consciousness (LOC), motor and sensory function, fontanels (in infants), pupils, cranial nerve function, vital signs, respiratory status, head dressing and drainage, seizure activity, fluid status

☐ PSYCHOSOCIAL CONCERNS/ DEVELOPMENTAL FACTORS

Age, developmental level, habits (e.g., what comforts child, bedtime routine, favored objects), usual coping strategies, family interaction patterns, acceptance of condition, anxiety/fears

☐ PATIENT AND FAMILY KNOWLEDGE

General and neurosurgical pre- and post-op care; probable and possible anticipated results (e.g., deficits, rehabilitation); readiness, willingness, and ability to learn

Nursing Care

☐ LONG-TERM GOAL

The child will remain neurologically stable postoperatively; the child will resume pre-op neurologic function or participate in rehabilitation as fully as possible within limitations; the child will resume normal or adjusted roles in family/school/society; OR the child will maintain vital functioning and sustain life with comfort and dignity until death.

NURSING DIAGNOSIS #1

Alteration in tissue perfusion: cerebral related to increased ICP

Rationale: Edema, bleeding, hydrocephalus, or cerebral infarction can cause cerebral ischemia. Increased drowsiness 24-96 hours postoperatively indicates cerebral edema. Depending on the site and nature of the procedure, bleeding can occur in the meninges, cerebrum, cerebellum, or ventricles. Hypotension (intraoperatively or postoperatively) as well as thrombotic or air emboli can cause an infarction in the brain.

☐ GOAL

The child will demonstrate adequate cerebral perfusion.

IMPLEMENTATION

- Monitor vital signs every 15 minutes to 1 hour and as necessary.
- Elevate head of bed 30°-45° unless otherwise specified.
- Position child to maintain venous outflow from the brain; (position may need to be flat following subdural evacuation, turning may be limited when bone flap removed or with posterior fossa surgery); maintain head/neck in proper alignment.
- Assess head dressing/drain for amount and type of drainage every 1-4 hours.

EVALUATION CRITERIA/DESIRED OUTCOMES

The child
- Maintains ICP of 0-15 mm Hg
- Has cerebral perfusion pressure (CPP) greater than 50 mm Hg
- Maintains or improves neurologic status

NURSING DIAGNOSIS #2

a. **Ineffective breathing pattern** related to increased ICP, alteration in LOC
b. **Ineffective airway clearance** related to alteration in LOC
c. **Impaired gas exchange** related to shallow respirations

Rationale: Refer to The Child with Increased Intracranial Pressure, Nursing Diagnosis #2, page 161. The long operative time required for some surgical procedures increases the risk for post-op complications. Shallow respirations lead to atelectasis, which may be indicated by a fever within the first 24-48 hours postoperatively.

GOAL

The child will demonstrate effective air exchange.

IMPLEMENTATION

- Refer to *The Child with Increased Intracranial Pressure*, Nursing Diagnosis #2, page 161.
- Monitor temperature and pulse every 2-4 hours (elevations may indicate atelectasis).
- Monitor LOC.
- Maintain a patent airway by correct positioning, suctioning, utilizing airway adjuncts.
- Monitor respiratory rate, rhythm, and depth every 15 minutes to 1 hour; auscultate breath sounds every 2-4 hours for adequate aeration and to detect adventitious sounds.
- Assess circulatory status (i.e., peripheral pulses, blood pressure, skin color) every hour to detect hypoxia.

- Monitor arterial blood gas values for acid-base abnormalities and decreased oxygen saturation.
- Administer oxygen as ordered; monitor effectiveness.
- Encourage deep breathing and limited coughing every 1-2 hours as appropriate.
- Assess color, amount, consistency of pulmonary secretions to determine need for sputum culture, treatments to break up secretions.

EVALUATION CRITERIA/DESIRED OUTCOMES

The child
- Maintains arterial blood gases within normal limits
- Breathes regularly with rate appropriate for age
- Has normal breath sounds

NURSING DIAGNOSIS #3

a. **Alteration in fluid volume: excess** related to steroid therapy, syndrome of inappropriate antidiuretic hormone (SIADH)
b. **Fluid volume deficit** related to diuretic therapy, diabetes insipidus, blood loss, undertransfusion in surgery, fluid restriction, inadequate intake

Rationale: Management of cerebral edema or increased ICP with drug therapy and/or fluid restriction can result in fluid and electrolyte imbalances. An altered LOC or loss of the gag reflex (cranial nerves IX and X) can contribute to problems with oral intake. SIADH can occur with a variety of brain disorders, the stress of surgery, anesthesia, and certain medications. Surgery in the pituitary-hypothalamic area can alter ADH secretion and cause diabetes insipidus.

GOAL

The child will maintain adequate fluid intake and output.

IMPLEMENTATION

- Refer to *The Child with Increased Intracranial Pressure*, Nursing Diagnosis #3, page 162.
- Assess child's LOC and cranial nerve function (gag reflex) before attempting oral feedings.
- Monitor intake and output to avoid fluid deficit or excess.
- Notify physician of urinary output under .05 cc/kg/hour or over 2 cc/kg/hour.
- Monitor laboratory findings indicative of fluid imbalance (e.g., electrolytes, osmolarity, BUN, creatinine).
- Monitor weight daily on same scale, at same time, in same clothes.

- Take vital signs every 1-2 hours to measure hemodynamic response to fluid imbalance.
- Monitor central venous pressure, pulmonary artery pressure, and pulmonary capillary wedge pressure if catheter present every 1-2 hours and as necessary for hemodynamic response to fluid imbalance.
- Assess skin turgor and presence of edema every 4 hours.
- Administer replacement fluids and medications if necessary; evaluate effectiveness.

☐ EVALUATION CRITERIA/ DESIRED OUTCOMES

The child
- Maintains electrolytes, osmolarity, specific gravity within normal limits
- Excretes at least 0.5-1 cc/kg of urine every hour

NURSING DIAGNOSIS #4

Potential for injury related to seizure activity, drug therapy (steroids), cranial nerve V dysfunction, absence of bone flap, cerebrospinal fluid (CSF) leak/infection

Rationale: Cerebral edema may alter neuronal functioning, leading to the development of seizures. Children requiring surgery for abscesses, arteriovenous malformations (AVM), and intracerebral hemorrhages are likely to experience seizures. Metabolic imbalances such as hypoxia, hypoglycemia, and electrolyte imbalances pre- or postoperatively can also contribute to the development of seizures. Corticosteroids such as dexamethasone (Decadron), used to treat/prevent post-op increased ICP, irritate the gastrointestinal (GI) tract and cause bleeding. Cranial nerve V dysfunction resulting from increased ICP or direct injury places the person at risk for corneal abrasion. Increased ICP may also necessitate the bone flap not being replaced to allow the brain to expand. Communication with the subarachnoid space as a result of surgery or a basilar skull fracture can cause a CSF leak. Secondary brain/brainstem damage can occur as a result of an infectious process.

☐ GOAL

The child will be free from physical injury or secondary brain/brainstem injury.

☐ IMPLEMENTATION

- Monitor for seizure activity; refer to *The Child with Epilepsy*, page 122
- Protect from potential injury related to seizures (e.g., keep bed in low position, side rails up and padded).

- Assess GI secretions for color and presence of blood.
- Administer medications (anticonvulsants, antibiotics, antacids, cimetidine) as ordered; evaluate effectiveness.
- Assess cranial nerve V function every 3 hours.
- Apply artificial tears and/or eye patches as needed to lubricate and protect the eyes.
- Position to avoid pressure on flap site; use donut ring as necessary to avoid undue pressure on the area.
- Observe incision site and change or reinforce dressing as necessary, maintaining sterility.
- Assess for otorrhea or rhinorrhea indicating CSF leak; do not pack ear or nose as this may cause an increase in ICP.
- Monitor temperature every 4 hours.
- Assess child's LOC at least every 1-2 hours to determine changes.

☐ EVALUATION CRITERIA/DESIRED OUTCOMES

The child
- Exhibits no indications of GI bleeding
- Is free from corneal abrasions
- Maintains baseline neurologic status

NURSING DIAGNOSIS #5

a. **Impaired physical mobility** related to decreased LOC, paresis/plegia
b. **Impairment of skin integrity** related to limitations in mobility

Rationale: Mobility may be limited postoperatively as a result of alterations in wakefulness/arousal, motor/sensory function. Immobility or limitations in mobility caused by an altered LOC and motor/sensory deficits places the child at risk for the development of skin problems.

☐ GOAL

The child will actively or passively participate in mobilization; will be free from injury.

☐ IMPLEMENTATION

- Refer to *The Child at Risk for Hazards of Immobility*, page 156.
- Inspect skin (e.g., capillary refill, color, warmth, blisters) every 4 hours for pressure areas.
- Monitor motor/sensory functions to determine abilities and limitations.
- Perform range-of-motion exercises every 4 hours while child is confined to bed; refer to *The Child Requiring Range-of-Motion Exercises*, page 237.
- Reposition or assist with repositioning every 2-4 hours to relieve pressure over bony prominences.

- Assist with ambulation as needed.
- Coordinate nursing efforts with physical therapy.
- Encourage child's participation in activities as appropriate.

☐ **EVALUATION CRITERIA/DESIRED OUTCOMES**

The child
- Maintains joint mobility
- Sits in chair, ambulates as able
- Is free from pressure sores

NURSING DIAGNOSIS #6

Impaired communication: verbal related to dysphasia

Rationale: Expressive or receptive aphasia in a previously verbal child may become evident postoperatively as a result of surgical manipulation of brain/cerebral edema.

☐ **GOAL**

The child will demonstrate improved ability to express self, increased ability to understand.

☐ **IMPLEMENTATION**
- Assess child's ability to express self and to understand communication.
- Speak in short, simple sentences in a calm, unhurried manner.
- Acknowledge understanding of child's difficulty with communication.
- Utilize alternative methods of communication (e.g., magic slate, picture/alphabet board) as needed.
- Utilize parents to help understand child's needs and communication abilities.
- Coordinate nursing efforts with speech therapy.

☐ **EVALUATION CRITERIA/DESIRED OUTCOMES**

The child
- Communicates basic needs
- Participates in speech therapy

NURSING DIAGNOSIS #7

Alteration in comfort: pain related to increased ICP, surgical manipulation

Rationale: Manipulation of intracranial tissue during surgery causes edema resulting in increased ICP; the child may subsequently complain of a headache. Preoperatively, the pathology alters the intracranial contents and pressure causing a headache.

☐ **GOAL**

The child will have a reduction in pain.

☐ **IMPLEMENTATION**
- Assess the child's level of discomfort using a subjective 0-10 point self-rating scale, if possible; refer to *The Child Experiencing Pain*, page 216.
- Administer analgesics; evaluate effectiveness.
- Promote a quiet, restful environment; position for comfort with head of bed elevated to promote venous drainage.
- Evaluate effectiveness of comfort measures.
- Assess for factors contributing to the pain experience (e.g., anxiety, unfamiliar environment, increased blood pressure, inadequate rest); provide alternate interventions (e.g., favored object, position of comfort, gentle touch, holding if permitted, guided imagery, distraction).

☐ **EVALUATION CRITERIA/DESIRED OUTCOMES**

The child
- Verbalizes reduction or absence of pain following interventions
- Displays decreased crying
- Sleeps for uninterrupted periods

NURSING DIAGNOSIS #8

Alteration in nutrition: less than body requirements related to NPO status, IV fluid restriction, altered LOC, dysphagia, difficulty sucking/chewing

Rationale: Postoperatively, the child may exhibit an altered LOC or cranial nerve dysfunction as a result of cerebral edema or direct surgical manipulation which can prohibit or reduce oral intake. In an effort to control ICP, fluids may be restricted. An IV may be necessary to keep the child NPO until the neurologic and GI status improves.

☐ **GOAL**

The child will maintain optimal nutritional status and fluid intake.

☐ **IMPLEMENTATION**
- Assess LOC and cranial nerves V, VII, IX, X, XII functions to determine ability to handle food and fluids.
- Monitor intake and output and dietary intake to determine deficit.
- Monitor electrolytes as poor oral intake and fluid deficit can cause electrolyte imbalance.

- Administer IV fluids as ordered; refer to *The Child with an Intravenous Catheter*, page 174.
- Administer nasogastric feedings and water if ordered; refer to *The Child Requiring Tube Feedings*, page 288.
- Assist with oral feedings when indicated.
- Advance diet as tolerated for condition and age (i.e., full liquids, soft or pureed, regular).
- Provide oral hygiene before/after each oral feeding to facilitate taste sensation.
- Monitor daily weights.
- Auscultate bowel sounds every 4-8 hours to determine presence or absence of peristalsis.
- Record and monitor number and character of bowel movements.

☐ **EVALUATION CRITERIA/DESIRED OUTCOMES**

The child
- Maintains weight, demonstrates long-term growth
- Tolerates parenteral or tube feedings
- Has increased oral intake without aspiration

NURSING DIAGNOSIS #9
a. **Sensory-perceptual alteration** related to brain damage, altered LOC
b. **Altered growth and development** related to imposed hospitalization, sensory deficits, altered LOC

Rationale: The child's ability to see, hear, and feel may be altered as a result of the condition necessitating surgery (e.g., a tumor pressing on the auditory nerve, hemiparesis). The child may be lethargic, confused, or disoriented pre- and postoperatively, limiting ability to accurately interpret the environment and attain developmental milestones.

☐ **GOAL**

The child will be able to accurately interpret incoming stimuli as age appropriate; will attain developmental milestones within limits of functional capabilities.

☐ **IMPLEMENTATION**
- Assess neurologic (LOC, cranial nerve function, motor/sensory function reflexes) and developmental status to determine abilities and deficits; refer to *Normal Growth and Development*, pages 300–314.
- Orient to environment every 1-2 hours; place familiar objects (e.g., toys, blanket, pictures) in bed; play audiotapes of parents reading (if no hearing deficits).
- Modify approach to child based on deficits and age.

- Avoid talking about the child in his/her presence as if child is not there.

☐ **EVALUATION CRITERIA/DESIRED OUTCOMES**

The child
- Is oriented to environment
- Responds appropriately to stimuli
- Attains age-appropriate developmental milestones as able

NURSING DIAGNOSIS #10
a. **Fear** related to perceptions of uncertain future, unfamiliar environment
b. **Ineffective individual/family coping** related to actual/perceived loss of well-being
c. **Alteration in family process** related to actual/perceived loss of well-being of child
d. **Knowledge deficit** regarding disease process, treatment, prognosis

Rationale: The condition necessitating surgery may be causing a temporary or permanent alteration in the child's neurologic status. This uncertainty and/or the unfamiliar hospital environment/procedures stress the coping abilities of the child/family. Inadequate preparation in regard to intracranial surgery may relate to insufficient pre-op teaching if surgery is sudden and unexpected. Prior to discharge, the parents will require information related to drug therapy and follow-up care.

☐ **GOAL**

The child/parents will effectively adapt to actual or potential altered abilities; will demonstrate adequate knowledge related to surgery, pre-op and post-op interventions.

☐ **IMPLEMENTATION**
- Assess understanding of condition and anticipated post-op outcomes.
- Explain tests/procedures, frequent assessments, treatments in simple, concrete terms; repeat as necessary.
- Inform at age-appropriate level about shaving of the head, head dressings, frequency of nursing assessments, use of invasive equipment, and the probable and possible anticipated results, including potential rehabilitation.
- Keep family informed of child's progress.
- Encourage expression of feelings, concerns, questions, verbally or through play.
- Assess child's/family's emotional reaction to child's condition.

- Inform child/parents of progress, prognosis, and plan of care.
- Utilize other personnel to assist child/family to cope with child's condition (e.g., child life worker, pastor, clinical nurse specialist, social services).
- Prior to discharge, instruct regarding wound care; dosage, route, and side effects of medications; follow-up appointment with physician; and therapy (speech, occupational, physical) schedule.

☐ EVALUATION CRITERIA/DESIRED OUTCOMES

The child/parents
- State type of surgery to be done and rationale (as appropriate)
- Describe what to expect in immediate post-op period
- Verbalize/play out feelings related to fears
- Discuss ways to adapt to child's changed status

The Child with an Intravenous Catheter

Definition/Discussion

The administration of intravenous (IV) fluids through a peripheral infusion site may be for water/electrolyte maintenance/replacement or medication infusion. Though some of the principles are applicable, this guide does not completely address the care of a child with a central line.

Nursing Assessment

☐ **PERTINENT HISTORY**

Any previous experience with IVs, reason for IV

☐ **PHYSICAL FINDINGS**

Location of good veins for infusions, sites of previous IVs/infiltrations, preference for right or left hand, hydration status, weight

☐ **PSYCHOSOCIAL CONCERNS/ DEVELOPMENTAL FACTORS**

Coping mechanisms for painful procedures, age/developmental level, previous experience with restricted activity, habits/routines (e.g., playing, sleeping, eating), what comforts child

☐ **PATIENT AND FAMILY KNOWLEDGE**

IV therapy, reason for IV, level of acceptance and knowledge, readiness and willingness to learn

Nursing Care

☐ **LONG-TERM GOAL**

The child will receive IV therapy free from complications.

NURSING DIAGNOSIS #1
a. **Alteration in fluid volume: excess** related to equipment malfunction, child/parent changing infusion rate, iatrogenic fluid overload
b. **Fluid volume deficit** related to equipment malfunction, child/parent changing infusion rate, inadequate fluid resuscitation

---

Rationale: IV administration is an artificial method of delivering fluids that bypasses the body's regulatory systems, thus making it easy to under/overhydrate the child.

☐ **GOAL**

The child will maintain appropriate fluid volume for age/size, diagnosis, and status.

☐ **IMPLEMENTATION**

- Calculate fluid requirements for child, check if they coincide with physician's order and with child's diagnosis (may be decreased in patients with neurologic, cardiac, or renal problems or increased in patients with other conditions, such as sickle cell anemia).
- Hang all tubing with an in-line burette (volume control chamber); fill chamber with no more than 2 hours' worth of fluid at one time.
- Use pediatric microdrip tubing for infants and young children.
- Use infusion device to monitor flow rate (a regulator or controller infuses fluid using gravity while a pump will infuse fluid against a certain amount of pressure).
- Keep infusion device positioned so that child cannot change rate, stop/start infusion.
- Check that IV is dripping, pump is on, rate is correct every time you come in contact with child, at least every hour.
- Monitor vital signs; maintain accurate intake and output; weigh daily at the same time, on the same scale, in the same clothes; assess for edema (e.g., fontanel, periorbital, dependent).
- Explain to child/parents importance of keeping infusion constant; caution them not to regulate IV (unless appropriate as in care-by-parent units, teaching for home IV).

☐ **EVALUATION CRITERIA/DESIRED OUTCOMES**

The infant
- Has normal fontanel (i.e., not sunken/bulging)
- Has eyes that are not sunken, no periorbital edema

The child
- Maintains normal blood pressure, heart rate, urine output for age and weight
- Has good skin turgor

NURSING DIAGNOSIS #2
Impaired physical mobility related to arm-boards, restraints

Rationale: Physical restraining devices are used in order to keep the child from moving too much, dislodging/picking/pulling the IV. When restrained the child has limited freedom of movement.

☐ **GOAL**

The child will maintain patent IV with minimal amount of restraint, free from neurovascular impairment.

☐ **IMPLEMENTATION**

- Bundle/mummy infant for IV insertion.
- Have another nurse help older child hold still for IV insertion.
- Have child help choose insertion site if old enough, use nondominant hand if possible.
- Use scalp veins in infant when possible; explain to parents this permits greater freedom of movement for infant, less chance of dislodging the IV, and easier insertion in infants who have a lot of subcutaneous tissue.
- Restrain extremities as necessary; explain reason to child/parents; release from restraints every 2 hours for 15 minutes.
- Assess restrained extremities for pulses, movement, sensation, temperature, and color every 2 hours and as necessary.
- Use armboard of appropriate size for child.
- Use medicine cup cut in half and padded or other covering device to protect IV site from child's touch.
- Check for pressure areas every 8 hours if using foot vein; use caution not to dislodge IV or let foot move when untaping IV board.
- Offer diversional activities appropriate to age/development.

☐ **EVALUATION CRITERIA/DESIRED OUTCOMES**

The child
- Maintains patent IV
- Requires minimal restraint
- Maintains strong, equal pulses, movement, sensation, temperature, normal neurovascular check in affected extremity

---

NURSING DIAGNOSIS #3
Fear related to pain, needles

Rationale: IV insertion is a painful and sometimes unfamiliar procedure. The child usually has no choice whether an IV will be inserted or not and usually does not want one.

☐ **GOAL**

The child will be appropriately prepared for the IV insertion; will experience a minimal amount of fear.

☐ **IMPLEMENTATION**

- Prepare child/parents as age/developmentally appropriate.
- Discuss why IV is necessary, probable length of treatment; show child/parents equipment and allow to handle.

Infant
- Give information to parents.
- Handle infant gently.
- Speak softly.
- Bundle for security and safety.
- Avoid inserting IV into same arm child uses for thumb/finger sucking if possible.
- Cuddle immediately after insertion.

Toddler and preschooler
- Give information to child/parents as appropriate.
- Speak softly; handle confidently.
- Prepare equipment out of sight; take to treatment room and insert IV promptly.
- Bundle for insertion.
- Cuddle immediately after insertion.

School-age child
- Explain procedure and ask for cooperation.
- Demonstrate equipment; give time for questions and venting of anxiety/fear.
- Allow choices as appropriate (e.g., right or left hand, type of tape).
- Give positive reinforcement after procedure.

Adolescent
- Explain procedure, elicit questions.
- Discuss fears related to procedure.
- Include in decisions (e.g., site, use of armboard, tape).

☐ **EVALUATION CRITERIA/DESIRED OUTCOMES**

The infant
- Has IV inserted with minimal trauma
- Quiets with comforting soon after procedure

The older child
- Describes/plays out procedure
- Verbalizes fear and attempts to control self during insertion

NURSING DIAGNOSIS #4

Diversional activity deficit related to restriction/limitation of movement

Rationale: The equipment set-up and restraining devices used for an IV limit a child's normal freedom of movement.

☐ GOAL

The child will receive adequate stimulation to meet normal growth and development needs.

☐ IMPLEMENTATION

- Take child for walks, to playroom, sit in hallway where activity is.
- Have developmentally appropriate toys, games, books in crib, at bedside; refer to *Normal Growth and Development*, pages 300–314; encourage activities that do not require use of the extremity that has IV (e.g., if IV is in right hand and child is right handed, read books or walk instead of coloring).
- Teach child/parents how to move IV pole, unplug infusion pump (if battery operated) for walks, and to plug it back in.
- Set up study schedule and encourage keeping up with lessons from school if appropriate.

☐ EVALUATION CRITERIA/DESIRED OUTCOMES

The child
- Demonstrates interest in environment
- Verbalizes no complaints of boredom
- Displays no listlessness, apathy from lack of stimulation
- Performs age-appropriate developmental tasks

NURSING DIAGNOSIS #5

Alteration in comfort: pain related to infiltration, phlebitis

Rationale: Children have small veins and often do not understand the need for limiting movement in the area of IV, so infiltration may occur easily. Phlebitis, as in any inflammation, may cause pain at the site.

☐ GOAL

The child will be free from pain associated with continuous IV therapy.

☐ IMPLEMENTATION

- Monitor site every time in contact with child (at least hourly)
  - check temperature of site
  - touch site above catheter to check if soft or taut
  - check symmetry of limbs or head
  - check for bogginess in scalp by pressing on scalp
  - question child if it hurts and where, note nonverbal signs of pain
- Dilute antibiotics in appropriate amount of fluid to prevent phlebitis.
- Ensure that child is properly restrained and that reasons for limiting movement are explained.
- Discontinue infusion if infiltration has occurred; elevate limb; apply warm, moist compresses (if no medication infusing at the time) and report; refer to hospital procedure manual for specific guidelines.

☐ EVALUATION CRITERIA/DESIRED OUTCOMES

The child
- Shows no evidence of discomfort at or around IV site
- Shows no favoring of site, no limitation of movement
- Experiences quick resolution of infiltration

NURSING DIAGNOSIS #6

Knowledge deficit regarding ongoing IV infusion and potential complications

Rationale: The child/parents need information and teaching in order to deal appropriately with IV equipment, to cope with limitations of movement, and to help prevent complications.

☐ GOAL

The child/parents will understand the need for and potential complications of IV therapy.

☐ IMPLEMENTATION

- Discuss with child/parents why infusion is necessary.
- Teach reasons for restraints (e.g., to avoid touching/picking at site; immobilize the area).
- Explore methods to maintain mobility.
- Explain to parents that an infant still needs holding and teach methods to pick up and hold infant with an IV.
- Tell to call nurse if IV not infusing (e.g., not dripping, alarm is sounding, or if site is painful, red swollen, cool or warm to touch).

☐ EVALUATION CRITERIA/DESIRED OUTCOMES

The child/parents
- State reason for IV
- Demonstrate how to move about room, halls with IV equipment
- Call nurse when infusion is not dripping, bottle is empty
- List potential complications and methods to avoid them

The Child with Leukemia

Definition/Discussion

Leukemia is a neoplastic disorder of the blood-forming system resulting in an overproduction of immature, white blood cells. Survival rates for this once fatal illness have improved dramatically in the past 10 years with the use of effective combinations of chemotherapeutic drugs and radiation therapy.

Nursing Assessment

☐ **PERTINENT HISTORY**

Course of illness (length, characteristics), prior treatment, previous infections, childhood illness, immunization history

☐ **PHYSICAL FINDINGS**

Signs of anemia (e.g., pallor, fatigability, tachypnea, dyspnea), leukopenia (e.g., fever, infections), or thrombocytopenia (e.g., petechiae, purpura, bruising, bleeding of mucous membranes); extramedullary invasion (e.g., lymphadenopathy, hepatomegaly, splenomegaly); central nervous system (CNS) involvement; testicular involvement (enlargement); renal involvement (e.g., hematuria, hypertension, renal failure); gastrointestinal (GI) involvement (e.g., mouth ulcers, oral and esophageal monilia, gingival hypertrophy, perirectal inflammation); bone and joint involvement; respiratory involvement; pain

☐ **PSYCHOSOCIAL CONCERNS/ DEVELOPMENTAL FACTORS**

Developmental level; coping mechanisms; habits (e.g., what comforts child, feeding/bedtime routines, favored objects); ability to accept diagnosis information

☐ **PATIENT AND FAMILY KNOWLEDGE**

Previous experience with cancer/leukemia/chemotherapy and death; components of blood and their functions, transfusions; level of knowledge, readiness and willingness to learn

Nursing Care

☐ **LONG-TERM GOAL**

The child will adhere to treatment regimen, living within minimum restrictions and discomforts while achieving appropriate growth and developmental tasks; the family will adjust to actual/potential losses.

NURSING DIAGNOSIS #1

Potential for infection related to disease process, immunosuppression

Rationale: The large number of immature white blood cells that proliferate in the body during the leukemic process do not provide a defense against infection, and at the same time drastically reduce the normal components of the blood. The treatment regimen of chemotherapy and radiation further reduces the bone marrow's ability to produce necessary blood components.

☐ **GOAL**

The child will be free from infections; the child/parents will carry out measures to prevent infections.

☐ **IMPLEMENTATION**

- Monitor the white blood cell count for decreases that indicate the child is at greater risk for infection.
- Isolate child from any persons with infectious diseases, especially chickenpox.
- Maintain good hygienic practices; ensure children wash hands after toileting.
- Monitor vital signs for signs of infection (e.g., increased temperature, pulse, and respiration) at least every 4 hours.
- Avoid rectal temperatures, suppositories, or enemas, as damaged mucosa promotes bacterial growth.
- Examine skin and mucous membranes daily for

any lesions or breaks; provide mouth care several times daily.

- Administer antibiotics as ordered; monitor for expected and toxic effects.
- Administer granulocytes as ordered; refer to *The Child Receiving Blood and Blood-Product Transfusions*, page 24.
- Provide balance between periods of rest and activity to avoid overtiring.
- Refer to *The Child Receiving Chemotherapy*, page 57 for additional care.

☐ EVALUATION CRITERIA/DESIRED OUTCOMES

The child/parents
- Carry out measures to prevent infection

The child
- Has stable vital signs within normal limits
- Is free from respiratory, other infection

NURSING DIAGNOSIS #2

Potential for injury (hemorrhage) related to altered coagulation

Rationale: Platelets are crowded out by the proliferation of white blood cells, putting these children at risk for hemorrhage.

☐ GOAL

The child will be monitored for early signs of hemorrhage; will be protected from bleeding.

☐ IMPLEMENTATION

- Inspect skin and mucous membranes daily to detect signs of bleeding; instruct to blow nose gently.
- Report any signs/symptoms of hemorrhage (e.g., decreased blood pressure, tachycardia, pallor, diaphoresis, increased anxiety).
- Examine all urine and stools for gross evidence of bleeding; hematest urine and stools; avoid rectal temperatures and medication.
- Use small-gauge needles for all injections and apply pressure dressing to puncture site after needle removal.
- Use a soft toothbrush to prevent gum bleeding; give frequent oral hygiene with a nonirritating mouthwash; monitor gums and oral mucosa for discomfort and bleeding; lubricate lips.
- Do not give aspirin or aspirin-containing products.
- Monitor child's blood studies for changes and abnormal results.
- Be alert for CNS symptoms (e.g., headache, blurring of vision) resulting from intracranial hemorrhage.

- Handle gently; change position carefully; refrain from pulling against bed sheets.
- Provide soft toys and books, avoid sharp objects.
- Pad crib/bed to minimize trauma.
- If blood component therapy is ordered, refer to *The Child Receiving Blood and Blood-Product Transfusions*, page 24.

☐ EVALUATION CRITERIA/DESIRED OUTCOMES

The child
- Has no bruising, petechiae, bleeding
- Has normal blood pressure and heart rate
- Is free from pallor, diaphoresis, increased anxiety
- Plays quietly with safe toys/activities

NURSING DIAGNOSIS #3

Leukemic children will often undergo radiation therapy and multiple courses of chemotherapy; refer to The Child Receiving Chemotherapy, *page 57, and* The Child Undergoing Radiation Therapy, *page 234, for additional nursing care as needed.*

NURSING DIAGNOSIS #4

Alteration in nutrition: less than body requirements related to cancer cachexia

Rationale: Children with leukemia may develop cancer cachexia, a general state of malnutrition in neoplastic disease caused by increased metabolic rate, anorexia, and alterations in taste perceptions. Treatment is more effective and better tolerated if the child is well-nourished.

☐ GOAL

The child will ingest adequate food and fluids to maintain and support normal growth and development.

☐ IMPLEMENTATION

- Weigh weekly.
- Include foods child likes in menu; involve child/parents in food selection; make mealtime a special occasion for children (e.g., a "picnic"); provide colorful foods/fluids to stimulate appetite.
- Make breakfast as high in caloric intake as possible (children often lose their appetite as the day progresses).
- Offer small amounts at frequent intervals; avoid foods that cause irritation to mucous membranes

(such as hot liquids, spicy and rough foods); give soft foods and cool, soothing drinks.

- Consult with physician and dietician regarding specific nutritional needs (e.g., increased protein as a protection against infection); discuss these with child/parents.
- Teach/reinforce basic nutritional principles (e.g., food groups, balanced diets, calorie requirements).
- Provide between-meal protein supplements (e.g., eggnogs, milkshakes).
- Schedule meals around chemotherapy, give oral hygiene prior to meals; control nausea with antiemetics.
- Avoid foods that the child finds unpleasant due to altered tastes.
- Chart food intake, as well as fluid intake and output.
- Administer parenteral nutrition if unable to ingest foods orally; refer to *The Child Receiving Total Parenteral Nutrition,* page 276.

☐ **EVALUATION CRITERIA/DESIRED OUTCOMES**

The child
- Has good skin color and turgor
- Shows normal growth and weight gain for age
- Has adequate urinary output with specific gravity less than 1.020

NURSING DIAGNOSIS #5

a. **Ineffective individual/family coping** related to diagnosis, changes in body image and usual role function, hospitalization, treatment, fear of death
b. **Disturbance in self-concept** related to changes in appearance, role disturbance
c. **Grieving** related to actual/potential losses

Rationale: Cancer is a life-threatening illness that engenders many fears and requires many changes. Fears of death or the side effects of treatment are common and must be addressed.

☐ **GOAL**

The child/family will express feelings/fears about the disease process and possible death; the child will deal adaptively with changes in body image, side effects of treatment.

☐ **IMPLEMENTATION**

- Refer to *The Child Who is Dying/Terminal,* page 116, *The Parent Experiencing Grief and Loss,* page 139, and *The Child Experiencing a Body-Image Disturbance,* page 30.
- Determine child/family stage of grieving and re-

sponses; support and encourage adaptive responses; assist in altering maladaptive responses (e.g., suicidal behavior).
- Support a realistic assessment of the child's condition; reinforce family for focusing on short-range planning, one day at a time.
- Help child maintain a positive self-image by experimenting with wigs or hair pieces and by meeting other children who have successfully handled body-image changes.
- Support the child's need for unique, personal adjustments to change.
- Point out any signs of progress or positive change.
- Reassure about benefits of treatment; support and comfort child undergoing severe side effects such as nausea and vomiting, fever.
- Encourage parents to provide care as much as possible.
- Spend time with the child encouraging expression of feelings, but do not push; let child set own pace; accept all feelings child/family express; share that others have expressed similar concerns/fears; accept negative feelings and know that this is part of the process of working through and dealing with the diagnosis.
- Be alert to children expressing feelings, fears through play with toys, or drawing pictures.
- Provide diversional play for child within safe limits; refer to *The Child Requiring Play Therapy,* page 226.
- Explain all treatments to child at age-appropriate level of understanding; encourage child to ask questions about treatment.
- Encourage parents to get adequate rest, to eat well, and to take time for self; initiate referral to social services for financial assistance as needed.
- Explain purpose/services of support groups; refer to available community resources.

☐ **EVALUATION CRITERIA/DESIRED OUTCOMES**

The child/parents
- Deal adaptively with changes in body
- Develop effective coping mechanisms
- Express fears and concerns with staff and each other

NURSING DIAGNOSIS #6

Knowledge deficit regarding diagnosis, treatment protocol, follow-up care

Rationale: Leukemia is a very complex disease with many treatments and treatment side effects that the parents must know in order to comply and be able to notify the physician/clinic if there are any problems.

☐ **GOAL**

The child/parents will understand the disease process, treatment regimen, and treatment side effects.

☐ **IMPLEMENTATION**

- Plan short sessions with child/parents.
- Give written and verbal instructions regarding infections, bleeding, diet, chemotherapy, radiation.
- Teach measures to help prevent infections (e.g., adequate nutrition, rest and sleep, protection from physical injuries, cleanliness, avoidance of large crowds).
- Instruct child/parents how to avoid injury; keep floor clear of objects that could cause a fall.
- Describe what happens when the child is in remission and provide a list of symptoms (e.g., fatigue, pallor, low-grade fever) that might suggest that the remission is ending; instruct to contact physician should symptoms occur.
- Explain the importance of laboratory studies as a means of evaluating the effectiveness of the treatment regimen; provide a written schedule of return appointments for continuation of therapy.
- Review intended action, dosage, scheduled administration, and side effects of all medications prescribed; instruct to notify physician of toxic effects.
- Reinforce dietary guidelines followed in hospital as appropriate for after discharge.
- Refer to home health nurse as needed.

☐ **EVALUATION CRITERIA/DESIRED OUTCOMES**

The child/parents

- Describe susceptibility of children with leukemia to infection; list signs and symptoms of infection
- List ways of avoiding injury/bleeding
- Know to promptly contact physician/clinic for any early signs of infection; report and properly treat any evidence of bleeding
- Select a diet specific to nutritional needs
- List medications, with times, dosage, and possible side effects
- State toxic manifestations of medication and methods to minimize them
- Have information/referral to a community support group or home health nurse
- Have follow-up appointment with physician/clinic

The Child with Meningitis

Definition/Discussion

Meningitis is an inflammation of the membranes of the brain and spinal cord. Encephalitis is an infection of the brain substance. Myelitis describes an inflammation or infection of the spinal cord. Overlap of these conditions is common and terms like meningo-encephalitis or encephalomyelitis may be used.

Nursing Assessment

☐ PERTINENT HISTORY

Birth history (in neonate), chronic illness, neoplasm, sickle cell anemia, immunosuppression, splenectomy; recent respiratory/middle ear infection, mastoiditis, sinusitis; recent surgery, lumbar puncture, skull fracture, or head trauma; exposure to mumps, meningitis, or travel out of the country; crowded living conditions; ingestion of poisons/toxins/drugs; complaints of behavior changes, fever, nausea, vomiting, headache, stiff neck, photophobia, diplopia, painful ocular movement, arthralgia, sore throat, backache

☐ PHYSICAL FINDINGS

(Physical findings are influenced by the age of the child and the causative organism), altered level of consciousness (LOC), irritability, lethargy, confusion, seizures (e.g., focal, generalized), ataxia, positive Brudzinski's and Kernig's signs/nuchal rigidity, opisthotonus, bulging fontanel, nystagmus, ptosis, diminished hearing; tachycardia, dysrhythmia, elevated blood pressure; altered breathing patterns; vomiting; diarrhea; petechial rash; abnormal lumbar puncture results

☐ PSYCHOSOCIAL CONCERNS/ DEVELOPMENTAL FACTORS

Age, developmental level, habits (e.g., what comforts child, bedtime routine, favored objects), family interaction, behavior patterns, coping mechanisms, previous experience with illness and hospitalization, religious beliefs

☐ PATIENT AND FAMILY KNOWLEDGE

Level of comprehension, understanding of condition, pathophysiology, relationship to symptoms, communicability, treatment, follow-up, home care, readiness, willingness, and ability to learn

Nursing Care

☐ LONG-TERM GOAL

The child will regain optimal health with minimal neurologic disability.

NURSING DIAGNOSIS #1
a. **Impaired gas exchange** related to increased intracranial pressure
b. **Ineffective airway clearance** related to fatigue, weakness, altered LOC
c. **Ineffective breathing pattern** related to depressed respiratory effort

Rationale: Altered consciousness, depressed cough and gag reflexes predispose the child to poor airway clearance and aspiration. Hypercapnia and hypoxia from increased intracranial pressure (ICP) result in reflex vasodilation further increasing pressure on sensitive brain tissue. Immobility and dehydration result in pooling and thickening of respiratory secretions.

☐ GOAL

The child will maintain adequate oxygenation.

☐ IMPLEMENTATION

• Auscultate breath sounds every 4 hours; report adventitious sounds (e.g., crackles, wheezes).
• Monitor respiratory rate, pattern, patency, exchange; observe skin, nail beds, mucous membranes for cyanosis.
• Monitor arterial blood gases (ABGs) for hypoxia, chest x-rays for infiltrates.
• Ensure position change at least every 2 hours; en-

courage activity to tolerance as ordered (e.g., sitting up, turning).
- Instruct to take 10 deep breaths an hour; use games, toys to encourage child.
- Maintain patent airway; set up properly functioning suction equipment; suction gently to clear secretions; utilize side-lying position, jaw thrust, head tilt.
- Check for depressed gag reflex.
- Administer oxygen as ordered; monitor effectiveness.
- Observe for increased confusion, irritability, restlessness; report any to physician.

☐ EVALUATION CRITERIA/DESIRED OUTCOMES

The child
- Maintains ABGs within normal limits
- Has no adventitious breath sounds
- Is alert and oriented as age appropriate
- Has unlabored respirations with good air exchange

NURSING DIAGNOSIS #2
a. **Alteration in tissue perfusion: cerebral** related to inflammatory processes, increased ICP
b. **Potential for injury** related to disorientation, restlessness, seizures, unfamiliar environment
c. **Alteration in thought processes** related to changes in LOC
d. **Impaired communication: verbal** related to disorientation and confusion

Rationale: Inflammatory processes cause tissue swelling that interferes with fluid movement within the cranium, increases ICP, and obstructs cerebral blood flow.

☐ GOAL

The child will maintain adequate cerebral tissue perfusion; will remain oriented with intact thought processes and communication as age appropriate; will be free from injury.

☐ IMPLEMENTATION

- Observe and record LOC on admission and with each contact (e.g., alertness, orientation, irritability, lethargy, inappropriate response, subtle changes).
- Check neurologic status every 1-2 hours and as necessary until stable (e.g., symmetry of movement, infantile reflexes, pupil response, ability to follow commands, motor ability, hand grips,

move and focus eyes, visual acuity, deep tendon reflexes, seizure activity, verbal response).
- Monitor for signs of increased ICP (e.g., increasing head circumference, bulging fontanel, increasing blood pressure, decreasing pulse, respiratory irregularities, irritability, high-pitched cry, restlessness, confusion, pupillary changes, focal deficits, seizures).
- Refer to *The Child with Increased Intracranial Pressure*, page 160, and *The Child with Epilepsy*, page 122.
- Note any seizure activity; record affected body parts, length of seizure, and aura if any.
- Institute seizure precautions (e.g., side rails up and padded, bed in low position, airway and bite stick at bedside, suction equipment ready, call bell within easy reach, night lighting, rectal temperatures).
- Administer anticonvulsants as ordered; monitor effectiveness.
- Elevate head of bed 30°.
- Maintain head and neck alignment to facilitate venous return.
- Administer antibiotic therapy on time to ensure maintenance of blood levels.
- Maintain quiet, restful environment (e.g., low lights, quiet hallway, child in position of comfort; avoid jarring the bed or unnecessary procedures).
- Minimize the number of caretakers.
- Teach older child to avoid Valsalva maneuver (e.g., straining, coughing, sneezing) and to change position slowly.
- Approach in a calm manner; be consistent, speak clearly and slowly to increase comprehension.
- Talk while providing care; use therapeutic touch and listening techniques.
- Verbally orient to person/place/time/situation; have toys, stuffed animals, favored objects, radio, television, and other familiar objects, (e.g., photographs, books, games).
- Use child's name; encourage visitation by family.
- Perform range-of-motion (ROM) exercises, (passive, active) as ordered; establish routines; refer to *The Child Requiring Range-of-Motion Exercises*, page 237.
- Avoid restraints if possible.
- Monitor any signs/symptoms of septic shock (e.g., hypotension, elevated temperature, increasing respiratory rate, confusion, disorientation, peripheral vasoconstriction).

☐ EVALUATION CRITERIA/DESIRED OUTCOMES

The child
- Maintains orientation and alertness
- Is free from seizure activity
- Has vital signs within normal limits
- Is free from injury
- Rests quietly

NURSING DIAGNOSIS #3

a. **Alteration in fluid volume: deficit** related to decreased fluid intake, abnormal fluid loss
b. **Alteration in fluid volume: excess** related to inappropriate secretion of antidiuretic hormone

Rationale: The hypermetabolic state of infectious processes combined with anorexia, nausea and vomiting results in increased sensible/insensible fluid losses, altering fluid and electrolyte balance. Hypothalamic dysfunction, which frequently accompanies central nervous system diseases, results in syndrome of inappropriate antidiuretic hormone secretion (SIADH).

☐ GOAL

The child will maintain adequate fluid and electrolyte balance.

☐ IMPLEMENTATION

- Measure vital signs at least every 4 hours.
- Monitor lab studies, specifically electrolytes, urine specific gravity every shift.
- Observe for signs of dehydration (e.g., tenting, dry mucous membranes, increasing pulse, increasing serum sodium, weight loss, increasing urine specific gravity, fluid loss greater than fluid intake).
- Inspect for signs of fluid retention and hypotonicity indicating SIADH (e.g., decreasing urine output, increasing urine specific gravity, decreasing serum sodium concentration, irritability, anorexia, nausea).
- Record intake and output every shift and as necessary; note and report imbalances.
- Weigh on admission and daily on same scale, in same clothes, at same time.
- Encourage oral fluids within ordered limits (children are frequently on fluid restrictions; ensure that total IV and oral intake do not exceed these limits).
- Give fluids frequently but in small amounts to minimize gastric distension.
- Maintain temperature less than 101°F (38.3°C); refer to *The Child with a Fever*, page 128.
- Administer IV therapy for hydration/delivery of antibiotics; refer to *The Child with an Intravenous Catheter*, page 174.
- Maintain and monitor central venous pressure if in place.

☐ EVALUATION CRITERIA/DESIRED OUTCOMES

The child
- Has vital signs within normal limits
- Maintains serum electrolyte values within normal limits

- Has moist skin with good turgor
- Maintains temperature below 101°F
- Excretes at least 1 cc/kg of urine/hour
- Maintains preillness weight

NURSING DIAGNOSIS #4

Alteration in nutrition: less than body requirements related to anorexia, fatigue, nausea and vomiting

Rationale: Infectious and healing processes increase metabolic and nutritional needs. Increased intracranial pressure stimulates nausea and vomiting, which can interfere with maintaining adequate intake.

☐ GOAL

The child will maintain an adequate nutritional level; will have minimal nausea and vomiting.

☐ IMPLEMENTATION

- Interview child/parents regarding food preferences.
- Provide diet as ordered and tolerated.
- Serve small, frequent, nutritious meals.
- Instruct to eat slowly and to avoid lying flat for 1 hour after meals.
- Allow family-prepared foods when therapeutic.
- Keep accurate record of nutrients consumed.
- Monitor daily weight.
- Provide pleasant environment for eating (e.g., eliminate odors, unpleasant sights, allow fresh air).
- Arrange for family member to eat with child if appropriate.
- Limit fluid intake during meals, 1 hour before and after eating to minimize distension.
- Provide good oral care.

☐ EVALUATION CRITERIA/DESIRED OUTCOMES

The child
- Consumes 75% of diet for age
- Participates in food selection
- Maintains preillness weight

NURSING DIAGNOSIS #5

Impairment of skin integrity related to immobility, diaphoresis, neurologic deficits

Rationale: Bedrest/immobility combined with poor nutritional intake and moist skin can result in breakdown from local irritation and ischemic changes over pressure-sensitive areas.

☐ GOAL

The child will maintain intact skin.

☐ IMPLEMENTATION

- Keep skin clean and dry; change soiled or moist linen immediately.
- Encourage active/passive ROM exercises as ordered (may increase ICP).
- Remind or help to turn at least every 2 hours.
- Use light covers/clothing to avoid excess moisture.
- Maintain fluid/nutritional balance.
- Observe bony prominences (e.g., occiput, heels, elbows, trochantors, scapula) and skin for signs of pressure injury (e.g., erythema, blanching, maceration, breakdown) at least every 8 hours.
- Massage skin, especially over bony prominences, at least every 4 hours; use sheepskin, heel pads, as needed.

☐ EVALUATION CRITERIA/DESIRED OUTCOMES

The child

- Maintains intact skin
- Changes position frequently
- Complies with ROM guidelines

NURSING DIAGNOSIS #6

Alteration in comfort: pain related to bedrest, meningeal irritation

Rationale: Meningeal irritation and increased ICP result in symptoms such as headache, photophobia, neck and back pain. Bedrest may cause muscle spasm/soreness.

☐ GOAL

The child will attain an adequate level of comfort.

☐ IMPLEMENTATION

- Assess level of discomfort using a 0-10 point self-rating scale for an objective measure of the pain; refer to *The Child Experiencing Pain,* page 216.
- Evaluate indicators of pain (e.g., facial expression, crying, movement), location, duration, radiation, intensity, precipitating/relieving factors.
- Implement comfort measures (e.g., soft voices, dim lighting, gradual position changes, guided imagery, repositioning, distraction, pillows, cool moist compresses, massage).
- Administer analgesics as ordered; evaluate one-half hour later for effect.
- Teach older child to avoid movements that increase ICP (e.g., bending, straining, coughing, sneezing, blowing nose).
- Limit visitors.

☐ EVALUATION CRITERIA/DESIRED OUTCOMES

The child

- Demonstrates behaviors of/verbalizes decreased pain
- Exhibits ability to rest
- Participates in activities as tolerated

NURSING DIAGNOSIS #7

a. **Ineffective individual/family coping** related to required adaptation to hospital environment
b. **Alteration in family process** related to hospitalization
c. **Anxiety** related to actual/potential changes in body functioning
d. **Fear** related to medical/nursing intervention, illness, risk of death
e. **Grieving** related to actual, potential, or perceived loss of child
f. **Altered growth and development** related to imposed hospitalization

Rationale: Illness produces changes in the body and its functioning. Separation from familiar surroundings and family causes stress and possibly regression. Hospitalization disrupts normal routines and practices, and fear and anxiety may result.

☐ GOAL

The child/family will demonstrate positive adaptation to illness and hospitalization.

☐ IMPLEMENTATION

- Orient to hospital routines and unit.
- Explain all procedures and rationale.
- Institute listening techniques (e.g., open-ended questions; unrushed, quiet atmosphere); provide parents opportunity to express feelings out of child's hearing range.
- Encourage verbalization/expression of thoughts/fears; use drawings, puppets, stories to help child elaborate; refer to *The Child Requiring Play Therapy,* page 226.
- Share indications of improvement with child/parents.
- Involve child/parents in care and decision making as able.
- Observe present coping mechanisms; support/guide the child/parents to new ones as needed.
- Reinforce independence as age appropriate.
- Support child/parents in adaptive process (e.g., allow touch, overnight visitation, phone calls).
- As child recovers, encourage diversional activities (e.g., going to playroom, hobbies, games, reading, watching television, VCR).

☐ EVALUATION CRITERIA/DESIRED OUTCOMES

The child/parents
- Participate in care and decision making
- Interact appropriately with staff
- Talk of illness, its impact, and potential outcome

NURSING DIAGNOSIS #8

Knowledge deficit regarding illness, hospitalization, treatment

Rationale: Children/parents harbor misinformation and misconceptions about body function, illness, and hospitalization. Understanding of the process, illness, and symptomology promotes compliance and adaptive behaviors.

☐ GOAL

The child/parents will demonstrate knowledge regarding the illness, hospitalization, and follow-up care.

☐ IMPLEMENTATION

- Encourage questions.
- Describe the illness and relate symptoms to disease state.
- Answer questions honestly and completely at appropriate level; reinforce previous teaching; refer to *Guidelines for Teaching Parents and Children*, page 316.
- Explain all procedures/treatments and rationale.
- Use age-appropriate teaching techniques (e.g., limit session time; use terms easily understood/ drawings; supply concrete examples the child can relate to; use reinforcement techniques).
- Discuss signs/symptoms of complications (e.g., headache, paresis/paralysis, seizures, hearing loss, blindness).
- Review follow-up care and complications needing physician referral.

☐ EVALUATION CRITERIA/DESIRED OUTCOMES

The child/parents
- Relate information about illness and care
- Verbalize complications requiring follow-up
- Relate specific information regarding home care and follow-up

The Child with Myelomeningocele

Definition/Discussion

Refer to *The Neonate with Myelomeningocele,* page 191.

Nursing Assessment

☐ **PERTINENT HISTORY**

Circumstances of repair at birth; problems/concerns regarding increased intracranial pressure (ICP), shunt obstructions or infections, UTIs, effectiveness of bladder management, bowel incontinence/constipation, ambulation, braces, wheelchair, weight management

☐ **PHYSICAL FINDINGS**

Level of consciousness, heart rate, blood pressure, respiratory changes, headache, vomiting, pupil changes, hand grasps; urine pH, specific gravity, residuals after voiding; stooling pattern, consistency of stool; range of motion of joints, ability to bear weight, scoliosis, lordosis; skin integrity; weight

☐ **PSYCHOSOCIAL CONCERNS/ DEVELOPMENTAL FACTORS**

Age, child's/parents' acceptance of defect and associated problems, progress with normal developmental tasks (e.g., language, school, peer group activities); ability to incorporate child's special needs into the family's life-style, habits/rituals (e.g., sleeping, eating, playing)

☐ **PATIENT AND FAMILY KNOWLEDGE**

Complications/treatment; community information, supportive, financial resources; level of knowledge, readiness and willingness to learn

Nursing Care

☐ **LONG-TERM GOAL**

The child/parents will adjust to the birth defect; the child will grow and develop to the fullest extent possible free from preventable complications.

NURSING DIAGNOSIS #1
a. **Potential for infection** related to surgical procedure, shunt
b. **Alteration in tissue perfusion:** cerebral related to impaired circulation of cerebral spinal fluid

Rationale: *The ventriculoperitoneal (VP) or ventriculoatrial (VA) shunt placed for hydrocephalus may become infected or obstructed resulting in meningitis or increased ICP. As the child grows, the shunt may become too short to drain effectively and require surgical revision.*

☐ **GOAL**

The parents will recognize signs of shunt infection, obstruction, and ineffectiveness; the child will be free from neurologic complications.

☐ **IMPLEMENTATION**

• Assess child for signs of increased ICP (e.g., headache, vomiting, ataxia, slowing of pupil reactivity to light, decreased heart rate, elevated blood pressure, altered respiratory rate) at least every 8 hours.
• Monitor for signs of shunt infection (e.g., signs of increased ICP, fever, neck stiffness, seizures).
• Note and report problems at the operative site (e.g., drainage, redness, warmth).
• Administer antibiotics as ordered; monitor effectiveness; ensure that IV medications are diluted in the appropriate amount of fluid and infused over the appropriate amount of time.

☐ **EVALUATION CRITERIA/DESIRED OUTCOMES**

The child
• Has normal temperature
• Shows no signs of increased ICP

NURSING DIAGNOSIS #2

Alteration in bowel elimination related to impaired innervation of the distal bowel

> **Rationale:** *Children with myelomeningocele are frequently incontinent and subject to constipation because of damage to the sensory/motor nerves.*

☐ **GOAL**

The child will maintain regular bowel elimination patterns.

☐ **IMPLEMENTATION**

- Develop home bowel management program (e.g., insert a bisacodyl suppository before breakfast, sit child on toilet following the meal accompanied by digital stimulation of the anal sphincter if necessary).
- Provide adequate fluid and fiber in diet.
- Encourage parents to discuss child's bowel management program with teacher so that it does not interfere with school activities.

☐ **EVALUATION CRITERIA/DESIRED OUTCOMES**

The child
- Has soft, formed stools at least every other day
- Is free from constipation or incontinence

NURSING DIAGNOSIS #3
a. **Functional incontinence** related to sensory deficit
b. **Total incontinence** related to impaired spinal nerves

Rationale: *Children with myelomeningocele experience incontinence and stasis of urine in the bladder because of damage to sensory/motor nerves. This predisposes the child to repeated UTIs and subsequent renal failure. Treatment may include medications, clean intermittent catheterization (CISC), or urinary diversions (e.g., ileal conduit, nephrostomy).*

☐ **GOAL**

The child will remain dry between bladder emptyings; will not develop UTIs; will maintain normal renal function.

☐ **IMPLEMENTATION**

- Send urine specimen to lab for analysis, culture and sensitivity with any sign of UTI (e.g., fever, urine is cloudy, has odor).
- Monitor intake and output, serum BUN, and creatinine routinely.
- Encourage intake of greater than normal amounts of fluids.
- Provide information regarding drugs used to en-hance bladder sphincter tone (e.g., cholinergics to increase tone, antispasmodics to relax the sphincter).
- Monitor administration of antibiotics/bacteriostatic medications; note and report side effects.
- Encourage intake of ascorbic acid (vitamin C) to acidify urine.
- Discuss clean intermittent self-catherization (CISC) with child/parents if appropriate; demonstrate proper techniques of CISC for child/parents if it is to be done at home; provide for return demonstration.
- Monitor ability to manage the external appliance; do peristomal skin care if child has a urinary diversion; check the appliance for fit around the stoma.

☐ **EVALUATION CRITERIA/DESIRED OUTCOMES**

The child
- Establishes regular voiding pattern
- Has normal urinary pH, specific gravity, urinalysis
- Has normal serum BUN and creatinine

NURSING DIAGNOSIS #4
Impairment of skin integrity related to pressure on bony prominences, incontinence, altered sensory perception

Rationale: *Depending on the level of the spinal defect, the child may have little or no sensation of damage to the skin from pressure, friction, or changes in temperature. The presence of urine or stool on the perineal area also predisposes the skin to breakdown.*

☐ **GOAL**

The child will remain free from skin breakdown; the child/parents will take appropriate preventive measures to minimize skin breakdown.

☐ **IMPLEMENTATION**

- Establish a routine for monitoring the skin for areas of redness or breakdown.
- Clean and dry perineal area with each change of diapers or underwear.
- Caution to avoid very hot or very cold surfaces/liquids in order to prevent burns or frostbite; position legs and feet so they are not caught in bed frames, doors, or moving parts of a wheelchair.
- Ensure that braces fit well and that parts in contact with bony areas are padded.
- Teach the child who is wheelchair dependent to lift the torso every 30 minutes to release pressure.

EVALUATION CRITERIA/DESIRED OUTCOMES

The child
- Is free from skin redness or breakdown

The child/parents
- List steps to be taken to avoid skin breakdown

NURSING DIAGNOSIS #5

Alteration in nutrition: more than body requirements related to immobility, diversional activity deficit

Rationale: Because of the child's immobility, a normal age-appropriate diet may contain too many calories for the child's growth needs, resulting in obesity. Boredom may also cause the child to use eating as a diversionary activity.

GOAL

The child will take in sufficient calories for normal growth; will gain weight following a normal curve that has been adjusted for decreased lower extremity growth; will not use eating as a diversion.

IMPLEMENTATION

- Compare child's typical intake with intake recommended for growth.
- Assist to develop a diet plan that incorporates the child's food preferences; limit "empty" calories if diet contains more than adequate calories.
- Provide support for the child who must reduce intake; develop a reward system for adherence to the diet plan.
- Assist to develop interests (e.g., crafts, hobbies); reinforce participation in non-food-related activities.

EVALUATION CRITERIA/DESIRED OUTCOMES

The child
- Gains weight following adjusted curve
- Maintains recommended diet
- Does not eat when bored

NURSING DIAGNOSIS #6

Potential for injury related to muscle weakness/paralysis, lack of coordination, impaired judgment

Rationale: The child with myelomeningocele may experience other problems associated with the original diagnosis. Musculoskeletal difficulties (e.g., stress fractures, lower extremity weakness) requiring casts, braces, or assistive devices are common. Approximately 50% of these children have some degree of mental retardation in addition to the physical limitations.

GOAL

The child will be free from injury.

IMPLEMENTATION

- Observe and note the child's motor abilities.
- Utilize devices/equipment that are used at home.
- Provide opportunities that allow the child to do what s/he normally would do at home.
- Follow basic safety rules (e.g., discard toys with sharp/removable parts, remove obstacles from child's path, keep side rails up when child is in bed).
- Handle gently at all times; support lower extremities when moving/repositioning.

EVALUATION CRITERIA/DESIRED OUTCOMES

The child
- Plays safely
- Experiences no fractures

NURSING DIAGNOSIS #7

a. **Disturbance in self-concept: body image** related to inability to participate in some activities typical for age
b. **Altered growth and development** related to effects of physical disability

Rationale: The child with a myelomeningocele may be unable to participate in gross motor activities typical of age group, thereby potentially limiting his/her ability to accomplish developmental tasks. The child may be embarrassed about wheelchair dependence, use of braces, bladder/bowel incontinence, further limiting positive self-esteem and social interactions.

GOAL

The child will have a positive self-concept and value own strengths; will be comfortable expressing feelings regarding the handicapping condition/limitations imposed; will demonstrate accomplishments in areas of interest.

IMPLEMENTATION

- Assist to express (e.g., verbal discussion, play, drawings) feelings about self as an individual; refer to *The Child Requiring Play Therapy*, page 226; recognize strengths and accomplishments.
- Explore ways child can excel despite limitations imposed by defect.

- Provide opportunities for child to take an active role in planning and implementing the treatment regimen.
- Introduce child to other children who are coping effectively with myelomeningocele.
- Encourage achievable age-appropriate developmental activities; refer to *Normal Growth and Development,* pages 300–314.
- Prepare parents to allow child independence in choices and activities.
- Provide the child with accurate information regarding the future (e.g., career choices, developing intimate relationships, having children) when age appropriate.

☐ EVALUATION CRITERIA/DESIRED OUTCOMES

The child
- Expresses feelings about the defect
- Recognizes strengths and accomplishments
- Discusses realistic plans for the future

NURSING DIAGNOSIS #8

Knowledge deficit regarding prevention of complications

Rationale: Many of the complications related to myelomeningocele can be prevented by adherence to the treatment regimen and identification of early signs of complications.

☐ GOAL

The child will not experience complications; the child/parents will comply with the prescribed treatment regimen; the family will successfully incorporate management into daily routine.

☐ IMPLEMENTATION

- Include all family members in teaching sessions whenever possible.
- Teach/review signs of increased ICP, urinary infections, renal dysfunction, skin breakdown; review symptoms requiring immediate medical interventions.
- Discuss management of bowel/bladder incontinence, skin pressure prevention, correct use of braces, nutritional needs, and the plan for preventing obesity as necessary.
- Allow adequate time for the child/family to express questions, concerns, and feelings.
- Provide information regarding community, supportive, and financial resources.
- Provide phone numbers of persons to contact as questions or concerns arise; instruct regarding return appointment.

☐ EVALUATION CRITERIA/DESIRED OUTCOMES

The child/parents
- Demonstrate successful management at home
- Recognize signs of complications early and institute appropriate treatment
- Maintain regular follow-up schedule

The Neonate with Myelomeningocele

Definition/Discussion

Spina bifida is the failure of the vertebral column to close during fetal development; this defect is associated with varying degrees of tissue herniation. Myelomeningocele, a more serious form of spina bifida, is the protrusion of the meninges, spinal cord, and spinal fluid through the vertebrae, with disruption of normal sensory/motor stimulation of the lower extremities and the genitourinary (GU) tract resulting in paralysis, musculoskeletal defects, and GU dysfunction. The degree of involvement depends upon the location of the spinal cord defect and the amount of neural tissue involved. An associated defect in myelomeningocele is the Arnold-Chiari malformation, an obstruction of the normal flow of CSF. Hydrocephalus can result from this obstruction and lead to neurologic damage. Occurring in approximately 2 of every 1,000 births, myelomeningocele may cause early death due to central nervous system infection, urinary tract infection (UTI), renal failure, or pulmonary disease. Most children can survive with surgical correction and long-term rehabilitative care.

Nursing Assessment

☐ PERTINENT HISTORY

Prenatal history, family history of spinal cord defects

☐ PHYSICAL FINDINGS

Presence of myelomeningocele at birth, increased head circumference, hypoplasia of lower extremities, joint dislocations/contractures, voiding pattern, stooling pattern, response to stimulation, leakage of cerebrospinal fluid (CSF); white blood cell count (WBC), cerebrospinal fluid culture and sensitivity; computerized tomographic (CT) scan

☐ PSYCHOSOCIAL CONCERNS/ DEVELOPMENTAL FACTORS

Parents' response to neonate, guilt, ability to make decisions related to immediate treatment, ability to communicate with each other

☐ PATIENT AND FAMILY KNOWLEDGE

Previous experience with myelomeningocele; prenatal diagnosis of defect; parents' understanding of disease, need for immediate treatment, normal neonatal care, and long-term needs of neonate; level of knowledge, readiness and willingness to learn

Nursing Care

☐ LONG-TERM GOAL

The parents will adjust to the birth defect of the neonate; the neonate will grow and develop to the fullest extent possible free from preventable complications associated with the congenital defect.

NURSING DIAGNOSIS #1

a. **Potential for infection** related to spinal malformation, operative site, shunt
b. **Alteration in tissue perfusion: cerebral** related to increased intracranial pressure

Rationale: The thin sac covering the exposed meninges may rupture, resulting in a loss of protective CSF and allowing bacteria to enter the spinal column. Surgical procedures are performed to repair the myelomeningocele and reduce pressure. Operative sites are susceptible to infection until healing occurs. The ventriculoperitoneal (VP) or ventriculoatrial (VA) shunt placed for hydrocephalus may become infected or obstructed, resulting in meningitis or increased ICP.

☐ GOAL

The neonate will be free from infection; will have a normal neurologic response.

☐ IMPLEMENTATION

- Monitor vital signs, observe for signs of infection (e.g., temperature or skin color change, poor feeding, irritability; change in color or characteris-

tic of sac/incision/shunt; drainage from sac/incision/shunt; increased WBC) at least every 4 hours.
- Measure occipital-frontal circumference (OFC) every 8 hours and as necessary; observe fontanels for bulging; palpate cranial sutures for separation.
- Observe feeding behavior; observe for irritability or lethargy; monitor for high-pitched cry that may be indicative of increased intracranial pressure (ICP).
- Turn neonate's head frequently to prevent skin breakdown; cushion head with a sheepskin, egg-crate mattress, or miniature waterbed made of a loosely filled plastic ice collar bag.
- Maintain prone or side-lying position to avoid pressure on sac/surgical incision/shunt; use sandbags, rolled towels, or foam wedges.
- Cover sac with moist, sterile dressing; do not allow dressing to dry.
- Maintain sterile technique (e.g., sterile gloves, linen) when caring for defect; maintain good handwashing technique at all times.
- Observe for signs of infection and obstruction if shunt is placed; maintain pressure dressing at site of insertion; position so that no pressure is placed on shunt.
- Protect sac/post-op incision from stool and urine (e.g., maintain a prone position, tape a sterile drape between the anus and sac/incision; clean perineal and anal areas with each stool and as needed).
- Observe incision/shunt for any change (e.g., color, drainage, approximation); clean incision with half-strength hydrogen peroxide and apply bacteriostatic ointment as ordered.

☐ EVALUATION CRITERIA/DESIRED OUTCOMES

The neonate
- Maintains normal temperature and vital signs
- Has clean incision
- Has normal OFC with no sudden increases

NURSING DIAGNOSIS #2
a. **Grieving** related to birth of child with a spinal malformation
b. **Alteration in parenting** related to hospitalization, loss of "perfect" child

Rationale: Most parents anticipate the birth of a normal, healthy child. Parents must resolve their grief over the loss of the "perfect" child in order to assimilate the neonate into the family unit. They need to make decisions regarding the treatment, compounding the confusion and despair they are already experiencing.

☐ GOAL

The parents will exhibit bonding behaviors; will make decisions about treatment of the neonate; will demonstrate acceptance of the neonate as part of the family unit.

☐ IMPLEMENTATION

- Refer to *The Parent Experiencing Grief and Loss,* page 139.
- Listen; be nonjudgmental.
- Encourage expression of feelings and concerns about neonate; discuss feelings in relation to treatment.
- Offer information regarding what to expect in terms of treatment.
- Assist to identify the normal aspects of the neonate; reinforce need for neonate to be treated like any other baby.
- Assist to develop strategies for holding and feeding child despite the need for neonate to maintain prone position.
- Model and reinforce acceptance behaviors (e.g., making eye contact with, talking to, soothing neonate).
- Discuss methods of altering family routine to incorporate the neonate.
- Support informed decisions made by parents regarding treatment.

☐ EVALUATION CRITERIA/DESIRED OUTCOMES

The parents
- Demonstrate acceptance by holding, feeding, and making eye contact with neonate
- Make informed decisions about treatment
- Adapt family routines to incorporate care and treatment of neonate

---

NURSING DIAGNOSIS #3

Altered growth and development related to required positioning, stimulation deficiencies, separation

Rationale: A neonate with myelomeningocele must be positioned in specific ways to decrease pressure on the sac/incision/shunt. Freedom of movement is restricted. Developmental stimulation needs are the same as for any healthy child but less easily available.

☐ GOAL

The neonate will achieve maximum potential; will achieve developmental milestones if no mental retardation exists; the parents will provide appropriate stimulation activities.

IMPLEMENTATION

- Teach parents that child has same need to be touched and nurtured as other neonates.
- Position neonate on abdomen or side.
- Use tactile stimulation while giving skin care.
- Turn from side to side, cuddle, talk with neonate every 2 hours.
- Talk to and touch neonate during feeding; hold neonate on side for feeding after surgery if possible.
- Put music box/tape of parents' voices near neonate.

EVALUATION CRITERIA/DESIRED OUTCOMES

The neonate
- Is as alert as condition allows
- Responds to appropriate stimuli by quieting, focusing
- Does not cry excessively

The parents
- Implement appropriate methods of stimulating development in neonate

---

NURSING DIAGNOSIS #4

Knowledge deficit regarding care of neonate with special needs

Rationale: Parents will need to consider both typical neonate care as well as the special needs of the child. These special needs may overwhelm parents who have limited experience with a neonate.

GOAL

The parents will express comfort with caring for neonate; will deal effectively with problems that arise; the neonate will grow and develop to the fullest extent possible.

IMPLEMENTATION

- Use diagrams and actual equipment to explain the pathophysiology of myelomeningocele, the expected effects on body systems (e.g., musculoskeletal, urinary, gastrointestinal), and shunt functions.
- Review potential complications (e.g., signs of infection, increased ICP, renal dysfunction).
- Review administration of medications; discuss potential side effects.
- Demonstrate normal neonatal care (e.g., feeding, bathing, stimulation, holding, sleep/activity patterns); provide for return demonstration.
- Arrange for contact with other parents of children with a myelomeningocele; inform of other available resources (e.g., public health nurse).
- Reinforce concept of team approach to health care; describe roles of the various team members.
- Provide parents with phone numbers of persons to contact for questions or concerns; instruct regarding return appointments.

EVALUATION CRITERIA/DESIRED OUTCOMES

The parents
- Care for the neonate appropriately
- Identify signs of potential complications

The neonate
- Grows and develops within the limitations imposed by the defect

The Child Requiring Nasogastric Intubation

Definition/Discussion

Nasogastric (NG) intubation involves the insertion of a tube into the stomach through the nasal passage for the purpose of feeding, instilling medication, irrigating the stomach, or initiating gastric suctioning. Various conditions and situations (e.g., ingestion of toxic substances, GI bleeding, chemotherapy, cerebrovascular accidents, eating disorders), may require the insertion of an NG tube for gastric gavage or lavage purposes.

Nursing Assessment

☐ **PERTINENT HISTORY**

Medical/surgical history, history of gastrointestinal (GI) disorders/congenital defects; medical diagnosis; onset of symptoms; allergies or conditions affecting the sinuses, nasal passages, and oropharynx; medication history

☐ **PHYSICAL FINDINGS**

Weight, height, head circumference (in infants), nutritional intake, gastric/rectal bleeding, paralytic ileus, presence of toxic substances in the blood/urine, level of consciousness, status of oral and pharyngeal mucosa and structures

☐ **PSYCHOSOCIAL CONCERNS/ DEVELOPMENTAL FACTORS**

Age, developmental level, previous experience with NG tube, available coping mechanisms/support system, habits/rituals (e.g., playing, sleeping, eating)

☐ **PATIENT AND FAMILY KNOWLEDGE**

Purpose, procedure for insertion, side effects, potential complications, level of knowledge, readiness and willingness to learn

Nursing Care

☐ **LONG-TERM GOAL**

The child will have an NG tube inserted with safety, privacy, and a minimum of discomfort; the child will be free from complications associated with the tube.

NURSING DIAGNOSIS #1

Potential for injury related to incorrect insertion/care of NG tube

Rationale: *Correct insertion and maintenance of the NG tube will provide a safe and more comfortable treatment situation for the child.*

☐ **GOAL**

The child will cooperate with insertion as developmentally able; will experience minimal discomfort.

☐ **IMPLEMENTATION**

- Check the orders to verify type and size of tube to be inserted.

Older Child

- Provide sufficient light, working space, and privacy.
- Explain tube's purpose and procedure for passing it; stress child's active role in the procedure; arrange a signal that child can use to direct pauses during procedure; explain sensations child will experience.
- Arrange all necessary equipment and supplies in a readily accessible place
  - facial tissues
  - glass of drinking water, if not contraindicated, with a flexible straw
  - basin of water for lubrication (if using Enteriflex tube)
  - 50- or 60-cc syringe with irrigating tip
  - water-soluble lubricating jelly (unless using Enteriflex tubes)
  - paper tape
  - stethoscope
  - suction equipment
- Have the conscious child sit in high-Fowler's position; place a clean towel over child's chest.
- Give child a tissue to hold in one hand and a glass of water in the other.
- Measure length to be inserted by extending tube from tip of child's nose to the earlobe, and then to

xyphoid process; mark tube with piece of tape at this spot.
- Lubricate tube liberally to tape mark; if using an Enteriflex tube, place entire tube in basin of tap water to lubricate.
- Insert lubricated tube into 1 nostril and advance it to posterior pharyngeal wall using gentle, persistent pressure; ensure that child's head is slightly flexed to facilitate swallowing; when tube reaches pharynx, have child lean forward slightly and either take sips of water or swallow air repeatedly to keep trachea closed, suppress gag reflex, and facilitate passage of tube into the stomach; the tube may need to be gently rotated to move into the esophagus.
- Continue to pass tube until tape mark is at nostril; keep telling child how s/he is doing, how the procedure is progressing, and remind to continue swallowing.

Infant/Younger Child
- Prepare as developmentally appropriate, gather equipment, measure for placement as above, and mark site with tape; insert lubricated tube into nares directed straight back towards the occiput; gently hyperflexing the head decreases the chance of entering the trachea.
- Be sure to advance tube quickly when passing the gag reflex if child is conscious but unable to assist; assess constantly for signs and symptoms of respiratory distress.

Unconscious Child
- Turn on right side.
- Place an airway in mouth to depress tongue (older child).
- Advance tube between child's breaths and while swallowing; stroke throat and neck to help passage of tube.
- Remove tube quickly if child chokes, becomes cyanotic, or has any difficulty breathing.
- After placement is verified and stomach contents have been aspirated, turn child onto left side.

All Children
- Verify correct placement of tube
  - aspirate stomach contents using a syringe; return contents
  - place stethoscope over gastric region and introduce a small amount (1-10 cc depending on size of child) of air quickly into tube with a syringe; listen for crackling or gurgling as air exits tube into the stomach; be sure to plug free end of tube at all times, except when checking position, feeding, or irrigating to prevent air from entering the stomach
- Secure tube with tape to the cheek; in younger children, secure further by taping tube to upper lip; use caution not to occlude opposite nostril with tape or tape tube in such a way that it distorts or puts pressure on nares; restrain from pulling on tube if necessary.
- Attach proximal end of tube to low intermittent

suction if ordered; if tube feedings are ordered, refer to *The Child Requiring Tube Feedings*, page 288.
- Remove guide wire if using an Enteriflex tube after placement has been verified and tube is secured.
- Record amount and type of suction drainage, irrigation solutions, tube feedings, and medications administered.
- Chart insertion procedure, child's response, and periodic function of tube (e.g., patency, drainage, irrigations).

☐ EVALUATION CRITERIA/DESIRED OUTCOMES

The child
- Describes tube insertion procedure correctly
- Verbalizes/indicates minimal discomfort from tube insertion and placement
- Maintains tube in correct position

NURSING DIAGNOSIS #2
a. **Alteration in oral mucous membrane** related to placement of tube for several days
b. **Ineffective breathing pattern** related to nonpatent nares
c. **Alteration in tissue perfusion: GI** related to excessive negative suction pressure
d. **Alteration in comfort** related to placement of NG tube

Rationale: The tube can cause laryngitis, esophagitis, or pharyngitis when left in place for several days; traumatic gastric ulcers can occur if tube is connected to suction and the suction pulls gastric mucosa into the lumen of the tube; oral mucous membranes can become dry and ulcerated; the nostril without the tube can become plugged causing respiratory distress (young infants are obligatory nose breathers).

☐ GOAL

The child will be free from side effects/complications from the NG tube.

☐ IMPLEMENTATION

- Change tube every 3 days and as necessary, alternating nares to decrease chance of ulceration; pinch end of tube when pulling it out.
- Provide mouth care at least every 4 hours; have child gargle and rinse mouth 3 times daily with mouth wash, water, or saline; have child brush teeth (if present) and massage gums 3 times every day.
- Suggest sucking on hard candies, if permitted and child is old enough.

- Provide anesthetic spray, lozenges, or rinses for sore throat if ordered; monitor effectiveness.
- Apply cream or ointment to lips and nose.
- Administer analgesics as ordered; evaluate effect.
- Monitor for gastric bleeding and respiratory distress every 8 hours and as necessary; check appearance of gastric secretions, hematest secretions and stools; monitor respiratory pattern every 4 hours.

☐ EVALUATION CRITERIA/DESIRED OUTCOMES

The child
- Maintains intact nasal and oral mucosa
- Appears comfortable with tube in place

NURSING DIAGNOSIS #3

Knowledge deficit regarding maintenance and care of NG tube

Rationale: If child is going home with the NG tube, child/parents need instruction regarding the care of the tube, suction equipment, and feedings at home.

☐ GOAL

The child/parents will verbalize an understanding of care of the tube, equipment, and feedings to be performed at home.

☐ IMPLEMENTATION

- Instruct how to check for correct placement of tube.
- Review signs/symptoms of respiratory distress.
- Instruct on irrigation of tube
  - verify tube placement in stomach
  - slowly instill 2-10 cc normal saline with a syringe
  - gently aspirate; if bleeding occurs, stop and call physician
- Instruct regarding tube feeding procedure; refer to *The Child Requiring Tube Feedings*, page 288.
- Instruct on use of suction equipment (e.g., how to attach it, turn it on, assess for gastric bleeding).
- Instruct in care of mucous membranes and in comfort measures; avoid food/fluids of extreme temperature (e.g., hot, cold).

☐ EVALUATION CRITERIA/DESIRED OUTCOMES

The child/parents
- Demonstrate irrigation of the tube and tube feedings
- Verbalize principles behind gastric suctioning; use suction equipment correctly
- Verify placement of NG tube correctly
- List signs/symptoms of gastric bleeding and respiratory distress
- Describe techniques to protect mucous membranes and to provide comfort measures

The Child with Nephrotic Syndrome

Definition/Discussion

The nephrotic syndrome is the result of an alteration of the glomerular membrane making it more permeable to the passage of protein. It is characterized by marked proteinuria, hypoproteinemia, hyperlipidemia, edema, and hypovolemia. Idiopathic nephrotic syndrome (also known as minimal change nephrotic syndrome, childhood nephrosis, and lipoid nephrosis) is the most common form in children. Ninety percent of nephrotic syndrome is idiopathic in origin. Resolution of the disease process usually occurs within 28 days of beginning prednisone at a dose of 2 mg/kg/day. One month of daily steroid therapy is followed by one month of alternate-day therapy; 2/3 of these children will have relapses and will be treated with another course of steroids. Approximately 10% of children will not respond to any form of therapy, and will progress to chronic renal failure.

Nursing Assessment

☐ **PERTINENT HISTORY**

Congenital anomalies, previous illness (especially recent respiratory infections), medications, heroin use, neoplasms, systemic disease, diabetic nephropathy, allergies, primary renal disease, home treatment (e.g., diet, fluids, rest), usual weight

☐ **PHYSICAL FINDINGS**

Edema (generalized, labial, or scrotal); ascites; weight gain; pallor; fatigue; urinary output, character; respiratory function; nutritional status; skin integrity; blood pressure; temperature; heart rate; signs of infection; specific gravity and urine protein; serum BUN and creatinine, albumin and cholesterol, hemoglobin and hematocrit; estimated sedimentation rate

☐ **PSYCHOSOCIAL CONCERNS/ DEVELOPMENTAL FACTORS**

Developmental level, coping mechanisms, usual routines/habits, acceptance of disease

☐ **PATIENT AND FAMILY KNOWLEDGE**

Pathophysiology of disease, treatment, prognosis; level of knowledge, readiness and willingness to learn

Nursing Care

☐ **LONG-TERM GOAL**

The child will decrease excretion of urinary protein thus decreasing edema; the child will continue normal growth and development.

NURSING DIAGNOSIS #1

Alteration in fluid volume: excess related to altered kidney function resulting in edema

Rationale: The altered glomerular membrane is more permeable to protein, especially albumin; the excretion of protein in the urine lowers oncotic pressure, which causes fluid to shift out of the intravascular to the interstitial space resulting in edema and hypovolemia. Intravascular hypovolemia may cause an increase in pulse rate or a pulse that is thready in quality. As a compensatory mechanism, the renin-angiotension mechanism and anti-diuretic hormone are activated to increase reabsorption of water and sodium, thus increasing edema.

☐ **GOAL**

The child will regain/maintain fluid and electrolyte balance, be free from protein in the urine and from edema.

☐ **IMPLEMENTATION**

- Assess pulses in all extremities every 4 hours, note quality.
- Maintain a strict intake and output record, weigh daily at same time, on same scale, in same clothes.
- Test specific gravity and protein of every voided specimen.
- Restrict salt and fluid as ordered.
- Measure abdominal girth at umbilicus daily.
- Administer albumin IV as ordered; note response.
- Administer medications as ordered (e.g., predni-

sone, diuretics, antihypertensives); monitor for side effects.
- Monitor electrolytes; observe for decrease in potassium when on diuretics.
- Observe for signs of edema (e.g., puffy eyes, ankles, feet; congestive heart failure).

☐ **EVALUATION CRITERIA/DESIRED OUTCOMES**

The child
- Has normal pulse rate, rhythm, and strength
- Maintains balanced intake and output
- Shows no increase in weight
- Has normal urine specific gravity and protein
- Maintains or reduces abdominal girth
- Shows no periorbital edema, swelling of extremities, respiratory distress

---

NURSING DIAGNOSIS #2

Potential for infection related to the use of steroids, decreased immune response, bedrest

Rationale: Massive proteinuria leads to malnutrition and a decrease in the production of antibodies. Malnutrition plus administration of steroids causes a decreased immune response predisposing the child to infections, especially cellulitis, peritonitis, pneumonia, and septicemia. Edematous tissue provides an excellent medium for growth of microorganisms. Bedrest may also predispose the child to developing pneumonia.

☐ **GOAL**

The child will remain free from infection.

☐ **IMPLEMENTATION**
- Monitor vital signs for increased temperature, respiratory and heart rates, blood pressure every 4 hours; notify physician of any abnormal findings.
- Know that prednisone masks signs of infection.
- Monitor visitors for presence of contagious illness; avoid contact with infected persons.
- Use good handwashing and aseptic techniques for all invasive procedures.
- Administer antibiotics as ordered; monitor for side effects.
- Observe for peritonitis (e.g., increased abdominal distension, pain, rigidity, vomiting, diarrhea).

☐ **EVALUATION CRITERIA/DESIRED OUTCOMES**

The child
- Is afebrile
- Has respiratory rate, heart rate, and blood pressure within normal limits
- Has no signs of peritonitis

NURSING DIAGNOSIS #3

Alteration in nutrition: less than body requirements related to poor appetite, loss of protein in urine, ulcers, gastrointestinal (GI) bleeding

Rationale: Alteration in the glomerular membrane renders it permeable to plasma proteins, which are ultimately excreted in the urine. Malnutrition and muscle wasting can occur as a result of protein depletion and may not be noticed until the edema disappears. The child has a decreased appetite because of increased abdominal pressure from ascites. Steroid treatment potentiates ulcers and GI bleeding.

☐ **GOAL**

The child will eat 3 meals plus 2-3 supplemental snacks a day that are high in protein and carbohydrate.

☐ **IMPLEMENTATION**
- Consult with dietician to plan a high-protein (2-3 gm/kg/day), high-carbohydrate diet.
- Offer small quantities of foods or liquids frequently to increase interest in eating.
- Provide sodium-restricted or no-added-salt diet during edematous phase (1-2 gm/day); explore non-sodium seasonings.
- Offer special and preferred foods as allowed.
- Administer supplementary vitamins as ordered.
- Offer additional high-potassium foods if on diuretics (e.g., orange, grapefruit, or grape juice).
- Provide a pleasant and relaxed atmosphere at mealtimes.
- Make eating a special occasion, such as a picnic.
- Encourage family/friends to eat with child.
- Maintain usual mealtime rituals as possible.
- Administer antacids in conjunction with steroids.
- Test stools and vomitus for the presence of blood daily and as necessary.

☐ **EVALUATION CRITERIA/DESIRED OUTCOMES**

The child
- Ingests high-protein/high-carbohydrate diet of sufficient calories for age
- Demonstrates normal growth for age
- Shows no evidence of blood in stools/vomitus

NURSING DIAGNOSIS #4

Impairment of skin integrity related to prolonged bedrest, edema

Rationale: Pressure from lying in bed and edema may interfere with the blood and oxygen/nutrient supply to the skin resulting in increased susceptibility to skin breakdown. A break in skin integrity along with an altered immune system may easily lead to infection.

☐ GOAL

The child's skin will remain intact; the child will be free from skin discomfort.

☐ IMPLEMENTATION

- Provide conscientious skin care: keep skin surfaces clean, apply lotion to edematous areas every 2-4 hours; allow child to participate; massage skin gently.
- Use sheepskin next to skin.
- Support edematous organs (e.g., the scrotum) with T-binder.
- Place an alternating air mattress on the child's bed; avoid contact with hard surfaces.
- Reposition at least every 2 hours; maintain a chart or schedule of positions and times.
- Bathe, dry, and separate skin folds with cotton.
- Cleanse eyelids with warm saline.
- Change diapers often if child is not toilet trained; let buttocks and perineum air dry if possible; do not close diapers if increase in scrotal or labial edema.
- Use clothing that is nonbinding.
- Use heat lamp 18 inches from skin for 15-20 minutes to promote healing if breakdown is present.

☐ EVALUATION CRITERIA/DESIRED OUTCOMES

The child
- Has intact skin
- Is free from reddened areas on skin

NURSING DIAGNOSIS #5
a. **Impaired physical mobility** related to fatigue, edema, imposed bedrest
b. **Diversional activity deficit** related to imposed bedrest
c. **Altered growth and development** related to condition, immobility, hospitalization

Rationale: Children at the toddler/preschool age level may have difficulty understanding that bedrest allows edema to recede. They also may resist the imposed bedrest because of boredom. Children on forced bedrest have restricted activities, thereby limiting routine opportunities for growth and development.

☐ GOAL

The child will maintain bedrest; will participate in appropriate diversional activities to prevent boredom.

☐ IMPLEMENTATION

- Maintain bedrest if child has edema, hypertension, hematuria; allow child to increase activity as tolerated when asymptomatic.
- Explain reasons for bedrest and isolation at age-appropriate level.
- Offer quiet, age-appropriate play activities (e.g., coloring, reading, writing).
- Involve child development specialist in planning quiet games and activities.
- Organize nursing care so child has periods of uninterrupted rest.
- Encourage child to rest when tired.
- Encourage parents to participate in quiet activities with child.

☐ EVALUATION CRITERIA/DESIRED OUTCOMES

The child
- Maintains activity restrictions
- Is not fatigued by allowed activities

NURSING DIAGNOSIS #6

Ineffective individual/family coping related to diagnosis, changes in body image and usual role function, hospitalization, treatment, fear of long-term complications

Rationale: Nephrotic syndrome and steroid therapy cause changes in body image (e.g., edema) while hospitalization limits normal coping mechanisms. The possibility that the child may have long-term complications (e.g., repeated relapses, possible renal insufficiency) may produce increased stress and interfere with family functions.

☐ GOAL

The child/family will deal adaptively with changes in body image and usual role functioning; will express feelings about the disease process, treatment, hospitalization, and change in body image.

☐ IMPLEMENTATION

- Allow family members to express their feelings both individually and in groups about the disease, treatment, and hospitalization.
- Provide opportunities for family members to participate in care of child as much as possible.
- Explain all treatments to child at age-appropriate level; encourage child to ask questions about treatment.
- Be sensitive to child's body-image problems re-

lated to increased weight/size caused by edema and decreased growth related to steroid therapy.
- Encourage child to express feelings through therapeutic play, drawing of pictures, or verbalizations according to the developmental level; refer to *The Child Requiring Play Therapy*, page 226.
- Identify current coping mechanism; use role playing to explore alternative coping strategies.
- Help child maintain a positive self-image by emphasizing positive aspects of character; point out positive signs of change, such as weight loss or receding edema.
- Reassure child/family as to usually favorable prognosis.

☐ EVALUATION CRITERIA/DESIRED OUTCOMES

The child/family
- Deals adaptively with changes in body image
- Develops effective coping mechanisms
- Expresses fears and concerns about disease process, treatment, prognosis, hospitalization, and change in body image

---

NURSING DIAGNOSIS #7

Knowledge deficit regarding disease process, home management

Rationale: If knowledge deficit exists the child/parents cannot appropriately manage treatment of nephrosis or detect signs of complications early.

☐ GOAL

The child/parents will understand disease process and necessary treatment regimen.

☐ IMPLEMENTATION

- Teach proper procedure for testing urine protein, provide written instructions; obtain return demonstration; document all teaching.
- Ensure that parents know signs/symptoms of relapse; teach how to measure urine output, check for edema, monitor weight gain.
- Teach to record urine testing values and daily weights for use when seen as an outpatient.
- Tell parents not to have child immunized while receiving steroids.
- Describe all medications and side effects, including the reasons they are being given; tell parents that steroids must be discontinued slowly under physician supervision.
- Provide important phone numbers so physician can be contacted if problems arise.
- Reinforce importance of protecting child from infection; stress necessity for prompt treatment should one occur.

☐ EVALUATION CRITERIA/DESIRED OUTCOMES

The child/parents
- Describe nephrotic syndrome in own words
- Demonstrate urine testing
- List signs/symptoms of relapse
- Identify all medications, actions, administration schedules, possible side effects, dosages, and route of administration
- Verbalize importance of avoiding exposure to infections
- State importance of adhering to therapeutic regimen in an effort to prevent chronic renal disease
- Describe outpatient routine and importance of follow-up care with physician

The Normal Neonate

Definitions/Discussions

The normal neonate is a full-term newborn infant of 38-42 weeks gestation with an Apgar score of 7-10, and no anomalies, injuries, or need for special procedures. This group excludes the neonate 38 to 42 weeks gestation who is small for gestational age (SGA) or large for gestational age (LGA). SGA neonates weigh less than the tenth percentile and LGA neonates weigh greater than the ninetieth percentile when compared to the normal growth curve. Neonatal refers to the period of an infant's life from birth to 1 month.

Nursing Assessment

☐ **PERTINENT HISTORY**

Maternal medication/anesthesia, maternal pathology, length of labor, fetal tolerance of labor, length of time between rupture of membranes and delivery, previous experience of parents with neonates

☐ **PHYSICAL FINDINGS**

Weight, length, head circumference, heart rate, respirations, temperature, hematocrit, general appearance, condition of cord, reflexes and responses to environmental stimuli, muscle tone, seizures or atypical movements, activity pattern, presence of meconium, sensory/motor responses, behaviors (see table 8)

☐ **PSYCHOSOCIAL CONCERNS/ DEVELOPMENTAL FACTORS**

Sleep states; parental preparation for/expectations of neonate, available support systems

☐ **PATIENT AND FAMILY KNOWLEDGE**

Physical care needs of the neonate, growth and development, anticipated/actual parental life-style changes, readiness and willingness to learn

Nursing Care

☐ **LONG-TERM GOAL**

The neonate will function adaptively to extrauterine existence as a new member of a family without complications or the need for special support measures.

NURSING DIAGNOSIS #1
Ineffective airway clearance related to oropharyngeal secretions

Rationale: Extrauterine adjustment requires the clearance of amniotic fluid/secretions from the airway to allow optimal pulmonary function.

☐ **GOAL**

The neonate will maintain an open, clear airway; will breathe without difficulty; will be adequately oxygenated.

☐ **IMPLEMENTATION**

- Do Apgar score immediately at birth and 5 minutes later; repeat every 20 minutes until stable.
- Monitor cardiopulmonary status carefully to detect any cardiac anomalies/respiratory distress at least every 2-4 hours; observe, report, and record presence of breath sounds, cyanosis, pallor, choking, grunting, nasal flaring, retraction, shallow or irregular respirations, asymmetric chest expansion, and respiratory rates below 35 or above 50/minute, and periods of apnea greater than 10 seconds.
- Keep bulb syringe or DeLee mucous trap readily accessible at cribside; have mechanical suction equipment with oxygen and resuscitation equipment readily available and in good working order.
- Position on side or stomach; elevate foot of bassinet between 15° to 30° to promote gravity drainage.
- Know that position should be flat and prone if there has been a difficult passage of head or forceps delivery.

☐ **EVALUATION CRITERIA/DESIRED OUTCOMES**
The neonate
- Has easy respirations
- Has pink mucous membranes, no circumoral cyanosis

NURSING DIAGNOSIS #2
a. **Alteration in nutrition: less than body requirements** related to poor sucking reflex
b. **Fluid volume deficit** related to poor sucking reflex

Rationale: Extrauterine adjustment necessitates the independent acquisition of food, which may be complicated by an uncoordinated suck/swallow reflex, excessive secretions, anomalies, or maternal medications. Rapid metabolic rate predisposes neonate to fluid and electrolyte imbalance and hypoglycemia. The stomach empties in 2-4 hours, necessitating frequent feedings around the clock. Parents may not know what to expect regarding feeding behaviors/needs of neonates and thus inadvertently provide inadequate nutrition. The neonate requires approximately 24 oz fluid/day for adequate weight gain (120 kcal/Kg/day), commercial formulas and breast milk contain approximately 20 calories/oz. Following an initial weight loss of 5%-10%, the average weight gain during 10th to 30th day of life is approximately 1 oz/day.

☐ GOAL

The neonate will demonstrate rooting behavior, effective grasp of nipple, satisfactory sucking/swallowing behavior for adequate nourishment; the parent-neonate feeding pattern will be successfully and satisfactorily established.

☐ IMPLEMENTATION

- Observe and record neonate's feeding behavior readiness (e.g., reflexes, level of arousal when hungry, ease in burping, and pattern of regurgitation); explain and demonstrate these behaviors to both parents.
- Demonstrate how to hold, feed, and burp neonate; have parents give return demonstration; provide positive feedback and encouragement; provide support for the parents of a difficult feeder.
- Support parent's decision to feed via breast or bottle; provide information as needed or requested.
- Have breast-fed babies nurse shortly after delivery; assist mother to position neonate to suckle without having to turn head by cradling baby on its side so they are tummy to tummy; encourage to gently stroke the area around the neonate's mouth to elicit the rooting reflex; ensure that neonate latches on to the areola while feeding.
- Provide frequent (often every 2 hours) and on-demand feedings; assist mother to relax before each feeding (anxiety, fear, and fatigue will interfere with milk production).
- Prevent neonate from sleeping during feedings; if

neonate falls asleep while latched on, instruct mother to gently break the suction by placing her finger in corner of baby's mouth.
- Assess maternal-neonate interaction during feeding; help mother to interpret cues and achieve success in feeding; reinforce mother's optimism, positive feelings about self and nurturing behavior; know that mothers feel guilty and inadequate when neonates fail to feed satisfactorily, even though it may not be their fault.
- Hold neonate for all bottle feedings and let neonate set the pace; ensure nipple provides a slow, steady stream of milk; burp after every ounce taken (some babies will not allow this interruption).
- Stress importance of maintaining 1 feeding method (the neonate uses different skills for breast-feeding and bottle-feeding).
- Place on side or abdomen with head turned to side after feeding to prevent aspiration (mild regurgitation is common because of swallowed air and temporary incompetence of cardiac sphincter); report vomiting of any kind to physician.

☐ EVALUATION CRITERIA/DESIRED OUTCOMES

The neonate
- Has steady weight gain
- Feeds comfortably on a regular schedule
- Sleeps well between feedings

NURSING DIAGNOSIS #3
a. **Ineffective thermoregulation** related to neonatal status
b. **Alteration in tissue perfusion** related to hypothermia

Rationale: Adaptation to a cool, dry, drafty environment from a warm, moist, intrauterine existence stresses the immature thermoregulatory mechanisms of the neonate. Axillary temperatures reflect cold stress before a rectal temperature and do not carry the risk of rectal perforation.

☐ GOAL

The neonate will maintain a normal body temperature.

☐ IMPLEMENTATION

- Prevent exposure and chilling; keep neonate snugly wrapped in a lightweight blanket; accomplish care and treatments quickly in a draft-free, warm environment.
- Maintain nursery/mother's room temperatures within recommended range of 22.2°-23.3°C (72°-76°F) with 40%-60% humidity.

- Measure axillary temperatures at least every 2-4 hours.
- Postpone bathing for 4-6 hours after birth until axillary temperature stabilizes at 36.5°-37°C (97.7°-98°F).
- Provide extra warmth until body temperature stabilizes but prevent overheating (neonates cannot sweat to lower body temperature).

☐ EVALUATION CRITERIA/DESIRED OUTCOMES

The neonate
- Achieves/maintains body temperature between 36.5°-37°C

NURSING DIAGNOSIS #4

Potential for infection related to lack of normal flora, open wounds

Rationale: Neonatal immunologic function is not mature. In addition to the umbilical cord stump, the neonate may have impaired skin integrity resulting from a circumcision or removal of electrodes following monitoring.

☐ GOAL

The neonate will have a dry cord and clean intact skin; will be free from infection.

☐ IMPLEMENTATION

- Employ hospital's standard nursery infection control procedures.
- Scrub hands for 3 minutes in disinfectant solution before entering nursery environment; wash hands for at least 15 seconds before and after handling each neonate.
- Keep neonates in separate isolettes (especially when an airborne organism is known to be causing infection problem).
- Enforce practice of caring first for noninfected neonates before moving on to infected neonates if unable to divide staff between infected and uninfected neonates.
- Exclude nursing staff with illnesses from all nursery duty.
- Keep the cord clean and dry; know that Bacitracin ointment, triple dye, or other medications may be used prophylactically; keep diaper folded below umbilicus until healing occurs; advise parents to avoid tub baths until umbilical stump falls off.
- Cleanse neonate per hospital procedure; cleanse buttocks area with each diaper change; apply prescriptive cream or ointment if indicated to protect from moisture, rashes, and skin breakdown.
- Use prophylactic drug per state law in neonate eyes within one hour of birth (if not previously done in delivery room); do not rinse eyes, gently blot excess solution on lids to prevent discoloration.
- Discard and do not reuse formulas once feeding is finished.
- Avoid kissing or holding neonate close to face.

☐ EVALUATION CRITERIA/DESIRED OUTCOMES

The neonate
- Has a drying, intact cord
- Maintains intact skin

NURSING DIAGNOSIS #5
a. **Knowledge deficit** regarding care requirements of a neonate
b. **Alterations in parenting** related to the birth of a child

Rationale: The care of a neonate requires techniques and knowledge that may be new to the parent. The addition of a child to a family unit requires adjustments to previous life-style patterns.

☐ GOAL

The parents will demonstrate safe techniques of caring for neonate; will express an understanding of the bonding process; the neonate/parents will display attachment behaviors.

☐ IMPLEMENTATION

- Promote rooming-in practices and liberal father-visiting policies; observe for eye contact, gazing at, talking to, stroking, cuddling, and fondling of neonate.
- Describe the characteristics of the neonate to both parents in an informative, nonjudgmental manner; keep parents informed of neonate's activity and progress.
- Explain the bonding process, its gradual development, and the role of reciprocal interaction.
- Teach normal hygienic practices of handwashing, providing a clean environment for neonate, proper cord care, circumcision care, skin care following diaper changes, protecting neonate from others with colds or infections, and preparing formula safely.
- Teach to observe for and report immediately signs of illness (e.g., fever, weight loss, poor feeding, vomiting, diarrhea, excessive irritability and crying, lethargy, respiratory distress).
- Teach normal bathing procedures using mild, nonmedicated soap; explain common skin lesions and assure that they will disappear without special treatment; tell them to report all rashes and lesions that do not disappear in a few days.

- Demonstrate, observe, and teach safe handling techniques to all who handle neonate (e.g., providing firm support to all body parts especially head, keeping a controlling hand on neonate while weighing or giving care, placing a hand between skin and diaper when pins are used).
- Discuss environmental needs of the neonate (e.g., room temperature, clothing, visitors, trips outside, car seats).
- Teach that neonate may go a day or 2 without stools if breast-fed, and that very soft stools are common, they are not diarrhea.
- Review new information with every parental contact; take care to point out developmental changes of the baby.
- Teach to identify neonate's reasons for crying (e.g., hunger, wetness, loud noises, strong odors, wish to be held) and to meet needs satisfactorily.
- Teach comfort measures (e.g., diaper changes, burp, rock, and singing to baby); play soft music near baby's crib; give pacifier to meet needs for more sucking time than feedings allow.
- Show objects and smiling, friendly faces to neonates at a distance of 12" when possible; hang bed mobiles 7"-9" from baby's eyes; use homemade mobiles made with bright, colorful objects, dark/light contrasts.
- Talk to baby often; expose to normal household sounds, but protect from unduly loud noises.
- Teach to play with baby, keep nearby as much as possible so it is convenient to touch often; swaddle in soft clothing and blankets; vary positions from time to time when awake or when sleeping; teach that cloth carriers that hold neonate next to the parent's body help meet tactile needs; teach how to ensure head support at all times.
- Discuss sleep states and their implications with parents; allow neonate to sleep as desired; sleep patterns and the amount needed vary greatly (10.5-23 hours during first 3 days).

☐ **EVALUATION CRITERIA/DESIRED OUTCOMES**

The parents
- Verbalize developmentally appropriate behavioral expectations of neonate
- Demonstrate safe care practices
- State when to report signs of illness and whom to call with questions

The neonate/parents
- Demonstrate attachment behaviors

Table 8
The Normal Neonate

Vital Signs/Physical Growth

Temperature	36°-37°C (96.8°-98.6°F) axillary
Heart rate	120-160 beats/minute
Respirations	30-60 breaths/minute
Weight	2,500-3,850 gm (5.5-8 lb); initial weight loss may be 5%-10% of body weight in first 10 days
Length	47.5-53.75 cm (19-21 in)
Head circumference	34-35 cm (13-14 in)
Anterior fontanel	5" × 4" in, diamond shaped, soft, flat
Posterior fontanel	May be closed
Hematocrit	40-70 gm
Dextrostix	Greater than 40

General Appearance

Skin	Dry, elastic with firm turgor; milia (tiny cyst of obstructed sebaceous glands) may appear across the bridge of the nose (disappear without treatment)
Color	Pale (physiologic jaundice may occur 48 hours after birth and disappear within 7 days); Mongolian spots (discolorations frequently occurring on the buttocks of dark-skinned neonates, generally fade by the preschool years)
Head	Slightly misshaped (a result of vaginal delivery), eyes puffy; head sags when unsupported

Chest	Round, may have slightly enlarged breasts with discharge
Abdomen	Rises and falls with respirations; slightly distended after feedings
Genitalia	Females may have bloody discharge, swollen labia and vagina; males may have swollen scrotum, undescended testicles
Extremities	Symmetrical movements; strong muscle tone with extension; may have brief, spontaneous, rhythmic tremors
Elimination	Meconium (greenish-black stools) for 2-4 days; become golden mustard color (if breast-fed) or yellow (if bottle-fed)

Sensory/Motor

Reflexes	Sucking, rooting, palmar grasp, startle, tonic neck, stepping/dancing, Moro, blinking
Swallow	Persistent, strong, noisy
Sight	Sees objects within 8"-12", follows objects, interested in faces, prefers black-and-white contrast, sensitive to bright lights, closes eyes
Hearing	Turns head to follow voices; prefers female, high-pitched, and falsetto-type voices; loud noises cause startle reflex
Taste	Discriminates between sweet and nonsweet, prefers sweet
Smell	Discriminates between odors; strong odors will cause babies to cry, turn head, and become active; sneezing and sniffles are common
Touch	Keeps hands in a fist but drops objects placed in them

Behaviors

Crying	The only way for the neonate to have needs met; vigorous, involving entire body; "colic" crying occurs with expulsion of flatus, starts and stops without reason
Activity pattern	Quiet or active sleep; relaxed, inactive or alert; active waking periods

The Child with Neuroblastoma

Definition/Discussion

Neuroblastoma is a tumor that arises from immature sympathetic nerve cells. The primary site of occurrence is in the abdomen near the adrenal gland, followed by the neck and chest. This tumor most commonly occurs in very young children, with 90% of the cases diagnosed in children under 5 years of age. Neuroblastomas are classified based on the extent of disease.

- *Stage I*: localized primary tumor that is completely resected
- *Stage II*: disease extends beyond the organ or structure of origin but does not cross the midline of the body
- *Stage III*: tumor that extends beyond the midline of the body
- *Stage IV*: remote disease involving distant metastasis
- *Stage IV-S*: infants who would otherwise be stage I or II but with metastatic disease limited to liver, bone marrow, or skin

The treatment regimen for neuroblastoma varies according to the stage of disease. It may include any combination of surgical removal, chemotherapy, and radiation therapy.

Nursing Assessment

☐ PERTINENT HISTORY

Medical and surgical history, primary site of tumor, presenting symptoms, date discovered/diagnosed, metastatic disease, family history

☐ PHYSICAL FINDINGS

General health status, height, weight, nutritional status, pain (particularly abdominal), bowel and bladder function disturbances, paralysis due to spinal cord compression, stage of tumor

☐ PSYCHOSOCIAL CONCERNS/ DEVELOPMENTAL FACTORS

Age, developmental level/tasks, sex, family structure, available support systems, usual coping mechanisms, roles and responsibilities, experience with cancer and cancer treatment (self and others), cultural/religious beliefs

☐ PATIENT AND FAMILY KNOWLEDGE

Prognosis, course of treatment, level of knowledge, readiness and willingness to learn

Nursing Care

☐ LONG-TERM GOAL

The child/family will adapt effectively to the diagnosis and treatment of neuroblastoma and the biopsychosocial changes that will occur; the child/family will return to normal or near-normal roles in the family and community after a reasonable period.

NURSING DIAGNOSIS #1

Anxiety related to diagnosis, treatment regimen

Rationale: The diagnosis of cancer will evoke anxiety in the child/parents due to its aggressive treatment and potentially fatal outcome. Extensive testing is necessary to stage the disease, and this can be very frightening.

☐ GOAL

The child/parents will express fear, anxieties, feelings, and questions associated with the diagnosis and its treatment regimen; will use appropriate coping mechanisms to manage anxiety.

☐ IMPLEMENTATION

- Know what physician has told child/parents regarding diagnosis, treatment, and prognosis; clear up any misconceptions, answer questions.
- Allow time for parents to express emotions and concerns without child present.
- Allow child (if appropriate) opportunity to express emotions and concerns without parents present; use puppets/drawings as appropriate; refer to *The Child Requiring Play Therapy*, page 226.
- Assess previous coping mechanisms and support systems; encourage child/parents to utilize them;

introduce new coping mechanisms if none are used or appropriate (e.g., methods of information seeking, clergy, active participation in care).

- Identify resources available to assist with the development/exploration of new coping strategies; provide a list of support groups/agencies available.
- Arrange for a meeting with another with a similar diagnosis if possible.
- Discuss life-style/role changes.
- Encourage continued expression of questions and concerns.
- Be honest; keep information and communication continuous, current, and consistent; refer to *The Child Receiving Chemotherapy*, page 57, and *The Child Undergoing Radiation Therapy*, page 234 for specifics regarding treatment.
- Refer for counseling as needed or requested.

☐ EVALUATION CRITERIA/DESIRED OUTCOMES

The child/parents
- Express relief of or reduction in anxiety
- Identify support systems
- Utilize effective coping mechanisms
- Verbalize feelings about neuroblastoma, life-style and role changes, and coping mechanisms

---

NURSING DIAGNOSIS #2

Alteration in comfort: pain related to surgical procedure

Rationale: The neuroblastoma will be either removed or staged by surgical procedure, causing post-op pain.

☐ GOAL

The child will experience relief of pain.

☐ IMPLEMENTATION

- Assess level of pain using a developmentally appropriate scale (e.g., color scale, 1-10 scale); refer to *The Child Experiencing Pain*, page 216.
- Assess for nonverbal cues of pain (e.g., flat affect, grimacing, not moving in bed, guarding).
- Administer analgesics as ordered; assess and chart their effectiveness frequently.
- Assist child to learn and utilize muscle- and total body-relaxation techniques as developmentally able.
- Provide diversional activities to enhance relief of pain (e.g., coloring, games, reading).
- Utilize effective nonmedication pain-relief techniques (e.g., massage, heat, cold).

☐ EVALUATION CRITERIA/DESIRED OUTCOMES

The child
- Expresses relief from pain
- Has minimal restriction of movement due to pain

NURSING DIAGNOSIS #3
a. **Urinary retention** related to location/effects of neuroblastoma, treatment
b. **Alteration in bowel elimination: constipation/diarrhea** related to location/effects of neuroblastoma, treatment

Rationale: Neuroblastoma involving the abdomen, as a space-occupying lesion, can cause alterations in normal bowel and bladder function; these changes can be reversed by tumor removal or shrinkage. Treatment of the neuroblastoma (e.g., chemotherapy, radiation) may also cause constipation or diarrhea.

☐ GOAL

The child will resume normal or near-normal bowel and bladder function.

☐ IMPLEMENTATION

- Assess pretumor bowel and bladder patterns.
- Assist in understanding why bowel and bladder function have been altered by the tumor and how treatment may reverse these effects.
- Keep an accurate intake and output; note any deviations from child's normal bowel and bladder function; assess the effects of therapy on bowel and bladder function daily.
- Assist with bowel and bladder function until the tumor effects can be terminated (e.g., Créde method, diapering, laxatives, manual stimulation).

☐ EVALUATION CRITERIA/DESIRED OUTCOMES

The child
- Voids regularly
- Has balanced intake and output
- Passes soft, formed stool at least every other day

NURSING DIAGNOSIS #4

Impaired physical mobility related to tumor effects

Rationale: In rare cases, neuroblastoma can cause spinal cord compression, resulting in problems ranging from pain or decreased function to complete paralysis of an affected extremity. Tumor shrinkage or removal may reverse these effects.

☐ GOAL

The child will maintain/regain physical mobility; will adapt effectively to any permanent alteration in mobility.

☐ IMPLEMENTATION

- Assess pretumor mobility level; monitor changes in mobility daily.
- Assist child/parents to understand effects of tumor on child's physical mobility.
- Assist to maintain physical mobility as able when function has been impaired (e.g., wheelchair, crutches, self-help aids).
- Assist child in achieving optimal physical mobility; consult physical/occupational therapists; implement range-of-motion exercises; refer to *The Child Requiring Range-of-Motion Exercises*, page 237; provide age-appropriate developmental activities.
- Deliver meticulous skin care; use egg-crate/sheepskin mattresses as appropriate.
- Keep child/parents informed of impairments that are resolving and those that may become permanent.

☐ EVALUATION CRITERIA/DESIRED OUTCOMES

The child
- Resumes pretumor physical mobility level
- Performs age-appropriate skills

NURSING DIAGNOSIS #5

Knowledge deficit regarding diagnosis, treatment regimen

Rationale: Neuroblastoma is a complex and unfamiliar disease. The child/parents must understand the treatment regimen and follow-up care to accomplish biopsychosocial adaptation.

☐ GOAL

The child/parents will understand the disease process, treatment regimen, and follow-up care for neuroblastoma.

☐ IMPLEMENTATION

- Arrange scheduled, uninterrupted sessions with child/parents.
- Give instructions at developmentally appropriate level (e.g., what child will see, hear, feel, taste, smell).
- Arrange for others with similar disease and treatment experience to share with the child/parents.
- Provide with names and phone numbers of physicians or appropriate individuals to contact for follow-up and emergency care.
- Refer to community support group or home health service as appropriate.
- Provide written materials supporting verbal instructions given (e.g., signs to watch for and report, medications to be given, appointments to be made, appropriate activity level).

☐ EVALUATION CRITERIA/DESIRED OUTCOMES

The child/parents
- Comply with instructions
- Verbalize understanding of neuroblastoma and its treatment
- Know when and how to contact appropriate person(s) for follow-up or emergency care
- Have information necessary to contact support groups or home health services

The Child with Nonaccidental Trauma

Definitions/Discussions

Child abuse is the nonaccidental injury or neglect inflicted upon children by their caretakers. It includes physical and emotional neglect, physical battering, psychologic attack, and sexual abuse. The presence of one physical or behavioral indicator (see Assessment) need not necessarily be viewed with alarm, but repeated "accidents" or multiple signs are a cause for suspicion and precautionary reporting. High-risk situations include presence of a child with a chronic illness, or family situations in which the parent has poor or nonexistent support systems.

In some cases, the abuse is unintended (e.g., the trauma is inflicted by someone who cannot cope or who has unrealistic expectations for the child). For others, the process of abuse may have to do with the sense of power it bestows upon the abuser. The aggressor may not be able to get these feelings of power from the peer/work environment, and so takes it out on the child who is dependent on the abuser for existence. Whether the abuse is intended or not, the consequences for the child are still the same.

Nursing Assessment

☐ PERTINENT HISTORY

Accident report of person(s) accompanying child, child's description of injuries, degree of agreement between accounts; person responsible for child's care at time of incident; probability that incident being described is feasible for the child's age/developmental stage; history of similar incidents for this child/sibling; history of abuse in extended family

☐ PHYSICAL FINDINGS

Vital signs; consciousness and orientation; general appearance (e.g., clean, dirty, clothing); bruises, locations and stages of healing; weight/height in relation to normal growth curve; untreated infections; dental hygiene; lumps on scalp; retinal hemorrhages, scars, lacerations, fractures (locations and quantity); multiple fractures, especially in children under age 2; burns (particularly from cigars or cigarettes) on soles of feet, palms of hands, buttocks, or genitalia; immersion or scalding burns of hands, feet and buttocks with line of demarcation and few splash marks, degree of tissue damage; human bite marks, dental injuries, or cuts around mouth or eyes; areas of hair loss, location and description; trauma to genital area

☐ PSYCHOSOCIAL CONCERNS/ DEVELOPMENTAL VARIATIONS

Child's developmental/cognitive level; actual support systems; social interactions, behavior pattern (e.g., unresponsive, shy, fearful at approach or touch of an adult, passive while being examined, apprehensive when hearing other children cry, ignores friendly overtures, performs self-stimulating activities, seeks attention with asocial or deliquent acts, misses school frequently or falls asleep in class); verbal expectations of punishment for minor, childish accidents (e.g., spilling milk, wetting bed)

☐ PATIENT AND FAMILY KNOWLEDGE

Feelings toward the child, understanding of child's cognitive abilities, reactions to the incident, interactions, readiness and willingness to seek appropriate medical and mental health follow-up

Nursing Care

☐ LONG-TERM GOAL

The child will be free from pain, injury, fear, and neglect. The parents/caretakers will limit the potential for abuse of the child. The parents will implement new coping mechanisms, will seek appropriate help, and will not abuse the child.

NURSING DIAGNOSIS #1
a. **Potential for injury** related to abuse, neglect
b. **Alteration in comfort** related to physical injuries from abuse

Rationale: The array of physical injuries that a child may experience are varied. The trauma/neglect is usually severe enough to cause the child physical discomfort. Psychologically, the older

---

child may be suicidal or put him-/herself in a position to be harmed (e.g., drug/alcohol abuse, sexual promiscuity).

☐ **GOAL**

The child will be free from injury, self-abusive behavior; will be free from pain.

☐ **IMPLEMENTATION**

- Suspect abuse in children with unexplained injuries, injuries with several explanations, spiral fractures or head injuries in children under 2, repeated accidents, or cases in which siblings have had similar accidents.
- Conduct a complete nursing assessment.
- Restrict visitors if necessary.
- Explain all actions to child/parents.
- Follow hospital/state policies regarding the reporting of suspected child abuse; call a child abuse hotline.
- Confront self-abusive behavior; inform child that you will protect him/her from injuring self.
- Assess for behaviors indicating pain (e.g., guarding of an extremity, not letting anyone touch a particular area).
- Refer to *The Child with Pain,* page 216.
- Position child for comfort.
- Administer analgesics as ordered; assess and document effectiveness.
- Refer to Nursing Care Planning Guide specific to injuries (e.g., head injury, burns).

☐ **EVALUATION CRITERIA/DESIRED OUTCOMES**

The child
- Is safe
- Is free from injury
- Does not engage in self-abusive behavior
- Verbalizes/demonstrates behaviors indicating comfort

NURSING DIAGNOSIS #2

Alteration in nutrition: less than body requirements related to neglect

Rationale: Child abuse may take the form of willful neglect (e.g., withhold needed nutritional nourishment) or unintentional neglect (e.g., lack of knowledge). The child may be underweight for height, or have failure to thrive or signs of starvation.

☐ **GOAL**

The child will gain weight according to the normal growth curve.

☐ **IMPLEMENTATION**

- Calculate caloric requirements appropriate for age; provide diet to meet these requirements.
- Weigh every other day, on same scale, in same clothes, at same time.
- Determine typical family activities associated with mealtime.
- Demonstrate appropriate mealtime behaviors; make mealtimes fun by socializing/eating with the child; have child eat with other children.
- Encourage regular mealtime intake as well as nutritious snacks.
- Provide positive reinforcement for appropriate mealtime behaviors.
- Refer to *The Child with Failure to Thrive,* page 125.

☐ **EVALUATION CRITERIA/DESIRED OUTCOMES**

The child
- Gains weight according to normal growth chart
- Associates pleasure, enjoyment, and satiation with mealtimes

---

NURSING DIAGNOSIS #3
a. **Anxiety** related to a betrayal of trust by caretaker regarding safety and protection
b. **Fear** related to potential for repeat physical injury, abandonment

Rationale: Children need to love and be loved. Once the child's trust has been betrayed, the child is likely to experience feelings of uneasiness. The child may fear that the abuser (particularly if it is a parent) will leave, or the school-age child may believe that the abuse is somehow deserved (i.e., punishment for some wrongdoing). Uneasy feelings about the abuser are generalized to all adults (e.g., hospital staff).

☐ **GOAL**

The child will be protected from continued abuse; will realize that the responsibility for the abuse lies with the abuser; will verbalize feelings of safety/security.

☐ **IMPLEMENTATION**

- Observe and describe suspicious behavioral characteristics (e.g., flinching and ducking when anyone reaches out to touch; withdrawn, continual scanning of environment; searching for potential danger).
- Reassure child of safety while in your care.
- Offer to hold, rock, hug child; note child's reactions to/tolerance of this physical closeness; do not try to force physical closeness; carry infant in front carrier as much as possible.

- Determine what activities comfort child; establish a routine and stick to it as much as possible.
- Encourage verbal child to talk about feelings; be a concerned, quiet, nonjudgmental listener.
- Provide play materials; refer to *The Child Requiring Play Therapy*, page 226.

☐ EVALUATION CRITERIA/DESIRED OUTCOMES

The child
- Discusses/plays out feelings
- Indicates comfort with staff verbally or through behaviors

NURSING DIAGNOSIS #4
a. **Disturbance in self-concept: self-esteem** related to parental abuse
b. **Ineffective individual coping** related to being unprotected and emotionally betrayed

Rationale: The basic relationship between child and parent is that of trust—to be protected, nourished, and loved. Children who are abused experience both physical and emotional traumas leading to a sense of worthlessness and feeling bad about oneself. In turn, the child may engage in self-deprecating statements and self-defeating behavior. Children are limited in their repertoire of coping mechanisms and trust their parents to keep them from harm. Abuse/neglect scars this trust and often pushes the child past the point of adaptive coping skills.

☐ GOAL

The child will begin to appreciate positive traits/aspects; will develop/implement adaptive coping skills.

☐ IMPLEMENTATION

- Observe for withdrawn behavior, and "setting self up" to get into trouble.
- Give positive reinforcement concerning appearance, participation in activities, abilities to complete projects; praise appropriately, not indiscriminately.
- Set appropriate limits; develop important task for child to do.
- Schedule time each day just for child; discuss perceived strengths/weaknesses; validate and reinforce strengths; assist to develop way to resolve weaknesses.
- Reinforce current adaptive coping skills; assist to develop new coping skills.
- Role play new coping skills with child to reinforce them.

☐ EVALUATION CRITERIA/DESIRED OUTCOMES

The child
- Makes positive statements about self
- Accepts praise
- Role plays use of new coping skills
- Uses old adaptive and new coping skills in daily interactions

---

NURSING DIAGNOSIS #5
a. **Alterations in parenting** related to inappropriate limit setting/expectations for child's developmental/cognitive level
b. **Knowledge deficit** regarding presence of abuse, reasons for it, normal growth and development

Rationale: The family may deny the abuse, may be unaware that the child's injuries are a result of abuse, or may feel a need to "protect" the abuser for financial reasons or out of fear of abuse themselves. Few abusive parents really want to hurt their child and afterwards feel guilty, embarrassed, and a failure as a "good parent." Inappropriate expectations of age-appropriate skills can also potentiate an abusive situation.

☐ GOAL

The family will acknowledge abusive activities; the parents will understand normal child growth and development; will relate to their child on an appropriate developmental/cognitive level.

☐ IMPLEMENTATION

- Listen; be aware of your own nonverbal messages and feelings; maintain composure and compassion.
- Communicate support; refrain from criticism or rejection.
- Discuss abuse as a family problem; reinforce that everyone has a responsibility to protect the child.
- Explore alternative financial support/resources; connect with resources in community.
- Teach parents regarding their child's current developmental level; refer to *Normal Growth and Development*, pages 300–314.
- Give anticipatory guidance on the next level of development and appropriate expectations for that level; provide a list of resources for information about future developmental tasks; encourage follow-up to reinforce this learning.
- Role play with parents to help them internalize concepts of growth and development; allow them to identify with current cognitive level of child.
- Teach parents how to fulfill their wish to be good parents and "to do the right thing"; teach them to

enjoy their child, pointing out lovable attributes and features.

- Ask parents to join you and child in playing; role model for parent how to praise child; praise parent for participation; see *The Child Requiring Play Therapy*, page 226, and *Guidelines for Teaching Parents and Children*, page 316.
- Demonstrate how limits can be set and enforced; discuss how discipline can be given with consistency, fairness, and without physical force or uncontrolled anger; reinforce with praise and encouragement any parental attempts to nurture, comfort, cuddle, or express affection to the child.
- Help parents explore feelings; assist in defining stressors and help develop alternative methods of managing them.
- Assist parents to recognize behaviors that indicate increasing frustration/lack of coping; discuss actions to take to avoid abusing child.
- Explain that a child whose only emotional contact with parents is via abuse may provoke the parent deliberately in order to gain attention.

- Teach that the child will respond more positively and be better controlled if productive, emotionally satisfying activities are done together.
- Reassure parents that they have rights and needs also; provide them with names of organizations (e.g., Parents Anonymous) that assist parents who have abused their child; encourage involvement in follow-up visits.

☐ EVALUATION CRITERIA/DESIRED OUTCOMES

The parents

- Recognize abuse, own high-risk behaviors
- Describe how they will protect the child(ren)
- Manage future stressful situations without resorting to abuse
- State appropriate developmental tasks, behaviors to expect of child
- Set appropriate limits on child's behavior
- Role play actions to take when high-risk behaviors/situations occur
- Contact community support groups

The Child with Osteogenic Sarcoma

Definition/Discussion

Osteogenic sarcoma, the most common bone tumor in the pediatric age group, arises from bone-producing mesenchymal cells. It most often occurs among adolescents and is found predominantly in rapidly growing bones, such as the distal femur; other likely sites of disease include the humerus, ilium, and proximal femur. The primary treatment, depending on tumor size, location, and evidence of metastatic disease, is surgery, which may include amputation at the joint above the involved bone or limb-salvage procedures. Chemotherapy and radiation therapy are often used in conjunction with surgery.

Nursing Assessment

☐ PERTINENT HISTORY

Medical and surgical history; primary site of tumor; date discovered/diagnosed; metastatic disease; normal activity level

☐ PHYSICAL FINDINGS

General health, height, weight, nutritional status, pain, impaired activity, limp, swelling at site of tumor

☐ PSYCHOSOCIAL CONCERNS/ DEVELOPMENTAL FACTORS

Age, sex, developmental level/tasks, available support systems; usual coping mechanisms, roles and responsibilities, experience with cancer and cancer treatment (self and others), family structure, cultural/ religious beliefs

☐ PATIENT AND FAMILY KNOWLEDGE

Disease, prognosis, course of treatment, previous exposure to cancer and treatment regimen education, level of knowledge, readiness and willingness to learn

Nursing Care

☐ LONG-TERM GOAL

The child will adapt effectively to the diagnosis, treatment, and resulting biopsychosocial changes; the child will return to normal or near-normal roles in the family and community after a reasonable period.

NURSING DIAGNOSIS #1

Alteration in comfort: pain related to cancerous invasion of the bone and surrounding soft tissue

Rationale: Osteogenic sarcoma is a bulky tumor that invades the bone. Due to the dense, nonexpandable nature of the bone, rapidly produced tumor cells create pain in the bone. These tumor cells also extend into the soft tissue encircling the bone and produce pain.

☐ GOAL

The child will experience relief from or control of pain.

☐ IMPLEMENTATION

- Assess level of pain using developmentally appropriate scale to obtain objective measure (e.g., color scale, 1-10 scale); refer to *The Child Experiencing Pain*, page 216.
- Administer analgesics as ordered, assess frequently and chart effectiveness in terms of quality and duration.
- Adapt activities to accommodate non-weight bearing on the affected area.
- Assist to learn and utilize muscle and total body relaxation techniques.
- Provide diversional activities to enhance relief of pain (e.g., coloring, games, reading).

☐ EVALUATION CRITERIA/DESIRED OUTCOMES

The child
- Rates pain as less than 3 on a 10-point scale
- Participates in diversional activities

NURSING DIAGNOSIS #2

Anxiety related to diagnosis, treatment regimen

Rationale: The diagnosis of cancer will evoke anxiety in the child/parents due to its aggressive treatment and potentially fatal outcome. Amputation and limb salvage are both extensive surgical procedures that necessitate life-style changes.

☐ GOAL

The child/parents will express fears, anxieties, feelings, and questions associated with diagnosis and treatment regimen; will use appropriate coping mechanisms to manage anxiety.

☐ IMPLEMENTATION

- Know what physician has told child/parents regarding diagnosis, treatment, and prognosis; clear up any misconceptions; answer questions.
- Refer to *The Child Receiving Chemotherapy*, page 57, and *The Child Undergoing Radiation Therapy*, page 234, for specifics regarding those treatments.
- Allow time for child to verbalize feelings and concerns without parents present.
- Allow time for parents to express feelings and concerns without child present.
- Assess previous coping mechanisms and support systems; encourage child/parents to utilize these.
- Arrange for another child of similar age and diagnosis to talk with child if possible.
- Be honest with child/parents; keep information and communication continuous and current.

☐ EVALUATION CRITERIA/DESIRED OUTCOMES

The child/parents
- Express relief of or reduction in anxiety
- Identify and utilize effective coping mechanisms and support systems

NURSING DIAGNOSIS #3

Grieving related to loss of limb, limb function, possible death of child

Rationale: The grieving process starts when the child is diagnosed and the treatment alternatives are made known. Although limb salvage procedures allow retention of the affected limb, its function will be impaired to some extent. The fear of death must also be dealt with.

☐ GOAL

The child/parents will express grief and the personal meaning of the loss as developmentally appropriate.

☐ IMPLEMENTATION

- Assess child's/parents' stage in the grieving process being aware of the usual stages, including denial; assist to progress through the grieving process; refer to *The Parent Experiencing Grief and Loss*, page 139, and *The Child who is Dying, Terminal*, page 116.
- Recognize and help child/parents to see that feelings of depression, hostility, resentment, frustration, helplessness, and hopelessness are normal.
- Allow adequate and frequent time to verbalize feelings, ask questions, and express concerns; do not challenge or discourage any expressions; help to focus on adaptive feelings after allowing adequate time for grieving.
- Arrange for another child with similar disease to talk with child/parents to share experiences and present life-style changes and coping.
- Be honest and open regarding expected outcome of treatment, being realistic about impairments to expect while offering alternatives to deal with loss.
- Initiate referral for counseling if grieving is interfering with normal functioning.

☐ EVALUATION CRITERIA/DESIRED OUTCOMES

The child/parents
- Express grief and move towards resolution
- Identify effective coping patterns and appropriate support systems for continued resolution of loss

NURSING DIAGNOSIS #4

Impaired physical mobility related to adaptation to loss of limb, limb function

Rationale: Amputation or limb-salvage procedures of the affected upper or lower extremity will result in altered physical mobility. The child must compensate for the lost extremity through adaptation by other muscles and limbs. The use of prosthetic limbs will also require adaptation by the child. Fittings for prostheses should be done as soon as the physician allows.

☐ GOAL

The child will demonstrate adaptation to impaired physical mobility, using prosthesis, wheelchair, adaptive devices; will maintain or increase strength and endurance of unaffected limbs.

IMPLEMENTATION

- Assist child/parents to understand treatments of amputation/limb salvage and why this is treatment of choice for osteogenic sarcoma; discuss expected physical mobility impairment, use of prosthetic limb when indicated.
- Assess pretumor mobility level; help set realistic goals for return of function.
- Observe the prosthetist's teaching session; know how the prosthesis should be worn, handled, and maintained in order to reinforce teaching realistically and knowledgeably.
- Allow child/parents opportunity to observe and discuss with another child a prosthetic limb.
- Check stump daily for signs of skin irritation, redness, warmth, or tenderness; clean skin with mild soap and water daily, taking care to dry skin thoroughly.
- Utilize physical/occupational therapy to assist child in achieving optimal physical mobility.
- Encourage exercises designed to strengthen unaffected limbs and support muscles.

EVALUATION CRITERIA/DESIRED OUTCOMES

The child

- Uses prosthesis, wheelchair, or adaptive device satisfactorily
- Achieves maximal physical mobility with adaptations for impaired function
- Maintains or increases strength in unaffected limbs and accessory muscles of affected limb

---

NURSING DIAGNOSIS #5

Disturbance in self-concept: body-image related to the loss of limb, limb function
Refer to *The Child Experiencing a Body-Image Disturbance*, page 30.

NURSING DIAGNOSIS #6

Knowledge deficit regarding diagnosis, treatment regimen

Rationale: *Osteogenic sarcoma is a complex and unfamiliar disease. Both the disease and its ongoing treatment regimen must be understood to permit adaptation in life-style, emotional preparedness.*

GOAL

The child/parents will understand the disease process, treatment regimen, and follow-up care.

IMPLEMENTATION

- Give instructions at developmentally appropriate level (e.g., what child will see, hear, feel, taste, smell); provide written material to enhance and review verbal instructions.
- Detail ongoing treatment regimen; include schedule of chemotherapy and methods to reduce, avoid side effects.
- Provide written instructions of signs to watch for and report, additional medications to be given, appointments to be made, activity level.
- Arrange for other children/families with similar disease and treatment experience to share with child/parents.
- Provide names and phone numbers of physicians or appropriate individuals to contact for follow-up and emergency care.
- Refer to community support group or home health service.

EVALUATION CRITERIA/DESIRED OUTCOMES

The child/parents

- Comply with instructions
- Verbalize understanding of diagnosis and treatment
- Know when and whom to contact for follow-up or emergency care
- Verbalize some feelings about diagnosis, life-style and role changes, and coping mechanisms
- Have information about support groups or home health services

The Child Experiencing Pain

Definition/Discussion

Pain is a sensation of discomfort, distress, or agony resulting from a single stimulus or a class of stimuli. Emotions of anxiety, anger, depression, fear, loneliness, feelings of abandonment, and fear of body intrusion can alter perception and expression of pain. Research indicates that children experience as much pain as adults yet clinical studies show that physicians and nurses underestimate pain in children and tend not to offer pain medication or teach skills to cope with pain.

Nonverbal communication and changes in physiologic measures are present before verbal expression of pain in children; children may deny pain to be "good" or to avoid a "shot" or may fake pain to avoid school or unpleasant procedures, so observation of nonverbal and physiologic changes becomes important in differential diagnosis. Behavioral reactions to pain correlate with the age of the child. Pain reactions are subjective and individual, depending on individual life experience, maturity, and culture as well as type of pain, location, and stimuli.

Nursing Assessment

☐ PERTINENT HISTORY

Duration of pain; noxious stimuli: mechanical (trauma, friction), chemical (microorganisms, toxins, drugs), thermal (heat, cold), electrical; prior painful experiences and responses to them; use of pain medication (type, amount, time)

☐ PHYSICAL FINDINGS

Flushed skin; increased pulse, respirations, blood pressure; dilated pupils; vomiting; loss of appetite; favoring/guarding body part, location of pain; nature of pain (e.g., superficial, deep, referred), if able to differentiate; *newborn:* total body movement with brief, loud crying; *infant and toddler:* rolling head from side to side, pulling on ear for pain in ear or head, tense body postures, widely opened eyes, flexing knees for abdominal pain, refusing to move body part; *preschool/school-age child:* clenching teeth and fist, rigid posturing; *adolescent:* psychosomatic complaints

☐ PSYCHOSOCIAL CONCERNS/ DEVELOPMENTAL FACTORS

Cultural differences in expressing pain; ability to localize; words used to describe pain ("hurt," "owie," "boo-boo"); emotions, mood, affect; activity level; usual response to pain, coping mechanisms; *infants:* no memory of painful experience prior to 6 months, association of environment with painful experience; *toddlers:* fear of body intrusion; *preschooler:* magical thinking or fantasies (e.g., something they did/ thought caused the pain experience), increased verbal skills to communicate pain, poorly developed concept of body integrity, no understanding of temporal relationship, faking symptoms, *school-age child:* fear of body injury, exaggeration; *adolescent:* importance of body image, overconfidence compensating for fear

☐ PATIENT AND FAMILY KNOWLEDGE

Causes of pain, techniques for coping; level of knowledge, readiness and willingness to learn

Nursing Care

☐ LONG-TERM GOAL

The child will have pain recognized and treated; the child will be free from any pain that impairs day-to-day functioning or interferes with the attainment of life goals.

NURSING DIAGNOSIS #1

Alteration in comfort: pain related to condition

Rationale: Pain affects children's ability to cope with illness/hospitalization, interfering with their ability to reach their developmental potential.

☐ GOAL

The child will verbalize (or exhibit behaviors that indicate) a decrease in pain; will be free from pain-related immobility; will demonstrate an increased ability to cope with pain and discomfort; the parents/child will discuss feelings and concerns about pain and measures to relieve them.

☐ IMPLEMENTATION

- Help child talk (if able) about pain and relief measures.
- Discuss child's discomfort with parents; encourage them to carry out selected nursing care; ask to express their concern to you; explain rationale for comfort measures and pain medication.
- Administer analgesics as ordered; monitor frequently for effectiveness; report to physician if child's pain is not effectively relieved.

Infant/toddler

- Touch, comfort, hold; use soft voice or music.
- Observe for physiologic changes; monitor vital signs; examine part of body child pulls, rocks, or favors.
- Utilize distraction; rock, sing, carry, play peek-a-boo or other games that child enjoys.
- Maintain parent/child contact and do procedures as quickly as possible if distraction does not help; hold if restraints are needed; protect from injury (e.g., falling, breaking off the injection needle).
- Pay attention to toddler's complaints (can communicate verbally, localize their pain [e.g., "owie on my knee"], rarely fake pain).
- Ask parent what words, behaviors, and methods precipitate a response of intense physical resistance and emotional upset, and which methods of coping with pain are likely to be helpful.
- Listen to parents' feelings and concerns; include pertinent information from parents in care plan.
- Avoid intrusive procedures (e.g., rectal temperature, injections) as much as possible as these are threatening whether painless or painful; ask physician for oral medications, axillary temperature, or other alternatives.
- Accept regression (e.g., becoming incontinent even if toilet trained); give permission to cry.
- Have comfort objects available (e.g., bottle, blanket).
- Offer pain medication in forms that toddler will take (e.g., crush and put in gelatin or ice cream).

Older toddler/preschooler

- Monitor for self-imposed limitation of activity.
- Avoid use of heat, cathartics, or laxatives when abdominal pain is present.
- Report change of pain to physician.
- Do not take verbal attacks personally; understand that child is afraid; allow parent to do as much as possible for child.
- Tell child "It's OK to cry;" offer comfort; listen to child's concerns and feelings.
- Cover injection sites, abrasions, cuts with Band-Aids to give security that body injury is "fixed" and body integrity maintained; use progressively smaller dressings as size of dressing will be interpreted as progress in healing.

- Know that child may have exaggerated fears about body injury (e.g., worries about bleeding, insides falling out, needle punctures, mutilation, and castration); use term "fixed" rather than "removed."
- Measure axillary or oral rather than rectal temperature if child is able to cooperate.
- Use therapeutic play to prepare child for procedures and to discuss pain as part of illness/accident; use dolls, puppets, stuffed animals to demonstrate a procedure or to encourage a child to talk about an experience; refer to *The Child Requiring Play Therapy*, page 226.
- Clarify that child is not to blame for pain; magical thinking leads to guilt, shame, and idea that pain is punishment for wrongdoing.
- Desensitize to threatening equipment (e.g., needles, oxygen mask) by introducing it in pleasant, familiar surroundings, using play (e.g., dress a stuffed bear with an OR mask, cast, or give the bear a "shot"); if child shows fear, move equipment far away in room and reintroduce with play at a later time; allow child to touch and play with the equipment under supervision.
- Have child rate pain with a range of happy to sad faces or utilize colors to demonstrate discomfort; ask child to color or place an "x" in location of pain on a picture of child's body; give choice of comfort measures.
- Encourage child to draw pictures or use toys or dolls to tell stories about pain and hospitalization experience; allow child to project feelings onto dolls to learn child's perceptions and concerns.

School-age child

- Teach relaxation using imagery
  - "take deep breath and blow out slowly; let arms and legs be as limp as a wet noodle"
  - "breathe into painful area; let your breath blow out the pain; slowly breathe out and imagine pain is blowing away with the breath"
  - "put your hand or pillow over the 'hurt' and softly breathe into that area; as you breathe out, imagine that the tightness is melting away and that the hurt feels better"
- Observe nonverbal cues of fear or pain and offer support; know that crying or losing control may cause embarrassment; reassure as necessary.
- Limit procrastination and bargaining as delaying a dreaded event often increases anxiety.
- Ask preference as to presence of parents; discuss choice with parents.
- Tell child about available pain medications; explain that the sting of an injection or bad taste of medicine only lasts a moment, but will help take away some of pain for longer period of time.
- Allow child to plan and problem solve within reasonable limits for situation and condition, utilizing present cognitive skills.
- Use humor to distract or teach (e.g., comic books,

funny songs, stories) if child likes humor, jokes, and puns.
- Be extremely sensitive when examining genital area as touching the school-age child's genital area is very threatening.

Adolescent
- Approach with respect; ask what helps with pain/discomfort and use these coping methods (e.g., pillow, hot tea, earphones with music, icepacks); offer privacy.
- Avoid authoritarian attitude; do not try to be "hip" or use adolescent jargon.
- Assess learning needs and offer information on techniques to distract or decrease pain; give something positive to do as well as to restore feelings of control (e.g., relaxation with imagery or cutaneous stimulation [e.g., rub skin in rhythmic pattern with lotion, powder, menthol, or cream; use pressure, heat, cold, electric vibrator set at moderate intensity]).
- Listen to and accept adolescent's concerns and feelings; use open-ended questions and be nonjudgmental.
- Assess knowledge and offer small amounts of information about pain, medications, and pain management as adolescent shows interest.
- Work with adolescent to find effective methods of coping with pain.
- Assess effectiveness of pain medications and techniques to distract or decrease pain.

☐ EVALUATION CRITERIA/DESIRED OUTCOMES

The child
- Is relieved of pain
- Displays no physical behaviors indicating presence of pain
- Has no complaints of pain when asked (if verbal)

- Expresses feelings about pain and its relief at age-appropriate level
- Uses effective pain-relief measures at age-appropriate level

---

NURSING DIAGNOSIS #2
Knowledge deficit regarding cause of pain and pain management

Rationale: If knowledge deficit exists child/parent cannot appropriately manage treatment of pain. A lack of understanding increases anxiety and tension, further increasing pain.

☐ GOAL
The child/parents will adhere to pain management treatment at home and verbalize its importance.

☐ IMPLEMENTATION
- Answer questions using nonthreatening, brief, and honest information at child's level of understanding.
- Give child/parents verbal and written instructions regarding list of medications, dosages, schedule, possible side effects and when to report them to physician/clinic; where and how to obtain refills.
- Have child/parents demonstrate techniques to distract from or decrease pain.
- Make appointment for follow-up care.

☐ EVALUATION CRITERIA/DESIRED OUTCOMES
The child/parents
- State appropriate administration of medications, side effects, and when to contact physician concerning problems
- Utilize techniques to distract or decrease pain
- Keep appointment for follow-up care

The Child Requiring Peritoneal Dialysis

Definition/Discussion

Peritoneal dialysis is the diffusion of solute molecules through a semipermeable membrane (the peritoneum) from the side of higher concentration (the child's blood) to that of lower concentration (the dialysate). Fluids pass through the semipermeable membrane by means of osmosis. The purpose is to remove toxic substances, body wastes, and fluids that the kidney normally excretes, and to maintain life until kidney function is restored, if possible.

Peritoneal dialysis (PD) is based on two principles

- *diffusion:* the random movement of molecules, ions, or small particles in solution or suspension toward a uniform concentration throughout the available volume
- *osmosis:* the diffusion of a solution through a semipermeable membrane

The dialysate is removed repetitively and replaced with fresh solution in order to maintain a high mean diffusion gradient between body fluids and dialysate. The rate and amount of water removed from the child depends on the osmotic pressure generated by the dextrose in the dialysis solution (dialysate). Solutions of 1.5%, 2.5%, and 4.25% are commonly available.

Prior to dialysis, a catheter is inserted into the peritoneal cavity by a physician under strict aseptic technique (a signed operative permit is necessary). A Teflon catheter is used in acute PD and is removed following the PD treatment; for chronic PD, the catheter is made of silastic with a Dacron felt cuff (bacterial barrier) and can last for many years if cared for correctly.

Dialysis (exchange) is accomplished by repeating a 3-phase cycle. Each cycle includes

- *inflow:* the time it takes for the dialysate to flow into the peritoneal cavity by gravity (usually 5-10 minutes)
- *diffusion or dialysis (dwell):* the time that the dialysate is in contact with the peritoneal cavity; length of dwell time is determined by the amount of fluid and serum waste products that need to be removed
- *outflow:* the time it takes the dialysate to drain from the peritoneal cavity by gravity (usually 10-15 minutes)

Three common methods may be used

- *manual single-bottle method:* the catheter is attached to Y-tubing and prescribed fluid (usually 10-50 ml/kg sterile dialyzing solution warmed to body temperature) is run in by gravity; the tubing is clamped just before the bottle or bag is empty (inflow phase); the dialysate remains in the peritoneal cavity until a degree of equilibrium between the dialysate and body fluids is achieved (diffusion or dialysis phase); the bottle or bag is lowered to the floor, the tubing unclamped, and the fluid drains out (outflow phase)
- *continuous ambulatory peritoneal dialysis (CAPD):* a prescribed amount of dialysate is connected to the *permanent* catheter and allowed to flow into the abdomen (inflow phase); the catheter is then clamped and the dialysate allowed to dwell for 2-4 hours (diffusion or dialysis phase). During this time the empty dialysate bag is folded and kept on the child. After diffusion, the empty dialysate bag is lowered to a clean surface (usually a paper towel on the floor), unclamped, and the dialysate is allowed to flow out by gravity (outflow phase). The process is then repeated with new dialysate 3-5 cycles a day, 7 days a week. During the night cycle the dialysate is allowed to dwell 7-8 hours.
- *continuous cycling peritoneal dialysis (CCPD):* this method is basically a reversal of CAPD exchanges. CCPD does cycles during the night with a simple cycling machine and the long dwell (diffusion or dialysis phase) during the day, which affords the child much more personal freedom for day activity. This method is also called intermittent peritoneal dialysis (IPD).

Peritoneal dialysis is superior to hemodialysis in that it requires a simple technique with no sophisticated equipment. However, it takes longer than hemodialysis and has increased risks for peritoneal and pulmonary infection and large albumin/protein loss. Peritoneal dialysis is contraindicated with bleeding or recent abdominal surgery.

Peritoneal dialysis can be done at home using CAPD or CCPD. The choice of home dialysis depends on the child/parent motivation, absence of medical problems that interfere with safety or performance of procedures, and the child's/parents' ability to learn required information and procedures. Advantages of home dialysis are economic (the cost is less than half that of other treatment in other centers), relative convenience (child/family can set up schedule that will accommodate work/school, social life), fewer medical complications, psychosocial health (preservation of family life, a greater degree of independence and confidence). The major disadvantages are disruption of family schedule and the fact that success or failure depends a great deal on the abilities of the child/parents. The parents may often feel directly responsible for the life of their child leading to strained relationships.

Nursing Assessment

☐ PERTINENT HISTORY

Hyperkalemia, hypertension, fluid overload, severe acidosis, severe edema, uremia, mental confusion, acute or chronic renal failure, drug poisoning, fatigue, headache, sleep difficulty, pruritus

☐ PHYSICAL FINDINGS

Congestive heart failure, pulmonary edema, hypotension/hypertension, rales, dyspnea; anorexia, metallic taste in mouth, ascites, uremic breath; anuria, oliguria, proteinuria, increased urinary specific gravity and osmolality; anemia; short attention span, confusion, possible convulsions and coma; peripheral neuropathy (numbness, twitching, paresthesia); nystagmus; periorbital edema, rash, petechiae, ecchymosis; dryness, yellow bronzing, pallor of skin; uremic frost; decreased resistance to infection; delayed wound healing; joint pain, loss of muscle mass; increased BUN, creatinine, serum ammonia, uric acid, potassium, phosphorus, magnesium, albumin/casts in urine; acidosis; abnormal glucose tolerance, clotting times, serum sodium; decreased serum albumin levels, lipids; abnormal liver function tests

☐ PSYCHOSOCIAL CONCERNS/ DEVELOPMENTAL FACTORS

Denial, anxiety, depression, personality changes, irritability, intermittent changes in memory/attention span (associated with elevated blood ammonia levels) may be particularly distressing to the child/family, adaptation to body-image change in adolescents, changed role in family, finances

☐ PATIENT AND FAMILY KNOWLEDGE

Disease and prognosis, support systems, treatment options, complications, home health maintenance regimen, level of knowledge, readiness and willingness to learn

Nursing Care

☐ LONG-TERM GOAL

The child/parents will adhere to prescribed regimen to aid recovery from the acute renal failure and to return to usual

roles; OR the child will adapt to the reality of long-term dialysis and will live within its accompanying limitations.

NURSING DIAGNOSIS #1

Anxiety related to fear of unknown procedure

Rationale: Lack of knowledge leads to increased anxiety. Preprocedure explanation and question/answer periods have a calming effect on the child/parents and promote comfort.

☐ GOAL

The child/parents will verbalize statements or demonstrate behaviors reflective of decreased anxiety.

☐ IMPLEMENTATION

- Explain each step of procedure; answer all questions as honestly as you can, and appropriately for age and level of child's development.
- Use teaching doll and allow child to handle equipment similar to that used during dialysis.
- Assess affect and mental status before dialysis; know that a dependence on the health team is established and that child/family may respond with a variety of feelings; all can be considered adaptive except suicidal tendencies; refer to *The Child with Chronic Renal Failure*, page 66.
- Recognize that questions about the procedure and necessary life-style changes are a sign of adaptation; when these occur, provide information and work with the child/parents to bring about changes.
- Plan care with child/parents, encourage involvement as much as possible; if child has been dialyzed previously, ask what you can do to enhance comfort during this dialysis.
- Assess child's/parents' support system, knowledge of procedure; provide as much information as requested and needed; speak in calm, reassuring tones; let child/parents know how long and at what times a nurse will be at the bedside.
- Emphasize that a variety of feelings and emotions are usual and expected in the adaptation process.
- Help child/family select clothing that will minimize appearance of dialysis bags and tubing.
- Consult social worker, clergy, or mental health worker as needed.

☐ EVALUATION CRITERIA/DESIRED OUTCOMES

The child
- Verbalizes or demonstrates age-appropriate behaviors showing reduced anxiety about treatment

NURSING DIAGNOSIS #2

Alteration in comfort: pain related to dialysate in abdomen

Rationale: The volume of dialysate may cause abdominal distension and create a feeling of pressure on abdominal organs. The dialysate may cause a chemical irritation; the peritoneal catheter may be malpositioned. Infection in the peritoneum (peritonitis) will also cause pain.

☐ GOAL

The child will demonstrate behaviors (verbal and nonverbal) of relative comfort during procedure.

☐ NURSING IMPLEMENTATION

- Assess for pain or discomfort during inflow and diffusion phases; have child describe the timing and type of pain; assess nonverbal behaviors in the infant and toddler (e.g., crying, irritability); in older child, ask "Where does it hurt?"; use pain self-rating scales (faces, numeric), and human figure drawing.
- Administer frequent back rubs, massage pressure areas, and change child's position as needed; (during infusion, child is usually supine with head slightly elevated to decrease discomfort of abdominal organs pushing up against diaphragm).
- Warm dialysate to core temperature before instilling into peritoneum.
- Provide age-appropriate toys or other diversions.
- Assure child that feeling of fullness lessens after first few exchanges.
- Administer analgesic when indicated; monitor for effectiveness and side effects.
- Make certain that complete solution drainage is occurring; check for abdominal distension.
- Notify physician for continuing pain.

☐ EVALUATION CRITERIA/DESIRED OUTCOMES

The child
- States absence of or decreasing discomfort during procedure
- Tolerates procedure comfortably
- Demonstrates behaviors that indicate comfort

NURSING DIAGNOSIS #3

Potential for injury (bowel, bladder, vessel perforation) related to catheter insertion, accidental removal or displacement of temporary catheter

Rationale: The insertion site of the peritoneal catheter is 1-2 inches below the umbilicus and may perforate the bowel, bladder, or a blood vessel. The temporary (straight) peritoneal catheter is secured by a purse-string suture and covered with a tight dressing. It can easily be dislodged if the child is very active.

☐ GOAL

The child will remain free from or be promptly treated for any potential complications of peritoneal catheter insertion; will maintain catheter in the correct position.

☐ IMPLEMENTATION

- Have child void before catheter insertion or catheterize if unable to void; monitor for indications of bladder perforation (e.g., large amounts of urine output [urine + dialysate] with high glucose level, strong urge to urinate frequently).
- Be alert to signs of bowel perforation (e.g., fecal material in returning dialysate fluid, strong urge to have bowel movement; sudden decrease in blood pressure, tachycardia).
- Assess for vessel perforation by checking returning dialysate fluid for blood; the first few returns may have some blood because of rupture of superficial capillaries during catheter insertion, but then should be clear.
- Keep child in bed and restrain limbs as necessary; provide age-appropriate diversional activities.
- Observe catheter for leaking around exit site or change in its length or position at least every 2 hours.
- Contact physician immediately should any of the above noted signs/symptoms be present.
- Monitor vital signs at least every 2-4 hours.

☐ EVALUATION CRITERIA/DESIRED OUTCOMES

The child
- Exhibits no signs of bowel, bladder or vessel perforation
- Drains clear dialysate solution
- Maintains catheter in correct position

NURSING DIAGNOSIS #4

a. **Fluid volume deficit** related to rapid removal of intravascular fluid
b. **Alteration in fluid volume: excess** related to fluid retention

Rationale: Dialysate solutions are hypertonic (1.5%, 2.5%, and 4.25% glucose), causing an osmotic gradient for fluid through the peritoneal membrane and may result in too rapid removal of fluid from the blood volume. Mechanical problems with catheter drainage (e.g., kinks, blockages) may cause fluid retention and fluid overload.

GOAL

The child will maintain fluid balance.

IMPLEMENTATION

- Record baseline assessment of weight, blood pressure, and pulse; check blood pressure and pulse when each outflow begins and ends; weigh after each exchange to check on fluid loss.
- If child is slightly hypotensive, turn on side to decrease pressure on vena cava.
- Assess and record hydration status prior to each exchange; select tonicity of dialysate, as ordered, according to physician's or agency's protocol.
- Keep accurate recording of fluid exchange balance; for each exchange, record essential exchange times on flow sheet (time infusion started and ended, time outflow begins and ends, amount of solution infused and returned, computed balance—usually a plus or minus amount).
- Describe and record dialysate color and clarity; report any cloudy outflow to physician.
- Apply firm pressure to lower abdomen and ask child to turn from side to side if fluid does not drain in a steady stream.
- Check with physician regarding amount of oral fluids permitted; accurately record intake and output.

EVALUATION CRITERIA/DESIRED OUTCOMES

The child
- Has normal vital signs
- Has good skin turgor, moist mucous membranes, and no edema
- Maintains adequate urine output for age

NURSING DIAGNOSIS #5

Potential for infection related to possible contamination through direct access of peritoneal cavity, chemical irritation from dialysate solution

Rationale: *Peritonitis is the major complication in peritoneal dialysis. There may be contamination during catheter insertion, during instillation of dialysate, or around catheter insertion site. Chemicals in the dialysate may also irritate the peritoneum significantly to start an infection leading to peritonitis (sterile peritonitis).*

GOAL

The child will remain free from peritonitis.

IMPLEMENTATION

- Maintain strict aseptic technique at all times (e.g., dressing, peritoneal catheter care, skin care).

- Monitor continuously for signs of infection (e.g., increased temperature, increased white blood cell count, cloudy dialysate, persistent abdominal pain).
- Check site for redness and drainage every 8 hours; assess catheter care technique of child/parents.
- Administer antibiotics as ordered; monitor for effectiveness and toxicity.
- Observe for septic shock (e.g., tachycardia, decreased blood pressure, narrowing pulse pressure, tachypnea).
- Obtain cultures of dialysate and catheter exit site as necessary.

EVALUATION CRITERIA/DESIRED OUTCOMES

The child
- Has a normal temperature, vital signs
- Returns clear dialysate
- Is free from significant pain
- Practices aseptic exit site care

NURSING DIAGNOSIS #6

Alteration in bowel elimination: constipation related to decreased peristalsis secondary to abdominal distension during dwell time

Rationale: *Peritoneal catheter and chemicals in dialysate may cause enough irritation to decrease or stop bowel activity.*

GOAL

The child will have normal bowel activity.

IMPLEMENTATION

- Assess for bowel sounds, bowel movements, abdominal distension, increased nasogastric output prior to dialysis and during inflow and diffusion phases.
- Keep child NPO if ileus is present.
- Have child change positions and/or ambulate to decrease distension.
- If medications given to encourage peristalsis, evaluate effectiveness.

EVALUATION CRITERIA/DESIRED OUTCOMES

The child
- Has at least 1 soft, formed bowel movement/day
- Maintains normal bowel sounds

NURSING DIAGNOSIS #7

Alteration in nutrition: less than body requirements related to excessive protein loss through dialysis outflow, anorexia secondary to abdominal distension, vomiting after too rapid instillation of dialysate

Rationale: One of the disadvantages of peritoneal dialysis is the excessive protein loss through the semipermeable membrane. The presence of the dialysate in the peritoneal cavity may cause abdominal distension and feelings of fullness with resultant decreased appetite. Rapid instillation of dialysates, especially after meals, may cause vomiting with further loss of nutrients.

☐ GOAL

The child will maintain adequate nutrition..

☐ IMPLEMENTATION

- Monitor serum albumin levels.
- Administer salt-poor albumin if prescribed.
- Consult dietician for dietary teaching; reinforce instructions and plans.
- Provide protein supplements to diet.
- Plan meals to allow for approximately 2 hours absorption time prior to instillation of dialysate.
- Encourage family involvement during mealtimes.
- Review foods allowed on diet; instruct as needed.

☐ EVALUATION CRITERIA/DESIRED OUTCOMES

The child
- Has normal serum albumin levels
- Maintains appetite and adequate nutritional intake
- Is free from vomiting

NURSING DIAGNOSIS #8

a. **Ineffective breathing patterns** related to pressure on diaphragm while dialysate fluid in abdomen
b. **Impaired gas exchange** related to ineffective breathing pattern
c. **Potential for infection** related to ineffective breathing pattern, impaired physical mobility

Rationale: With dialysate fluid in the abdomen, there may be sufficient pressure on the diaphragm to decrease inspiratory depth. Atelectasis/pneumonia may develop; the likelihood for these complications is increased by the necessity for limited mobility during dwell time.

☐ GOAL

The child will remain free from respiratory complications associated with peritoneal dialysis.

☐ IMPLEMENTATION

- Place child in semi-Fowler's position.
- Turn and deep breathe every 2 hours.
- Have older child use inspirometer every hour while awake.
- Auscultate breath sounds, check vital signs every 2 hours.
- Administer oxygen if appropriate.
- Note amount, color of respiratory secretions.

☐ EVALUATION CRITERIA/DESIRED OUTCOMES

The child
- Has no dyspnea
- Exhibits normal respiration and breath sounds
- Expectorates clear respiratory secretions easily

NURSING DIAGNOSIS #9

Ineffective family coping related to disruption of usual family life-style

Rationale: While scheduling time for home dialysis is more flexible than meeting hospital-based appointments for treatments, planning time for dialysis may interfere with other family events and be a source of conflict within the family. The family member responsible for performing the treatment may become overwhelmed by the responsibility or may become dictatorial and increase the child's feelings of dependency. Other family members (especially siblings) may resent the time and attention afforded the child and may react with avoidance and withdrawal or anger and hostility.

☐ GOAL

The family will identify and use effective coping strategies in meeting the challenges of caring for a child receiving home dialysis.

☐ IMPLEMENTATION

- Discuss usual family routines; encourage to share feelings about child's condition, need for dialysis, and changes in life-style required by treatment regimen; assist in planning treatments at times that cause least interference.
- Explain home dialysis can either serve to bring families closer together or create problems of conflicts, frustration, depression, remorse, withdrawal; much of the success of a home dialysis program depends on the people involved and

their ability to deal with stress and long-term illness.

- Elicit feelings of the child periodically and discuss; share with child that these feelings are usual and expected, and may be intermittent.
- Ask about special events involving other family members (e.g., siblings); discuss importance of recognition of achievements of all family members; ask to identify ways of acknowledging accomplishments.
- Work with child/family to adjust dialysis schedule to accommodate work and social events, trying to maintain as normal a life as possible.
- Work with social worker on ongoing basis; discuss psychosocial needs of family as a unit as well as individual needs of family members.
- Discuss child's/family's participation in a community support group of other dialysis patients where feelings and problems can be handled on an on-going basis (this can help child/family deal with own feelings); if no dialysis group can be found, contact a social worker for referrals to other sources.

☐ EVALUATION CRITERIA/DESIRED OUTCOMES

The family
- Shares feelings about child's condition and need for dialysis with each other
- Identifies important aspects of daily living and schedules dialysis treatments to allow maximum participation
- Indicates awareness of community resources available for psychosocial support

---

NURSING DIAGNOSIS #10

Knowledge deficit regarding treatment procedure, care of the catheter, home dialysis procedure

Rationale: Cooperation is needed to promote compliance and to prevent complications. Lack of understanding of treatment interferes with compliance. Compliance requires a thorough explanation, demonstration plus return demonstrations of the skills and procedures specific to peritoneal dialysis self-care in the home.

☐ GOAL

The child/parents will verbalize understanding of procedure and possible complications; will demonstrate proper performance of self-care dialysis procedure and verbalize understanding of vital

information regarding home dialysis; will demonstrate aseptic technique with catheter care.

☐ IMPLEMENTATION

- Instruct in all potential complications; give telephone number of physician and dialysis center, and explain when to call.
- If child is on long-term dialysis, periodically review prescribed regimens to assess degree of compliance; praise all positive efforts and discuss areas for improvement.
- Teach aseptic catheter care and dialysis protocol to child who goes home with indwelling peritoneal catheter; have child return demonstration.
- Listen to child's explanations, problems, and feelings; work out solutions with child.
- Review *Guidelines for Teaching Parents and Children*, page 316, for educational principles in health teaching; review teaching program from your center/agency to ensure that it is set up and carried out in a logical, sequential manner.
- Reassure that it is normal to feel discouraged, overwhelmed, inadequate, anxious when "in training"; discuss these feelings (unresolved, suppressed feelings can hinder the learning process); reward child/family for all efforts at expressing and resolving feelings.
- Explain that motivation is the single most important factor in a successful dialysis program; to foster this, give a great deal of praise and many rewards for learning the essential skills.
- Begin training program when a decision is made to initiate CAPD or CCPD; teach one skill at a time, beginning with the simple and proceeding to the complex; assess child's/family's readiness and ability to learn and proceed at that pace, rather than at yours.
- Provide training in essential areas of operation and maintenance of dialysis equipment, purpose and functions of dialysis, monitoring and interpreting vital signs, managing complications, ordering supplies, fluid and electrolyte balance, dietary management, self-medication, and emergency actions according to agency protocols.
- Discuss potential complications (e.g., drop in blood pressure, ruptured dialyzer, line separation, air in lines, clotted dialyzer, machine malfunction) and immediate solutions; ensure that child has written instructions.
- Review and reinforce principles of fluid and electrolyte balance; ask child/parents to describe correlation between needs/restrictions and dialysis; show child how to keep own intake and output record; reinforce correct behaviors and provide repeat instructions to modify incorrect behaviors.
- Ask child to tell you about dietary restrictions; check menu planning; work to find new foods or

new ways of preparing old ones that will give some dietary variety; coordinate teaching with a dietician.

- Assess self-medication schedule and assist in adjustment as needed; show how to keep own medical record; review side effects of medications and reinforce instructions as to when to notify physician.

☐ EVALUATION CRITERIA/DESIRED OUTCOMES

The child/family
- Demonstrates proper catheter care
- Demonstrates proper self-care procedures
- States understanding of home self-care

The Child Requiring Play Therapy

Definition/Discussion

Play is the natural language of a child; it is the expression of a child's biopsychosocial being in relation to the environment. Therapeutic play is a supervised, semistructured play experience that is deliberately planned, observed, and evaluated in relation to its intended objectives.

Nursing Assessment

☐ **PERTINENT HISTORY**

Effective coping methods used by child in the past, prior experiences with stress/hospitalization, child's favorite play materials, changes/disruptions in routine or life-style

☐ **PHYSICAL FINDINGS**

Any physical limitations that would restrict child from certain activities

☐ **PSYCHOSOCIAL CONCERNS/ DEVELOPMENTAL FACTORS**

Developmental level of child, pattern of play at home

☐ **PATIENT AND FAMILY KNOWLEDGE**

Purpose, willingness to learn and participate in therapeutic play activities

Nursing Care

☐ **LONG-TERM GOAL**

The child will express ideas, feelings, and imagination through play; the child will adapt to the stress of illness/ hospitalization through play.

NURSING DIAGNOSIS #1
a. **Knowledge deficit** regarding hospitalization, treatments
b. **Ineffective individual coping** related to limited cognitive abilities, lack of available communication skills
c. **Diversional activity deficit** related to hospitalization, enforced activity restrictions

---

Rationale: *During hospitalization, clinic visits, or illness experiences in the home, a child's emotional outlets may be restricted and fears intensified; and maladaptive behaviors may occur. The child may "act out" fear by aggression toward others, crying, denying the need for medical attention, or by withdrawing from interaction with others. Young children lack the cognitive/social/communication skills necessary to make sense out of the confusion they are experiencing. Play provides the child with a safe means of communicating thoughts, fears, concerns, and stressors. Health professionals may use therapeutic or goal-directed play to assist the child to relate to the environment and cope with injury, illness, hospitalization, discomfort, and separation from loved ones.*

☐ **GOAL**

The child will communicate thoughts, feelings, concerns through play; will use play to decrease the stress of hospitalization; will cooperate with treatments and procedures.

☐ **IMPLEMENTATION**

- Refer to *Normal Growth and Development*, pages 300–314.
- Plan the specific purpose(s) of the play (e.g., to determine fears/concerns, relieve anxiety, express creativity, channel energy, distract from discomfort/pain, explain or teach a diagnostic or treatment procedure).
- Pepare a playroom for ambulatory children and a portable cart for children on bedrest; consult teachers, recreation specialists, parents, and children for suggested equipment and supplies; use your imagination; determine choice of equipment/ toys/supplies based on child's development and goal.
- Request consultative assistance and patient behavior information from coordinator/specialist.
- Be alert to behaviors/actions that reflect child's feelings.

- Validate impressions but do not restrict spontaneity; avoid interruptions.
- Be nonjudgmental; do not direct child or develop rules/guidelines that inhibit child's self-expression.
- Use up-coming special events as themes (e.g., "Tell a story about . . .").
- Encourage older children to write poems, stories, or plays; provide positive reinforcement for all accomplishments.
- Provide and encourage drawing, coloring, and water painting for self-expression; avoid use of "coloring books" and structured "art"; display if acceptable with child.
- Provide dolls, selected medical equipment so child can act out selected experiences (e.g., getting a shot, being anesthetized, removing sutures).
- Use age-appropriate books, drawings, models to demonstrate tests and procedures.
- Observe play; note failure to respond to age-appropriate toys and play materials; monitor types of play (e.g., solitary, parallel, interactional).
- Acknowledge feelings and encourage child to express them verbally; listen to what is and what is not revealed; share observations and findings with other health care professionals.
- Use community resource volunteers for entertainment (e.g., musicians, magicians, clowns, dancers, actors, puppeteers).
- Use tapes, records, books, and cartoon movies available on free loan from community libraries, schools, recreation centers; identify community resources.
- Ask parents to bring in child's favorite toys/activities if possible.
- Record pertinent observations regarding play experiences and responses, revealed fears, feelings, and indications of new insights.

☐ **EVALUATION CRITERIA/DESIRED OUTCOMES**

The child
- Cooperates with treatment
- Shares fears/concerns
- Describes tests and procedures in own words

NURSING DIAGNOSIS #2

Knowledge deficit regarding value of play

Rationale: Some parents are not aware of the benefits of play.

☐ **GOAL**

Parents will understand usefulness of play in allowing child to explore feelings of fear, anxiety, pain, and happiness.

☐ **IMPLEMENTATION**

- Teach the relationship of play to ability to master developmental tasks and to cope with experiences in everyday life.
- Reinforce information about child's developmental level and cognitive abilities.
- Explain need for positive play experiences to promote child's self-esteem and sense of well-being.
- Role model appropriate activities/responses to facilitate optimal play.

☐ **EVALUATION CRITERIA/DESIRED OUTCOMES**

The parents
- Verbalize an understanding of how play can assist child to resolve feelings of tension, bring life experiences into child's level of comprehension
- Assist child in creative play activities

The Child with Pneumonia

Definition/Discussion

Pneumonia is an inflammation of the lungs, caused by bacteria, virus, or mycoplasma organism. The alveoli and bronchioles of children with pneumonia become plugged with a fibrous exudate. Children with pneumonia may experience a high fever, cough, convulsions. Bacterial pneumonia is treated with antibiotics.

Nursing Assessment

☐ **PERTINENT HISTORY**

Fever, cough, nasal discharge, anorexia/feeding difficulties, listlessness, prior respiratory illnesses, home treatment attempted, others sick at home

☐ **PHYSICAL FINDINGS**

Fever, dyspnea, tachypnea, cyanosis, use of accessory muscles, diminished breath sounds, rales, elevated white blood cell count (bacterial pneumonia), abnormal arterial blood gases (ABGs), chest x-ray

☐ **PSYCHOSOCIAL CONCERNS/
DEVELOPMENTAL FACTORS**

Age, developmental level, ability to understand rationale for interventions, experience with separation from parents, previous coping mechanisms, habits (e.g., what comforts child, bedtime/feeding routines, favored objects)

☐ **PATIENT AND FAMILY KNOWLEDGE**

Prior experiences with respiratory illnesses, understanding of need for intervention for respiratory distress; level of knowledge, readiness and willingness to learn

Nursing Care

☐ **Long-Term Goal**

The child will recover free from preventable complications.

NURSING DIAGNOSIS #1
Ineffective airway clearance related to inflammation and obstruction of the lower respiratory tract

Rationale: Inflammation of lung tissue interferes with the normal flow of air into and out of the alveoli.

☐ **GOAL**

The child will inhale and exhale air without use of accessory muscles; will have clear breath sounds; will maintain/regain normal respiratory rate and color.

☐ **IMPLEMENTATION**

• Monitor respiratory and heart rates at least every 2 hours.
• Observe respiratory effort every 2 hours; auscultate breath sounds and observe color.
• Observe for signs of increasing airway obstruction and respiratory failure (e.g., tachycardia, tachypnea, increased use of accessory muscles, pallor, restlessness); have emergency equipment closely available (e.g., appropriately sized ventilation bag, nasotracheal tube, laryngoscope, emergency medications).
• Utilize cardiorespiratory monitor to assist observation of respiratory and cardiac patterns as necessary.
• Administer oxygen at ordered flow via hood, cannula, or high humidity oxygen tent (face masks are not well tolerated by children).
• Bulb suction nares as needed as young infants are obligatory nose breathers.
• Assist to cough up secretions; obtain sputum for culture and sensitivity; suction as needed if unable to raise secretions.
• Monitor ABGs and other bloodwork as ordered.
• Initiate chest percussion and drainage if tolerated; schedule chest physical therapy before meals and before bedtime.
• Assist to maintain upright position (e.g., place in-

fant in infant seat and support head, elevate head of crib mattress).
- Maintain quiet, calm environment; allow to rest/ sleep as often as possible.
- Administer antibiotics as ordered; monitor for effectiveness, side effects.

☐ **EVALUATION CRITERIA/DESIRED OUTCOMES**

The child
- Displays normal respiratory rate and effort with no use of accessory muscles
- Has clear breath sounds with free movement of air
- Maintains normal ABGs

NURSING DIAGNOSIS #2
Fluid volume deficit related to inadequate oral intake, tachypnea, fever

Rationale: Insensible water loss from tachypnea and increased metabolic rate from fever will deplete total body water. Increased oral liquids will help loosen and liquify secretions.

☐ **GOAL**

The child will ingest adequate fluids for age/weight, will return to preillness weight; will maintain adequate urine output, moist mucous membranes, good skin turgor; will expectorate secretions.

☐ **IMPLEMENTATION**
- Calculate maintenance fluid requirement for weight; provide additional fluids to compensate for insensible loss and fever.
- Maintain IV at ordered rate; decrease IV rate as oral intake increases; protect IV from infiltration or dislodgment; refer to *The Child with an Intravenous Catheter*, page 174.
- Offer fluids preferred by child frequently in order to meet daily fluid requirement; utilize novel approaches to drinking (e.g., playing tea party, using funny straws); have fluids at room temperature or warm as very cold fluids may precipitate coughing; avoid milk as it tends to thicken secretions.
- Encourage the nursing mother to continue breast-feeding even though infant may be fussy with feedings; supplement breast-feedings with 5% dextrose and water as needed.
- Monitor intake and output, mucous membranes, skin turgor, urine specific gravity, and vital signs.
- Weigh daily on same scale, in same clothes, at same time.

☐ **EVALUATION CRITERIA/DESIRED OUTCOMES**

The child
- Has adequate intake and output for age/weight
- Maintains moist mucous membranes, good skin turgor
- Has urine specific gravity of 1.003-1.020
- Regains preillness weight

NURSING DIAGNOSIS #3
Diversional activity deficit related to respiratory isolation

Rationale: The child in isolation is prevented from engaging in interaction with other hospitalized children and unit staff. Opportunities for working/playing through the stressors related to hospitalization are diminished.

☐ **GOAL**

The child will work/play through the stresses related to hospitalization; will engage in age-appropriate activities.

☐ **IMPLEMENTATION**
- Provide child with age-appropriate activities (e.g., visual, auditory, tactile); arrange crib/bed so child can observe activities going on outside room.
- Ascertain favorite activities and make them available within constraints imposed by isolation; provide toys that can be gas autoclaved or cleaned with bacteriocidal agents upon removal from room; encourage child to decorate room with cards and posters.
- Assign volunteer to spend time in room when parents are absent.
- Rearrange furniture in room as child's respiratory status improves to make space for age-appropriate gross motor activities.
- Provide siblings with masks and gowns; allow them to enter room if parents permit and siblings are not ill/have not been exposed to any communicable disease in past 3 weeks.
- Enter room frequently to assess needs and to assure child that s/he is not being ignored; spend time playing with child.
- Encourage parents to bring in school activities; structure time so some school tasks are accomplished as status improves.

☐ **EVALUATION CRITERIA/DESIRED OUTCOMES**

The child
- Has no boredom/lethargy/irritability related to inactivity
- Is involved in age-appropriate activities

NURSING DIAGNOSIS #4

Alteration in comfort related to fever, dyspnea, chest pain

Rationale: Fever, dyspnea, and chest pain will make the child uncomfortable and interfere with the ability to effectively cough up secretions.

☐ GOAL

The child will demonstrate relief from dyspnea and chest pain; will cough effectively; the child's temperature will return to normal.

☐ IMPLEMENTATION

- Check temperature every 4 hours or more frequently if elevated; change damp bed linens as needed; sponge child with tepid water; stop if chilling or shivering occurs.
- Medicate with antipyretics as ordered; monitor effectiveness.
- Elevate head of bed; assist child to assume a position of comfort.
- Avoid use of narcotic analgesics or sedatives that could interfere with adequate respirations/cough reflex.
- Assist to splint chest with pillow while coughing.
- Plan care to allow adequate rest/sleep periods.
- Encourage parents to stay with child but provide with relief as needed; reassure them that someone will remain with child.

☐ EVALUATION CRITERIA/DESIRED OUTCOMES

The child
- Expresses comfort
- Coughs adequately and expectorates secretions
- Breathes easily
- Maintains normal temperature

NURSING DIAGNOSIS #5

Knowledge deficit regarding care of child after discharge

Rationale: The child will be discharged as soon as respiratory status returns to normal, oxygen is no longer needed, and (if a bacterial infection) the course of antibiotics is completed. However, the child will require more time to convalesce before returning to normal daily activity.

☐ GOAL

The child will return to normal activity; parents will know the steps to take the next time a respiratory infection occurs.

☐ IMPLEMENTATION

- Assist parents to develop a plan for home care that includes a well-balanced diet, rest/sleep periods, and appropriate activities.
- Reinforce need to protect child from contagious illnesses until respiratory status has returned to normal (e.g., avoid crowds/crowded areas, teach handwashing, separate from siblings with upper respiratory infections).
- Instruct regarding administration of antibiotics if appropriate.
- Instruct regarding signs of recurrent illness (e.g., fever, shortness of breath, coughing, poor color, poor feeding, change in behavior).
- Assure parents that a temporary loss of recently acquired developmental skills is a normal response to hospitalization.
- Provide phone numbers of persons to contact if questions or concerns arise; instruct regarding return appointment.

☐ EVALUATION CRITERIA/DESIRED OUTCOMES

The child
- Returns to normal daily activities
- Has no recurrence of respiratory illness

The parents
Take appropriate measures to seek health care assistance if respiratory illness occurs

The Child with Pyloric Stenosis

Definition/Discussion

Pyloric stenosis is the obstruction at the pyloric sphincter caused by hypertrophy and hyperplasia of the pyloric muscle. It is characterized by projectile vomiting after feedings, an olive-shaped mass in right upper quadrant (RUQ), left-to-right gastric peristalsis. Surgical correction is achieved by a longitudinal incision through the anterior wall of the pyloric canal (pyloromyotomy).

Nursing Assessment

☐ PERTINENT HISTORY

Vomiting after feedings, weight gain, size and frequency of stools, crying/lethargy

☐ PHYSICAL FINDINGS

Nutrition/hydration status; metabolic alkalosis, olive-shaped mass RUQ, left-to-right peristalsis.

☐ PSYCHOSOCIAL CONCERNS/ DEVELOPMENTAL FACTORS

Birth history, prior physical status, developmental level, parents' comfort with child care, other children in the family, support systems, what comforts child

☐ PATIENT AND FAMILY KNOWLEDGE

Understanding of disease and need for immediate attention; level of knowledge, readiness and willingness to learn

Nursing Care

☐ LONG-TERM GOAL

The child will recover from surgery free from preventable complications; the child will feed normally and gain weight.

NURSING DIAGNOSIS #1

Fluid volume deficit related to vomiting/pre-op dehydration

Rationale: The vomiting characterizing pyloric stenosis depletes total body water and electrolytes.

The loss of chloride causes bicarbonate retention, which leads to metabolic alkalosis.

☐ GOAL

The child will gain weight with balanced intake and output.

☐ IMPLEMENTATION

- Weigh preoperatively and every day postoperatively on the same scale, in the same clothing, at the same time.
- Calculate fluid maintenance requirements for weight; add fluids to compensate for losses.
- Calculate expected urine output for weight; maintain accurate intake and output; weigh diapers and subtract dry weight from wet weight (1 gm = 1 cc); check urine specific gravity every 8 hours.
- Maintain patent IV line; refer to *The Child with an Intravenous Catheter*, page 174.
- Maintain patent nasogastric (NG) tube if present; irrigate tube with 3 cc normal saline every 2-4 hours; note how much irrigant can be withdrawn; subtract amount of remaining irrigant from total NG output before calculating replacement; measure NG output every 4-8 hours; replace with ordered IV solution over next 4-8 hours.
- Monitor every 4 hours for signs of dehydration (e.g., poor skin turgor, dry mucous membranes, sunken fontanel, elevated heart rate, decreased blood pressure).
- Offer small amounts of liquids when normal bowel sounds are heard and child is permitted oral fluids; increase slowly.
- Monitor serum electrolytes.

☐ EVALUATION CRITERIA/DESIRED OUTCOMES

The child
- Has adequate intake and output for age and weight
- Has moist mucous membranes, good skin turgor
- Maintains heart rate and blood pressure within normal limits for age

231

- Voids adequately with urine specific gravity of 1.003-1.020
- Gains weight

NURSING DIAGNOSIS #2

Alteration in nutrition: less than body requirements related to vomiting, NPO status

Rationale: The child with pyloric stenosis will present with a slowed pattern of weight gain or a weight loss caused by vomiting. If vomiting has occurred over a period of time, decreased intake may lead to poor wound healing and susceptibility to secondary infections.

☐ GOAL

The child will gain weight within normal growth/development curve; the child's incision will heal quickly.

☐ IMPLEMENTATION

- Weigh preoperatively and daily postoperatively on same scale, in same clothing, at the same time.
- Chart child's preillness height and weight on growth grid to establish normal pattern.
- Check urine daily for presence of ketones.
- Begin small, frequent feedings of glucose water when oral fluids are allowed, then breast milk or dilute formula and advance quickly to full-strength feedings if there is no abdominal distension or vomiting; feed in semi-upright position, burp frequently, handle gently during/after feeding.
- Encourage parents to participate in feeding.
- Assist mother to maintain breast-milk production and reestablish nursing if child has been breast-fed.
- Position on right side with head elevated after feeding to allow escape of gas and promote passage of fluid from stomach to duodenum.
- Assess incision every 4 hours for signs of problems (e.g., redness, drainage, dehiscence); report any changes.

☐ EVALUATION CRITERIA/DESIRED OUTCOMES

The child
- Ingests adequate amounts of formula or breast milk without vomiting
- Gains weight
- Is free from ketonuria
- Heals adequately

NURSING DIAGNOSIS #3

Alteration in comfort: pain related to operative incision

Rationale: The pyloromyotomy incision may be temporarily painful and interfere with effective breathing/adequate sleep.

☐ GOAL

The child will have normal sleep and quiet awake patterns; will demonstrate no behaviors indicating pain; will have a normal breathing pattern and vital signs.

☐ IMPLEMENTATION

- Refer to *The Child Experiencing Pain,* page 216.
- Be alert to nonverbal behaviors indicating pain (e.g., behavior, inability to sleep, changes in vital signs).
- Observe incision for inflammation and signs of infection, bleeding, wound healing.
- Position diapers low over abdomen to avoid rubbing incision.
- Monitor effects of analgesics.
- Position child so stress on incision is minimized.
- Encourage holding and cuddling of child by parent, volunteer, or staff member.
- Rub child's back and extremities; speak in soothing voice; play quiet music, offer pacifier.
- Provide for uninterrupted rest/sleep.

☐ EVALUATION CRITERIA/DESIRED OUTCOMES

The child
- Maintains vital signs within normal limits
- Sleeps comfortably for age-appropriate periods of time
- Has no excessive crying, irritability

NURSING DIAGNOSIS #4

Alteration in parenting related to feelings of inadequacy

Rationale: Frequent vomiting by the child may make the parents feel inadequate and question their parenting skills. Other people may have told parents they were feeding/holding/caring for the child inappropriately. Negative feeding/parenting behaviors may have developed by the time the child is hospitalized.

☐ GOAL

Parents will understand cause of pyloric stenosis; will feel adequate in their parenting skills.

☐ IMPLEMENTATION

- Explain the pathophysiology of pyloric stenosis.
- Assure that feeding difficulties occurring prior to surgery had a physiologic etiology and were not caused by poor feeding techniques.
- Encourage parents to verbalize feelings, ask questions.
- Observe parent-child interactions; teach new skills/behaviors as appropriate and observe return demonstrations.
- Involve parents in feeding and physical care; verbally reinforce positive behaviors.
- Support parents in all aspects of care, especially when introducing oral feedings after surgery (particularly stressful if negative feeding behaviors developed before surgery).

☐ EVALUATION CRITERIA/DESIRED OUTCOMES

The parents
- State physiologic cause of vomiting
- Verbalize comfort about caring for child
- Hold child closely and maintain eye contact

NURSING DIAGNOSIS #5

Knowledge deficit regarding care of child after discharge

Rationale: The child may take several days to return to a normal eating, sleeping, and activity pattern. Parents may also have questions/concerns related to normal child care and parenting.

☐ GOAL

The parents will understand care of child after discharge; will assimilate the child back into the family unit.

☐ IMPLEMENTATION

- Encourage parents to assume care of child prior to discharge.
- Explain care of incision; have parents demonstrate cleaning and dressing incision.
- Answer any questions parents may have regarding normal child care.
- Provide written materials to support verbal instruction.
- Provide phone numbers of persons to contact if questions or concerns arise; instruct regarding return appointment.

☐ EVALUATION CRITERIA/DESIRED OUTCOMES

The parents
- Demonstrate correct incisional care
- State plans for feeding and caring for child at home
- Contact appropriate resources if problems occur
- Return for follow-up appointment

The Child Undergoing Radiation Therapy

Definition/Discussion

Radiation therapy is treatment with an ionizing radioactive substance or with roentgen rays in order to destroy malignant cells or to make malignant cells incapable of further cell division.

Nursing Assessment

☐ **PERTINENT HISTORY**

Medical and surgical history; type, primary site of cancer, date discovered/diagnosed; metastatic disease; treatment history; family history; reason for therapy, site of treatment

☐ **PHYSICAL FINDINGS**

General health status; height, weight; nutrition and hydration status; integrity of skin, mucous membranes; vital signs

☐ **PSYCHOSOCIAL CONCERNS/ DEVELOPMENTAL FACTORS**

Age; sex; developmental level; child's/family's available support systems; usual coping mechanisms; roles and responsibilities; experience with cancer and cancer treatment (self and others); habits (e.g., bedtime/feeding routines, what comforts child, favored objects)

☐ **PATIENT AND FAMILY KNOWLEDGE**

Type of cancer, prognosis, course of treatment, radiation therapy; level of knowledge, readiness and willingness to learn

Nursing Care

☐ **LONG-TERM GOAL**

The child will respond therapeutically with maximum benefits to radiation therapy; the child will experience reduced pain, symptomatic relief, minimum side effects, and restoration of confidence; the child will accept/adapt to biopsychosocial aspects of cancer diagnosis with recommended radiation treatment and continuing care.

NURSING DIAGNOSIS #1

Alteration in nutrition: less than body requirements related to nausea, vomiting, anorexia

Rationale: Gastrointestinal (GI) reactions and nutrition problems are caused by physiologic response to radiation treatments, emotional stress, and disease effects on the GI tract. When the child has had previous weight loss, surgery, or chemotherapy, nutrition problems are compounded.

☐ **GOAL**

The child will ingest sufficient calories to meet the body's requirements; will maintain optimal nutrition.

☐ **IMPLEMENTATION**

- Weigh daily to monitor nutritional status.
- Review importance of maintaining optimal nutrition.
- Arrange for consultation with dietician.
- Administer antiemetic medications approximately 2 hours before mealtimes and as necessary; evaluate effectiveness.
- Control environmental factors to decrease nausea and vomiting (e.g., avoid strong odors or food, noise).
- Encourage high-calorie diet with smaller meals spaced throughout the day; arrange for larger meals when anorexia and nausea are less apparent (e.g., in the morning); offer blenderized, bland, high-protein foods (e.g., cream cheese, cottage cheese, gelatin salad with fruit, ice cream, puddings, and milkshakes); or serve high-protein, high-calorie commercial supplements between meals.
- Adjust diet prior to and immediately after treatment (e.g., clear, cool liquids; bland diet or NPO).
- Arrange for family/friends to be present during meals; encourage companionship to help stimulate appetite and intake.

- Administer vitamin and mineral supplements as ordered.
- Encourage food experimentation in meal planning and preparation.
- Discuss alternative feeding methods if weight loss should become severe (e.g., nasogastric tube, IV, gastrostomy).

☐ EVALUATION CRITERIA/DESIRED OUTCOMES

The child
- Consumes at least 75% of body's nutritional requirement
- Maintains weight within 10% of normal
- Maintains positive nitrogen balance
- Is free from nausea and vomiting

NURSING DIAGNOSIS #2

a. **Fluid volume deficit** related to nausea, vomiting, anorexia, diarrhea
b. **Alteration in bowel elimination: diarrhea** related to radiation therapy

Rationale: Increased fluids are required to eliminate toxic waste products. Dehydration, weight loss, and electrolyte imbalance are complications of diarrhea which result from irritation of the GI mucosa by radiation therapy.

☐ GOAL

The child will maintain normal hydration status; will return to normal bowel pattern/consistency.

☐ IMPLEMENTATION

- Monitor hydration status (e.g., skin turgor, mucous membranes); record intake and output.
- Monitor laboratory tests for negative nitrogen balance and dehydration (e.g., total proteins, electrolytes, hematocrit); report significant changes.
- Weigh daily on same scale, at same time, with same clothes.
- Assess character and frequency of stools.
- Calculate fluid requirements; encourage increased fluid intake.
- Encourage child to sip slowly to reduce cramping and enhance absorption.
- Serve very cold, half-strength, flavored liquid feedings.
- Offer low-residue, low-lactose foods that do not irritate the GI mucosa.
- Administer antidiarrheal medication; monitor effectiveness.

☐ EVALUATION CRITERIA/DESIRED OUTCOMES

The child
- Is not dehydrated
- Has soft-formed stool at least every second to third day

NURSING DIAGNOSIS #3

Impairment of skin integrity related to radiation therapy

Rationale: Some degree of skin reaction occurs with radiation therapy. Early reactions include blanching or erythema of the skin and mucous membranes; late reactions include dryness, pruritus, peeling, blistering, and loss of tissue (e.g., epidermis, hair) on/around the area targeted for radiation.

☐ GOAL

The child's skin will remain intact; will be soothed and healed.

☐ IMPLEMENTATION

- Explain to child/parents that the indelible dye markings delineating areas to be treated or blocked out of the radiation field will be made on skin and must not be altered or washed off.
- Review skin care
  - do not rub or use soap, lotions, deodorants, or heating pad on area
  - wear soft, loose clothing next to area; avoid clothing that rubs or constricts the area
  - apply recommended cream to area twice daily until skin has returned to normal; cornstarch may be used to help control dampness or pruritus
  - avoid sun exposure to area for 1 year after end of treatments
  - use sunscreen with protection factor of 15 or greater
- Observe and report skin problems (e.g., erythema, tautness, itching, dryness, blistering, and shedding).
- Dress draining areas with nonadhering dressings, tubular stretch bandages, and nonallergenic tape.

☐ EVALUATION CRITERIA/DESIRED OUTCOMES

The child
- Has no erythema, blistering, weeping, dryness, or pruritus
- Has soft, supple, intact skin

NURSING DIAGNOSIS #4

a. **Knowledge deficit** regarding radiation therapy
b. **Fear/anxiety** related to perception of radiation therapy
c. **Altered growth and development** related to long-term effects of radiation therapy

Rationale: Children and adults are frightened by situations and feelings they do not understand. The general population is not knowledgeable about radiation therapy. The child/parents will need information regarding the specific course of treatment, what they can expect, and what side effects to be aware of. As survival/cure rates increase, health care professionals are becoming more cognizant of the long-term effects of a cancer diagnosis and antineoplastic treatment on normal growth and development, including psychologic/cognitive functioning.

☐ GOAL

The child/parents will have adequate knowledge of the radiation therapy plan and its effects.

☐ IMPLEMENTATION

- Teach the purpose, possible side effects, and expected outcome of radiation therapy; assist to cooperate with treatment and care regimen.
- Instruct in what to expect, especially noises and sensations during the treatment.
- Arrange tour of radiation department; introduce to personnel and view equipment.
- Provide information booklet from radiation department, if available, to reinforce verbal teaching.
- Provide time for questions and expressions of fears/concerns.
- Correct misconceptions about radiation therapy.
- Arrange discussion with another child of similar age to share radiation treatment experience.
- Instruct in how to cope with/manage side effects.
- Provide written instructions on skin care, dietary modifications, appointment times for treatments, medications, and phone numbers to call for information.
- Provide a list of treatment dates/physician appointments.
- Discuss parental fears and concerns about possible long-term effects; correct misconceptions and reinforce correct perceptions.
- Emphasize the importance of maintaining normal family life, school schedules, and disciplinary routines as possible.
- Assist parents to identify the child's normal needs/experiences and integrate them with those imposed by the diagnosis and treatment.
- Provide a phone number to call for concerns regarding developmental needs.
- Refer to community agencies and supports.

☐ EVALUATION CRITERIA/DESIRED OUTCOMES

The child/parents
- Describe proposed radiation treatment plan and aims
- List side effects and their management
- List radiation treatment, physician appointment times and dates
- Verbalize strategies for maintaining near-normal family life

The Child Requiring Range-of-Motion Exercises

Definition/Discussion

Range-of-motion (ROM) exercises are those in which a nurse, child, or family member moves each joint through as full a range of movement as possible without causing pain. *Active* ROM is performed by the child without any assistance; *active-assistive* ROM is carried out by the child with assistance from the nurse/therapist/family member; *passive* ROM is performed by the nurse/therapist/family member without assistance from the child.

Nursing Assessment

☐ **PERTINENT HISTORY**

Musculoskeletal disease/injury/congenital defect, mechanism of injury (if applicable), degree of function, medical/surgical history, medication history, allergies

☐ **PHYSICAL FINDINGS**

Current level of ROM, level of consciousness, development of musculoskeletal structures

☐ **PSYCHOSOCIAL CONCERNS/ DEVELOPMENTAL FACTORS**

Age, sex, developmental level, living situation, ability to meet activities of daily living, previous level of activity, usual coping mechanisms

☐ **PATIENT AND FAMILY KNOWLEDGE**

Necessity and principles of ROM exercises, complications that can occur if ROM exercises are not regularly performed, level of knowledge, readiness and willingness to learn

Nursing Care

☐ **LONG-TERM GOAL**

The child will maintain joint mobility and will develop muscular strength and endurance; the child will not develop atrophy, weakness, contracture, degeneration.

NURSING DIAGNOSIS #1
a. **Impaired physical mobility** related to condition (specify)
b. **Potential for injury** related to immobility

Rationale: There are a number of conditions and situations that render children immobile and at risk for developing complications from immobility (e.g., congenital defect, degenerative neuromuscular disease, trauma, coma, injury requiring traction). Complications that can occur if ROM exercises are not correctly performed on a regular basis include contracture of the joints, muscle atrophy, weakness, and general degeneration of all body systems. The choice of active or passive ROM exercises is made based on physician preference and child's ability and tolerance.

☐ **GOAL**

The child will maintain joint mobility, muscular strength, and circulation.

☐ **IMPLEMENTATION**

* Explain at appropriate cognitive level what you will be doing and why.
* Reassure the child.
* Instruct to breathe normally during either passive or active exercises; holding the breath can place undue strain on the cardiorespiratory system.
* Perform ROM exercises on a firm surface when possible (not in bed) to increase child proprioceptive information.
* Start with joints nearest trunk (e.g., shoulders, hips); distal joints will loosen up and be easier to exercise.
* Support all joints involved during the exercises; stabilize proximal and distal joints.
* Go slowly and smoothly to let muscles work with you; do not use jerking movements.
* Shake a spastic muscle gently to pull muscle out.
* Incorporate ROM into other activities when possible (e.g., bath, games); make it a positive experience for child.

- Adapt ROM to the child's specific needs
  Neck
  - extension: position the head as if looking upward
  - flexion: position head as if looking at the toes
  - lateral flexion: move head from one side to the other, keeping the ear near the shoulder
  - rotation: use a twisting motion, move head side to side, chin to shoulder, as though the child were looking from one side to the other

  Shoulder: put your hand on child's shoulder with fingers on scapula to stabilize
  - flexion: raise the arm forward and overhead
  - extension: return the arm to the side of the body
  - hyperextension: raise arm backwards away from front of body
  - vertical abduction: swing the arm outward and upward from the side of the body
  - vertical adduction: return the arm to the side of the body
  - horizontal adduction: swing the arm up and across the chest
  - horizontal abduction: return the arm back to side of body and beyond midline
  - internal rotation: with arm at 90° angle to the body and elbow bent at 90°, rotate shoulder so forearm and fingers point towards toes
  - external rotation: with arm at 90° angle to body and elbow bent at 90°, rotate shoulder so forearm and fingers point up to head

  Elbow (these movements can be performed in conjunction with shoulder movements)
  - flexion: bend the elbow
  - extension: straighten the elbow
  - forearm separation: with elbow bent at 90° and touching side of body, have palm up
  - forearm pronation; with elbow bent at 90° and touching side of body, rotate forearm so palm faces down

  Wrist
  - flexion: grasping the palm and supporting the arm with your other hand, bend the wrist forward
  - extension: straighten the wrist
  - hyperextension: bend wrist backwards beyond midline
  - radial deviation: bend the wrist toward the thumb
  - ulnar deviation: bend the wrist toward the little finger
  - circumduction: move the wrist in circular motion

  Fingers and thumb
  - flexion: bend the fingers and thumb onto the palm
  - extension: return them to their original position and beyond
  - abduction: spread the fingers
  - adduction: return the fingers to the closed position
  - circumduction: move the thumb in a circular motion

  Hip and knee (may be exercised together; place one hand under the knee, with the other hand supporting the heel)
  - flexion: lift the leg, bending the knee as far as possible toward the child's head
  - extension: return the leg to the hard surface and straighten; with child lying on side, position yourself behind child with one hand on child's hip, the other supporting top leg with knee bent; while stabilizing hip, gently pull leg back
  - abduction: with the leg flat, move the entire leg out toward the edge of the surface
  - adduction: bring the leg back toward the midline or center of the surface
  - internal rotation: bend knee 90°, turn lower leg outward so hip rotates inward
  - external rotation: bend knee 90°, turn lower leg inward so hip rotates externally

  Ankle
  - dorsiflexion: cup the heel with your hand and rest the sole of the foot against your forearm; steady the leg just above the ankle with your other hand and put pressure against the child's toes with your arm to flex the ankle (in active ROM the child can do this by moving the toes toward the anterior leg)
  - plantar flexion: move your hand from above the ankle to grasp the ball of the foot; move the other arm away from the toes and push the foot downward to point the toes (in active ROM, the child can do this by pointing the toes downward)
  - inversion: grasp forefoot and point toes inward; stabilize above ankle with opposite hand
  - eversion: grasp forefoot and point toes outward; stabilize above ankle with opposite hand
  - circumduction: rotate the foot on the ankle, first in one direction and then in the other

  Toes
  - flexion: curl the toes downward
  - extension: straighten toes and carefully stretch back

  Isometrics: have cooperative child contract the abdominals, gluteals, quadriceps, and upper arms, hold for 2 or 3 seconds, then relax the muscles; rest and repeat
- Perform/instruct that each exercise should be done the same number of times on each side of the body to ensure balanced mobility and strength.
- Include rest periods between exercises, even with passive ROM, to avoid fatigue and undue exertion on the cardiopulmonary system.

☐ EVALUATION CRITERIA/DESIRED OUTCOMES

The child

- Participates in ROM exercises as appropriate
- Denies fatigue or cardiopulmonary distress
- Maintains joint mobility and muscle strength

NURSING DIAGNOSIS #2

Knowledge deficit regarding ROM exercises

Rationale: Children who are temporarily or permanently immobile are at risk for developing complications related to immobility and must perform or have someone perform ROM exercises on a regular basis. Children/parents need instruction and demonstrations to perform these exercises correctly at home.

☐ GOAL

The child/parents will correctly demonstrate ROM exercises; will understand the implications of not performing ROM exercises.

☐ IMPLEMENTATION

- Instruct in ROM exercises as outlined above to ensure that principles are correctly understood.
- Demonstrate the exercises and the movements for all joints; allow time for a return demonstration.
- Provide written instructions including pictorial representations of all the exercises to provide further guidance and a reference after discharge.
- Instruct regarding the implications of not performing ROM exercises regularly.

☐ EVALUATION CRITERIA/DESIRED OUTCOMES

The child/family

- Verbalizes principles of ROM exercises
- Performs ROM exercises correctly on all joints with minimal prompting and assistance
- Describes implications and potential complications that can occur if ROM is not performed correctly and on a regular basis

The Child undergoing Renal Transplantation

Definition/Discussion

Renal transplantation entails removing a functioning kidney from a living related donor or from a cadaver and transplanting it into the right or left fossa of the recipient. Renal vessels are anastomosed to the recipient's iliac artery and vein. The ureter is transplanted into the bladder or anastomosed to recipient's ureter. Renal transplantation is the treatment for end-stage renal disease (ESRD) and provides an alternative to dialysis with its increasing requirements, financial restraints, and needs for quality control. A successful renal transplant can allow a child to return to an almost normal life. Most potential kidney recipients have a long waiting period because of a lack of suitable and available kidneys.

Pre-op tissue typing ensures as histocompatible a transplant as possible. The highest degree of compatibility is with identical twins, then with a sibling, then parent, and, lastly, with a nonrelative. The transplant or allograft is a foreign body within the recipient that stimulates the antigen-antibody reaction, possibly leading to rejection. Types of rejection include
- *hyperacute rejection:* occurs on the operating room table
- *acute rejection:* occurs within the first year postoperatively
- *chronic rejection:* the rejection process continues despite repeated efforts to increase immunosuppression. A child can survive several bouts of acute rejection, but once chronic rejection begins, it can become an insidious, irreversible process resulting in loss of the transplant. About 30%-40% of cadaver organs and 10%-20% of kidneys from live, related donors are rejected.

Pre-op management aims to put the child in as normal a metabolic state as possible via dialysis and dietary measures. It also includes eliminating potential sources of post-op infection (e.g., extraction of carious teeth, removal of infected kidneys in those with chronic pyelonephritis or polycystic disease).

Nursing Assessment

☐ PERTINENT HISTORY

End-stage renal disease; history of chronic renal failure treated either by hemodialysis or peritoneal dialysis; age, presence of associated disease (e.g., diabetes, lupus, prune belly syndrome, nephrotic syndrome)

☐ PHYSICAL FINDINGS

As for chronic renal failure (refer to *The Child with Chronic Renal Failure,* page 66); normal lower urinary tract outflow; results of lab tests (e.g., BUN, creatinine, electrolytes), immunologic evaluation

☐ PSYCHOSOCIAL CONCERNS/ DEVELOPMENTAL FACTORS

Anxiety, fear about prognosis/possible rejection; possible body-image disturbance accepting donated kidney as part of self and physical changes from immunosuppressive medications; donor anxiety regarding danger to own health, possible rejection; habits (e.g., bedtime/feeding routines, what comforts child, favored objects)

☐ PATIENT AND FAMILY KNOWLEDGE

All options for treatment, risks/benefits of transplant versus continued dialysis, expectations of transplant, prescribed medications/side effects; home care and outpatient routine; level of knowledge, readiness and willingness to learn

Nursing Care

☐ LONG-TERM GOAL

The child/parents will adjust and adhere to a lifelong medical regimen imposed by the kidney transplant.

NURSING DIAGNOSIS #1

Anxiety related to fear of unknown, lack of understanding of procedure

Rationale: Lack of knowledge causes increased level of stress, discomfort, and anxiety.

GOAL

The child/parents will verbalize decreased anxiety and satisfactory knowledge of pre- and post-op instructions; will exhibit behavior consistent with decreased anxiety (e.g., uninterrupted sleep, decreased somatic complaints, engage in age-appropriate activities).

IMPLEMENTATION

- Ask the school-age child/adolescent how it feels now to finally approach the reality of receiving a new kidney (usual feelings include euphoria, moderate apprehension, and anxiety, and fear of failure); if child is an infant or toddler, discuss these issues with parents; share that these feelings are commonly experienced by others in same situation, and are normal and expected; know that the child/parents need you to help sort out, interpret, and suggest ways to cope with the many feelings, concerns, and questions.
- Assess current knowledge about the surgery and what the child/parents want and need to know; usual questions revolve around potential for rejection of transplant, the donor, the need for post-op dialysis, drugs, radiation, limited isolation, overview of surgical day, pain, and discomfort; teach as needed; have child return demonstrate turning, deep breathing, effective coughing, use of pillow splint; be aware that these children/parents are usually much better informed than most surgical children and tend to ask more questions; be honest; provide current information; tailor pre-op teaching to child's developmental level (e.g., play, pictures, discussion).
- Assess need to discuss potential post-op complications; be open, honest, and answer all questions.
- Provide tour of ICU.
- Reassure that a kidney can experience several bouts of acute rejection and still function.
- Reassure that feelings of euphoria and depression often result from taking steroids, and that these feelings will probably be short lived; help child to express feelings to you/parents, as a way of dealing with them.
- Introduce the school-age chid and/or adolescent to a peer who has had a transplant so they can discuss experiences.

EVALUATION CRITERIA/DESIRED OUTCOMES

The child/family

- Exhibits behaviors indicative of and verbalizes a decreased level of anxiety
- Indicates understanding of pre-op teaching

NURSING DIAGNOSIS #2

Alteration in urinary elimination (oliguria) related to kidney rejection

---

Rationale: *Following transplant the body may attempt to reject the foreign protein by a severe antibody reaction that may impair renal functioning and cause symptoms of acute renal failure and rejection.*

GOAL

The child will maintain appropriate urinary output; will be free from rejection.

IMPLEMENTATION

- Observe for signs of acute rejection of kidney transplant (e.g., fever, increased blood pressure, swollen tender kidney, decreased urine, proteinuria, weight gain, complaints of "getting the flu"); report significant findings.
- Explain any necessity for temporary post-op dialysis (especially with a cadaver kidney) until the transplant is functioning adequately.
- Keep accurate intake and output; weigh daily, at same time, on same scale, in same clothes.
- Assess indwelling urinary catheter for patency; irrigate as necessary; report a decrease in output.
- Check shunt or fistula frequently for patency (high incidence of thrombosis postoperatively); refer to *The Child Requiring Hemodialysis*, page 144.
- Observe child for signs of hyperkalemia (may develop if massive blood transfusions are required or stored blood is administered); monitor serum potassium level as ordered.
- Monitor acid-base balance (some base deficit will be present but pH should not fall below 7.4); check with physician as to parameters for notification.
- Monitor kidney function tests (e.g., BUN, electrolytes, creatinine, urinalysis, renogram).
- Administer immunosuppressive drugs as ordered; watch carefully for toxic effects, especially changes in white blood cell count, hemoglobin, hematocrit, liver studies, bleeding time, and lab tests indicative of extensive immunosuppressive activity (e.g., blastcell counts, antibody titers).

EVALUATION CRITERIA/DESIRED OUTCOMES

The child

- Maintains urinary output between 3-5 cc/kg/hour
- Has laboratory studies within physician or protocol designated limits
- Is free from symptoms of rejection

NURSING DIAGNOSIS #3

a. **Alteration in tissue perfusion: renal** related to fluid volume imbalance (deficit or excess)
b. **Alteration in cardiac output: decreased** related to effects of electrolyte imbalance(s) associated with fluid imbalance

Rationale: After receiving a donor kidney, the child may be anuric, oliguric, or experience a massive diuresis. While there does not seem to be a cause-and-effect relationship, in all possible outcomes the implanted kidney may experience altered tissue perfusion (e.g., inadequate blood flow to the kidneys with fluid volume deficit, fluid overload with fluid volume excess). The ability of the implanted kidney to excrete fluid affects the circulating blood volume (e.g., with massive diuresis leading to fluid volume deficit and anuria predisposing the child to fluid volume excess). In addition, adequate tissue perfusion is necessary to decrease the possibility of rejection of the implanted kidney. Prompt recognition and implementation of measures to correct the underlying fluid imbalance and its associated electrolyte imbalances (which may cause cardiac dysrhythmias leading to a decreased cardiac output) are post-op nursing priorities.

☐ **GOAL**

The child will maintain fluid and electrolyte balance and cardiac output adequate to perfuse the implanted kidney.

☐ **IMPLEMENTATION**

- Monitor vital signs, central venous pressure, peripheral pulses, and level of consciousness (LOC) every 1-4 hours; assess for signs of decreased cardiac output (e.g., dyspnea, decreased LOC, hypotension, pallor, peripheral edema).
- Record all fluid intake and measure urinary output every hour; report to physician if output falls more than 50% of the previous hour's output; adjust fluid intake as ordered by physician or unit protocol.
- Monitor serum electrolyte levels, BUN/creatinine, hemoglobin and hematocrit.
- Monitor cardiac rhythm; treat any dysrhythmias per physician's order or hospital protocol; monitor response to treatment.

☐ **EVALUATION CRITERIA/DESIRED OUTCOMES**

The child
- Has normal blood pressure, heart rate, respirations, and peripheral pulses
- Maintains urinary output of 3-5 cc/kg/hour
- Remains alert and free from symptomatic dysrhythmias
- Has stable serum electrolytes, BUN/creatinine, hemoglobin, and hematocrit

NURSING DIAGNOSIS #4

Potential for infection related to administration of immunosuppressive drugs

Rationale: Transplant children are given medications to suppress the immune system to prevent rejection. Resultant immunosuppression may render any infection life threatening. Children with chronic renal failure are at particularly high risk because the disease has already decreased the effectiveness of their immune system. Detection of infection is difficult as the immunosuppressive drugs impair the usual inflammatory response that produces the common symptoms associated with infection (e.g., increased temperature, swelling, redness).

☐ **GOAL**

The child will remain free from any infection.

☐ **IMPLEMENTATION**

- Limit contact with people outside the immediate family and hospital staff.
- Keep any infected persons away from child.
- Use scrupulous hygiene measures; provide good oral hygiene every 4 hours or as needed.
- Provide respiratory hygiene every 2-4 hours while awake
- Provide early ambulation, if possible.
- Encourage good nutrition to prevent infection and enhance healing process.
- Maintain dialysis access with aseptic technique.
- Keep indwelling catheter patent; irrigate using strict aseptic technique only on physician order; refer to *The Child with a Urethral Catheter*, page 294; discontinue as soon as possible.
- Monitor carefully for signs of any infection (e.g., slight increase in temperature, malaise, drainage, cloudy urine, frequency, lower back pain, cough).
- Obtain ordered specimens for culture and sensitivity studies promptly.
- Administer antibiotic therapy as ordered; monitor for expected and toxic effects, especially with drugs detoxified by the kidneys (e.g., gentamycin and tobramycin).

☐ **EVALUATION CRITERIA/DESIRED OUTCOMES**

The child
- Is free from nosocomial or iatrogenic infection
- Has negative bacterial cultures

NURSING DIAGNOSIS #5

a. **Alteration in nutrition: more than body requirements** related to stress, administration of steroids
b. **Fluid volume excess** related to elevated serum sodium level, associated water retention

Rationale: Steroid therapy leads to excessive sodium and glucose being retained by the body. The stress of the operation also causes increased levels of cortisone to be released, resulting in hyperglycemia and hypernatremia. Excess sodium causes a retention of body water as the body attempts to dilute the solute excess.

☐ GOAL

The child will maintain normal blood glucose and serum sodium levels.

☐ IMPLEMENTATION

- Monitor blood glucose and sodium levels daily or as ordered.
- Check vital signs at least every 4 hours, especially for hypertension, tachycardia, and increased respirations.
- Observe for signs of hyperglycemia (e.g., confusion, dry mucous membranes, increased blood sugar); initiate emergency measures as needed; refer to *The Child with Diabetes*, page 104.
- Observe for signs of edema (e.g., puffy eyes/ankles, rales, increase in weight).
- Observe for signs of hypernatremia (e.g., thirst, anxiety, restlessness, dry skin and mucous membranes); report any significant findings.
- Administer medications as ordered: insulin for glucose excess, diuretics for water retention; monitor for effectiveness and toxicity; inform physician of child responses.

☐ EVALUATION CRITERIA/DESIRED OUTCOMES

The child
- Has normal blood glucose and sodium levels
- Exhibits no signs of hyperglycemia/atremia

NURSING DIAGNOSIS #6

Knowledge deficit regarding post-op treatment regimen

Rationale: To promote compliance and foster child feelings of control, the child/parents require sufficient information regarding specific postdischarge plan.

☐ GOAL

The child/parents will verbalize understanding of possible complications of post-op course and necessary home care.

☐ IMPLEMENTATION

- Provide list of medications with dosage and schedule; list side effects of each; explain the im-

portance of adhering to prescribed dosages and where and how to obtain refills; advise to take no over-the-counter drugs unless prescribed.
- Reinforce that the immunosuppressive drugs inhibit the body's ability to cope with infections; review signs and symptoms of infection; teach strict infection-control measures; discuss ways to carry out infection control at home.
- Instruct to contact physician at first sign of cold, fever, decreased urinary output, jaundice, anorexia, weight changes, hematuria, tenderness over implant, edema, puffy eyes; provide important phone numbers and written materials.
- Reassure that as the immunosuppressive drug dosage is decreased, the body slowly learns to cope with some degree of infection.
- Explain that dosages of the immunosuppressive medications may be changed frequently as related to the child's blood level.
- Explain drug interactions and possible resultant complications; warn that severe rejection/death may occur if immunosuppressive drugs are stopped suddenly; encourage to keep accurate medication records.
- Demonstrate proper wound care; plan time for return demonstration.
- Explain food and fluid restrictions and allow child/parents to plan daily menus and intake; discuss the importance of maintaining an accurate intake and output record as an indicator of fluid balance and renal functioning; have child/parents record intake and output for several days prior to discharge.
- Instruct in daily weights, frequent blood pressure check, wearing of Medic-Alert bracelet.
- Suggest avoidance of lap seatbelts without shoulder harness as they put pressure on kidney area; advise to avoid heavy lifting.
- Allow to verbalize current feelings and anxieties; reaffirm that such feelings are usual and to be expected.
- Initiate referrals, appointments with community support groups, mental health clinics, etc., as needed for continued psychosocial support.

☐ EVALUATION CRITERIA/DESIRED OUTCOMES

The child/family
- Records daily intake and output accurately
- Identifies medications prescribed and discusses planned schedule
- Recognizes side effects of medications and signs and symptoms of infection
- Indicates intention of returning for follow-up care and contacting physician if untoward medication effects or signs/symptoms of infection occur
- Recognizes signs and symptoms of rejection and how to contact physician if these occur

The Child with Reye's Syndrome

Definition/Discussion

Reye's syndrome is an acute, life-threatening illness involving hepatic, metabolic, and neurologic dysfunctions. There is a buildup of ammonia in the blood and a rapid form of liver damage caused by fatty tissue degeneration. It generally follows a viral illness such as influenza or chickenpox.

Nursing Assessment

☐ PERTINENT HISTORY

Course of recent acute illness (e.g., varicella, influenza) followed by 2-5 days of relative improvement; extrinsic (e.g., aspirin, antiemetics)/environmental (e.g., herbicides, pesticides) toxins; other family members ill; usual weight

☐ PHYSICAL FINDINGS

Vital signs, neurologic status, fluid balance, skin integrity; SGOT/SGPT, lumbar puncture, glucose/blood ammonia levels, bilirubin, prothrombin, arterial blood gases, liver biopsy result; Lovejoy's clinical stage (based on the degree of encephalopathy and cerebral edema)
- *stage I:* anorexia; lethargy; persistent vomiting; increasing blood pressure, pulse, and respiratory rate; somnolence; elevated liver enzymes
- *stage II:* behavior changes (e.g., irritability, hostility, disorientation, confusion, moaning, screaming, or strange crying), hyperventilation, moderately abnormal EEG, inappropriate verbalization, sluggish pupils
- *stage III:* coma, decorticate rigidity, Cheyne-Stokes respirations, Babinski's sign, pupillary light reflexes, and oculocephalic reflex (doll's eyes)
- *stage IV:* deepening coma, decerebrate rigidity, opisthotonic posturing (arched back), fixed and dilated pupils, absent oculocephalic reflex
- *stage V:* loss of deep-tendon reflexes, flaccidity, papilledema, seizures, respiratory arrest, isoelectric EEG, no pupil reflexes or response to painful stimuli

☐ PSYCHOSOCIAL CONCERNS/ DEVELOPMENTAL FACTORS

Developmental level, coping mechanisms, habits (e.g., bedtime/feeding routines, what comforts child, favored objects), impact of sequelae or death, socioeconomic level

☐ PATIENT AND FAMILY KNOWLEDGE

Disease process, current cognitive abilities, critical care unit experience, level of knowledge, readiness and willingness to learn

Nursing Care

☐ LONG-TERM GOAL

The child will return to home and family with mimimal residual effects; OR the child will maintain stable vital functions throughout rehabilitation and convalescence; OR (if disease advances) the child will be sustained with compassion and dignity until life-support systems have been disconnected; the family will cope with grief and loss.

NURSING DIAGNOSIS #1
a. **Alteration in tissue perfusion: cerebral, cardiopulmonary, peripheral** related to disease process
b. **Ineffective breathing pattern** related to increased intracranial pressure (ICP)
c. **Potential for injury** related to seizures or combative, restless behavior

Rationale: Damage to the cellular mitochondria leads to cerebral edema and increased ICP resulting in the potential for seizures. Increased ICP leads to hyperventilation, irregular respiration patterns, and eventual respiratory arrest. Therapeutic coma may be induced with barbiturates to decrease brain metabolism and oxygen demand, thus reducing cerebral edema by enhancing cerebral vasoconstriction.

GOAL

The child will maintain/regain neurologic function; will maintain adequate respiratory function; will be free from injury.

IMPLEMENTATION

- Position child on side with head in neutral alignment and head of bed elevated 30°; turn gently every 2 hours.
- Institute seizure precautions; pad sides of bed and protect from injury; have oxygen, emergency drugs, intubation and suction equipment readily available; refer to *The Child with Epilepsy*, page 122.
- Monitor level of consciousness (LOC), reflexes every hour; refer to *The Child with Increased Intracranial Pressure*, page 160.
- Monitor vital signs continuously for increased blood pressure, decreased pulse, and irregular respirations.
- Monitor for cyanosis, increased restlessness, tachypnea; auscultate breath sounds every 2 hours; administer humidified oxygen as ordered; monitor blood gases and report abnormalities.
- Have endotracheal tubes and mechanical ventilator readily available; assist with establishment of endotracheal intubation and mechanical ventilation to control pCO_2 levels.
- Maintain pressure lines (e.g., arterial and central venous) as appropriate.
- Suction mucus and secretions from mouth and nares as needed; hyperoxygenate child before and after suctioning; limit suctioning to 5-10 seconds to avoid increasing ICP.
- Assist with insertion of ICP monitoring device if child progresses to stage III; keep lines patent; monitor ICP at least every hour and report sustained increases; employ aseptic technique at insertion site; hyperventilate if ICP increases over 15-20 mm Hg; explain procedures in smooth, calm manner.
- Administer osmotic diuretics (e.g., mannitol) as ordered; monitor for effectiveness, side effects; know that a rebound increase in ICP can occur with prolonged use.
- Know that a coma may be therapeutically induced with barbiturates if child has ICP greater than 20 mm Hg for 4 hours or longer; ensure all alarm systems or monitoring equipment are operational; monitor cerebral perfusion pressure (mean arterial pressure minus ICP).
- Taper barbiturate therapy gradually as ordered as child begins to improve and ICP normalizes.
- Eliminate or reduce noxious environmental/excessive stimuli (e.g., bright lights, loud noises, monitors, radios, talking, sudden or unanticipated movements) as possible; organize nursing procedures and activities to provide rest.
- Give soothing sensory stimulation (e.g., stroking, touching while talking or humming to child) (not appropriate in Lovejoy's stage II).

EVALUATION CRITERIA/DESIRED OUTCOMES

The child

- Has no seizure activity or recovers from seizures free from injury
- Maintains/regains LOC
- Has stable vital signs
- Maintains ICP at less than 15 mm Hg
- Has normal respiratory rate and pattern for age

NURSING DIAGNOSIS #2

a. **Fluid volume deficit** related to nausea and vomiting, NPO status
b. **Alteration in fluid volume: excess** related to metabolic dysfunction, aggressive management
c. **Ineffective thermoregulation** related to disease process, increased ICP

Rationale: The child may be dehydrated initially from nausea and vomiting. Hyperthermia resulting from increased ICP will further disrupt the fluid balance. Aggressive treatment can result in fluid overload coupled with metabolic dysfunctions of the disease.

GOAL

The child will reestablish acid-base/fluid and electrolyte balance; will maintain temperature within normal limits.

IMPLEMENTATION

- Maintain NPO status; keep nasogastric (NG) tube patent; refer to *The Child Requiring Nasogastric Intubation*, page 194; measure gastric drainage to calculate replacement fluids.
- Give mouth care every 4 hours; clean tongue and teeth; apply moisturizing cream to nostrils and lips.
- Initiate parenteral fluids as ordered; calculate caloric intake; monitor glucose levels; administer insulin as ordered; regulate drip precisely; refer to *The Child Receiving Total Parenteral Nutrition*, page 276.
- Monitor intake and output every hour; insert Foley catheter and record urine output hourly; measure urine specific gravity every 8 hours.
- Report temperature elevations over 38.5°C (101.2°F); maintain normal temperature with tepid sponge baths/hypothermia blanket.

EVALUATION CRITERIA/DESIRED OUTCOMES

The child

- Is free from vomiting or aspiration
- Has good skin turgor, moist mucous membranes

- Has urine output of at least 1 cc/kg/hour with specific gravity of 1.003-1.020
- Maintains blood glucose within normal range
- Maintains temperature between 36°-37°C

NURSING DIAGNOSIS #3

a. **Impaired physical mobility** related to altered LOC
b. **Potential for injury** related to impaired clotting mechanisms, altered LOC

Rationale: Immobility inhibits circulation of blood throughout the tissues, allowing for breakdown of tissue. Liver dysfunction leads to platelet coagulopathies and potential for hemorrhage. Unresponsiveness or coma predisposes the child to corneal abrasions as a result of the inability to blink.

☐ **GOAL**

The child will be free from skin breakdown, corneal abrasions; will be free from bruises, bleeding.

☐ **IMPLEMENTATION**

- Refer to *The Child at Risk for Hazards of Immobility*, page 156.
- Inspect and record skin every 8 hours; keep skin clean and dry.
- Avoid pressure, particularly on areas of bony prominence; use air mattress, alternating pressure mattress, or water bed.
- Turn carefully every 2 hours; maintain appropriate head elevation (usually 30°) and alignment; massage bony prominences with each turn and as necessary.
- Give passive range-of-motion exercises every 8 hours and as necessary.
- Inspect skin for petechiae and bruising; hematest stool and drainage daily; administer antacids as ordered.
- Administer vitamin K as ordered; be prepared to administer fresh-frozen plasma; inspect all injection sites for bleeding.
- Apply sandbag pressure to liver biopsy site, turn child on right side, examine dressings for bleeding and observe abdomen for changes in softness every 15 minutes.
- Irrigate eyes with artificial tears every 2 hours; apply eye patches; tape eyes shut if necessary.

☐ **EVALUATION CRITERIA/DESIRED OUTCOMES**

The child
- Demonstrates no reddened or broken areas of skin
- Is free from corneal abrasions
- Shows no evidence of bleeding

NURSING DIAGNOSIS #4

a. **Ineffective individual/family coping** related to seriousness of disease process, treatment
b. **Anticipatory grieving** related to possible loss of child

Rationale: Reye's syndrome occurs suddenly and progresses rapidly giving the child/family little time to adjust to the illness. The child may be mildly or seriously ill. The parents must also cope with the potential neurologic impairment or death of the child.

☐ **GOAL**

The child/parents will cope adaptively with stress of diagnosis, hospitalization, treatment and prognosis.

☐ **IMPLEMENTATION**

- Give realistic, consistent information; attempt to be present when physician discusses prognosis/progress so this information can be clarified or reinforced; accept crisis/grief responses; refer to *The Family Requiring Crisis Intervention*, page 85, *The Parent Experiencing Grief and Loss*, page 139, and *The Child Who is Dying/Terminal*, page 116.
- Allow parent(s) to provide care when appropriate; encourage touching, stroking, and comforting child to reduce fears.
- Give repeated explanations of test and treatments as required.
- Encourage to bring tapes/pictures of family/friends when they cannot visit.
- Encourage expression of fears, grief, feelings of helplessness, guilt, anger, and despair outside child's hearing range.
- Arrange for professional counseling/spiritual support as indicated.

☐ **EVALUATION CRITERIA/DESIRED OUTCOMES**

The child/parents
- Cope adaptively with stress and illness
- Participate in care as able

NURSING DIAGNOSIS #6

Knowledge deficit regarding disease process, home care, neurologic sequelae

Rationale: Many parents are not familiar with Reye's syndrome or may harbor misconceptions. If knowledge deficits exist, child/parents cannot appropriately manage long-term rehabilitation.

☐ GOAL

The child/parents will understand Reye's syndrome; will manage neurologic sequelae at home.

☐ IMPLEMENTATION

- Give written and verbal instructions regarding pathophysiology of Reye's syndrome; tell how to contact physician/hospital regarding behavioral changes or new signs of illness/infection.
- Tell parents to expect nightmares, restless sleep, dependent behavior, fear, and anxiety until child has adjusted to stress of illness and hospitalization experience; help them identify methods of gentle reassurance without harmful overprotectiveness.
- Have parents talk with schoolteachers about possible slowness to complete work, distractibility, inattention, and forgetfulness (normal functioning may not return for several weeks).
- Direct to counseling and support group if indicated.
- Help parents contact National Reye's Syndrome Foundation for additional information, location of nearest chapter.

☐ EVALUATION CRITERIA/DESIRED OUTCOMES

The child/parents
- Discuss pathology of disease in own words
- Contact health care provider regarding signs of illness
- State behavior changes to be expected

The Child with a Right Atrial Catheter

Definition/Discussion

A right atrial catheter (RAC) is an indwelling catheter made of polymeric silicone rubber that can be left in place for long-term use. The catheter is positioned in the right atrium, tunnels through the subcutaneous tissue of the chest, and exits between the nipple and the sternum. Two incisions are made, one below the right clavicle (entrance site) and the second between the right nipple and the sternum (exit site). A tunnel is made with long forceps through the subcutaneous tissue between the upper and lower incisions. The catheter is pulled through the tunnel and inserted into the selected vein. The catheter may enter the vein by cutdown or a percutaneous stick; in the latter case, there would only be one incision at the exit site. The catheter is then advanced into the right atrium. A Dacron cuff lies about midway between the entrance and exit sites to help anchor the catheter in place and also act as a protective barrier to prevent ascending infection.

The single, double, or multiple-lumen catheters are used to administer total parenteral nutrition (TPN), blood/blood products, and medications, and to draw venous blood samples. Multilumen catheters have the same uses as the double-lumen catheter with the advantage of an additional access line.

The catheters are inserted by a surgical procedure that lasts about one hour. They can be placed in the treatment room, intensive care unit, or in the operating room. Usually meperidine (Demerol), promethazine (Phenergan), and chlorpromazine (Thorazine) are administered for sedation. General anesthesia may be indicated (in the operating room), particularly for small children who have difficulty lying still. Right atrial catheter care includes changing the dressing and injection cap, irrigation, drawing blood samples, administering IV push medications. Each institution has specific procedures for the care of these catheters. Use the following guidelines, but follow the procedures that your institution has outlined.

Nursing Assessment

☐ PERTINENT HISTORY

Need for long-term chemotherapy (e.g., antibiotics, antineoplastics), TPN, frequent blood-product re-placement, frequent blood samples where repeated venipuncture presents a risk, frequent central venous pressures readings; date of catheter placement, indications for placement

☐ PHYSICAL FINDINGS

Immunologic/hematologic/nutritional status, age, weight, specific factors reflecting condition requiring catheter insertion

☐ PSYCHOSOCIAL CONCERNS/ DEVELOPMENTAL FACTORS

Interpretation/acceptance of catheter; body image; fear, anxiety, effect of disease on self-concept; family interaction

☐ PATIENT AND FAMILY KNOWLEDGE

Rationale for, function, care, and operation of catheter; site care; administration of medications and daily irrigation; reason for and expectations of therapy; level of knowledge, readiness and willingness to learn

Nursing Care

☐ LONG-TERM GOAL

The child's catheter will remain patent and in place, free from complications to allow proper, safe administration of nutrition/medications; the child will remain free from infection; the child/parents will learn catheter care; the child will continue regular life-style with the presence of the catheter.

NURSING DIAGNOSIS #1

Anxiety related to insertion of right atrial catheter

Rationale: The child/parents are likely to have concerns about the insertion procedure. Providing information can promote feelings of control and decrease anxiety.

GOAL

The child/parents will verbalize decreased anxiety about the insertion procedure.

IMPLEMENTATION

Pre-operatively
- Assess what is known about the catheter; elicit fears, concerns, questions; provide information.
- Explain procedure; use pictures, drawings, and written information to describe location and uses.
- Provide the child with a catheter of the same type to be inserted; allow the child to see and touch the catheter.
- Explain postprocedure routines (e.g., frequent inspection of insertion site, vital sign monitoring, dressing changes); answer specific questions.

EVALUATION CRITERIA/DESIRED OUTCOMES

The child/parents
- Verbalize decreased level of anxiety.
- Indicate understanding of insertion procedure, use of the catheter, expected post-op routine

---

NURSING DIAGNOSIS #2

Potential for injury related to catheter occlusion/disconnection, air embolism

Rationale: Air embolism and hemorrhage may result after the RAC is placed if it ruptures or becomes disconnected. In addition, the catheter may become occluded by clot formation if not properly irrigated when not in use or after drawing blood.

GOAL

The child will be free from complications of RAC insertion; will maintain a patent catheter.

IMPLEMENTATION

- Apply pressure dressings at the entrance and exit sites for the first 24 hours; observe dressings for drainage (the sites may produce serosanguinous drainage for several days, especially if child is thrombocytopenic, but this should be controlled with pressure dressings); notify physician if bleeding continues; expect some bruising and tenderness along the tunnel.
- Keep a flow sheet of intake and output including the blood sample volume withdrawn at the bedside.
- Assess for signs of venous thrombosis (e.g., tenderness and edema of the shoulder, neck, and arm, usually on the side of the catheter), unexplained difficulty infusing IV fluids, edema, subcutaneous fluid along the tunnel, or leakage around the catheter at least every 4 hours.

- Irrigate catheter as ordered with heparin flush (per hospital protocol and after drawing each blood sample) to prevent thrombosis; know that the frequency of irrigation and concentration of heparin used varies depending on the RAC, the child's vulnerability to the effects of heparin, and hospital/physician protocols; check product information literature for the specific volume the catheter holds.

Irrigation
- Gather supplies
  - povidone-iodine and alcohol swabs
  - 10 cc syringe
  - 1 inch, 21-25 gauge needles
  - heparin flush (usually 100 units heparin/cc; follow hospital policy for heparin concentration and irrigation volume)
- Wash hands; clamp catheter over protective tape if not already clamped.
- Cleanse top of heparin flush bottle with alcohol or povidone-iodine swab; allow to air dry.
- Prepare syringe with appropriate amount of heparin flush.
- Cleanse junction of catheter and IV tubing with 3 alcohol and 3 povidone-iodine swabs working around junction out to periphery; allow to air dry.
- Insert needle, unclamp catheter, and inject heparin flush.
- Clamp catheter while infusing the last 0.5 cc of solution to prevent backflow of blood.
- Connect IV tubing and unclamp catheter; loop the catheter and tape to chest dressing.
- Document type and amount of irrigation solution used and ease of flow into catheter.

Blood Sampling
- Draw a discard sample of 3-5 cc according to hospital protocol; then withdraw sample as ordered through a single-lumen catheter or through the proximal lumen of a multilumen catheter; irrigate using procedure outlined above; attach a sterile injection cap securely or reconnect the IV after withdrawing ordered blood sample; document amount of blood drawn and child's response to procedure.
- Ask what usually facilitates blood withdrawal if you have difficulty withdrawing blood (catheter may be lodged against the wall of the atrium) or have child try one or a combination of the following to facilitate obtaining desired blood sample:
  - change position (roll to side, sit upright, lie flat, etc.)
  - take a deep breath or cough
  - perform Valsalva's maneuver (unless contraindicated because of risk of bradycardia)
  - raise one or both arms overhead, or lower arms

IV Fluid Administration
- Infuse IV at ordered rate; flush catheter with normal saline (or dextrose if appropriate) before and after administering any medications not compatible with IV solution; double check that IV is re-

started after drawing blood or giving medication; ensure that solutions are monitored by electronic pumps (not controllers that just regulate amounts, do not infuse against pressure) and that the pumps are not inadvertently turned off.
- Teach child to help keep tubing unkinked.
- Prevent air embolism by taping all connections securely; remove air bubbles from IV tubing and syringes; clamp catheter before changing injection cap or tubing.

Injection Cap
- Know that when the RAC is not connected to continuous IVs (or one of the lumens is not connected), the lumens are capped like a heparin lock, enabling the child to move around freely while maintaining a closed, sterile system; because the cap may be punctured several times a day, change it at least every 3-7 days according to hospital policy and each time a blood sample is taken.
- Inspect the cap integrity every 8 hours.
- Cap change
  - gather supplies (irrigation supplies, new injection cap)
  - wash hands
  - clamp catheter over protective tape and prepare supplies
  - put on sterile gloves
  - cleanse cap-catheter junction with 3 alcohol and 3 povidone-iodine swabs; allow to air dry
  - remove old cap and replace with new cap, twisting securely but without force
  - unclamp catheter and irrigate if needed (withdraw needle slowly from cap while infusing the last 0.5 cc of heparin flush to prevent backflow of blood)
  - tape cap-catheter junction securely, folding ends of tape onto itself (creating tabs to facilitate tape removal)

Catheter Damage
- Prevent catheter damage
  - use toothless clamps (e.g., bulldog or rubber-tipped hemostats) on catheter
  - keep clamp attached in close proximity to child at all times for emergency use
  - do not use scissors to remove old dressings or tape
  - use 1-inch needles for irrigation and medication administration
  - clamp only over protective tape and rotate clamp sites routinely
  - when catheter is not in use, keep coiled and secured against chest wall
- Clamp catheter close to the child's chest immediately if catheter leaks or is damaged.
- Use aseptic technique; use 3 alcohol and 3 betadine swabs to prep catheter before repairing.
- Cut off the damaged portion of the catheter with sterile scissors or scalpel (as long as more than 4 cm of catheter remains intact).

- Insert a 2-inch appropriate gauge angiocath or blunt needle into the catheter end and remove the stylus; pull back stylus before inserting so that it does not damage catheter.
- Follow the irrigation procedure and replace the injection cap or reconnect the IV fluids.
- Tape connections securely.
- Obtain appropriate permanent repair kit and repair catheter per directions.
- Document procedure and child's response.
- Check if blood culture is indicated.

☐ **EVALUATION CRITERIA/DESIRED OUTCOMES**

The child
- Is free from hemorrhage, thrombosis, air embolism
- Has good blood return prior to catheter irrigation
- Has catheter irrigated without difficulty
- Maintains catheter integrity

NURSING DIAGNOSIS #3

Potential for infection related to entry into systemic circulation, impaired skin integrity at catheter insertion site

Rationale: Once a foreign object has been introduced into the body the risk of infection is increased. Some patients may reject the catheter itself. Signs/symptoms of systemic infection include fever and chills; exit site infection includes drainage, inflammation and redness of site.

☐ **GOAL**

The child will remain free from infection.

☐ **IMPLEMENTATION**

Exit Site Care
- Check hospital protocol regarding exit site dressing change procedures; use aseptic technique at all times; assess entrance and exit sites for signs of infection with each dressing change; report minor temperature elevations as neutropenic patients have a poor immune response.
- Gather supplies
  - clean gloves
  - bag for contaminated supplies
  - sterile towel and gloves
  - hydrogen peroxide (H_2O_2), sterile H_2O
  - sterile bowl
  - 3 povidone-iodine swabsticks
  - 3 cotton-tip swabs
  - alcohol swab
  - povidone-iodine or antibiotic ointment
  - 2 x 2-inch gauze
  - 2 isolation masks

- transparent dressing
- Place child in supine position with equipment on bedside or overbed table.
- Wash hands and put on clean gloves.
- Remove and bag old dressing; loosen the dressing with an antibacterial soap if the tape removal is painful (this has not been shown to increase infection rate).
- Inspect entrance and exit sites for indication of infection (e.g., redness, ecchymosis, swelling, exudate).
- Remove gloves and wash hands; prepare sterile field, open sterile supplies onto field; pour equal amounts of H_2O_2 and H_2O into sterile bowl, open alcohol swab; put on sterile gloves
- Cleanse a 2-inch area around the exit site with 3 alcohol swabsticks with a circular motion using 1 swabstick at a time; move each swabstick from the inner to the outer aspect of the circle; do not recleanse any area with same swabstick; allow to air dry.
- Cleanse the area with H_2O_2/H_2O on cotton tip swabs using the same procedure; allow to air dry; clean catheter with 3 betadine swabs, using 1 at a time, moving from chest outward; allow to air dry.
- Apply a small amount of povidone-iodone ointment to the exit site and cover with sterile 2 x 2-inch gauze; apply an occlusive transparent waterproof dressing that allows the skin to breathe.
- Permit child to bathe (with physician's order) with the dressing in place; redress site if dressing gets wet.
- Change tubing every 24-48 hours (depending on hospital policy); change dressing according to hospital policy and if wet or soiled.
- Monitor for any systemic manifestations of infection (e.g., fever, tachycardia, tachypnea, hypotension) every 4 hours; report significant findings.
- Administer antibiotics as ordered; monitor for effectiveness and toxic effects.

☐ EVALUATION CRITERIA/DESIRED OUTCOMES

The child
- Is afebrile
- Has no drainage, inflammation, or redness of exit site
- Has a negative blood culture

NURSING DIAGNOSIS #4

Disturbance in self-concept: body image related to catheter placement

Rationale: Having an artificial appliance such as an RAC may be psychologically disturbing to the child/parents and may alter child's body image related to physical appearance. The catheter's meaning to the individual, and the individual's perception of how others view the physical self are integral parts of body image.

☐ GOAL

The child will use appropriate coping strategies to promote adaptation to body-image change; the child/parents will express feelings about catheter placement (either verbally or through play), identify disturbing aspects of having catheter in place.

☐ IMPLEMENTATION

- Encourage child/parents to verbalize/play out concerns and feelings (refer to *The Child Requiring Play Therapy*, page 226); acknowledge that others have expressed similar feelings; correct any misperceptions; provide additional information as requested; provide parents opportunities to ventilate feelings without child present.
- Refer to *The Child Experiencing a Body-Image Disturbance*, page 30.
- Assess how child expects the RAC to impact upon illness, recovery, body; do not challenge unrealistic perceptions; rather, tell how you view the impact; listen and acknowledge feelings.
- Provide emotional support for feelings (e.g., "You look sad/down/anxious. Tell me what you are feeling.").
- Ask child to describe past experience(s) that may have required adjusting to a change in physical appearance; inquire as to how child coped at that time; suggest ways similar methods could be used at present; use puppet play to encourage verbalization.
- Provide a mirror so child can look at insertion site.
- Include parents and child, if age appropriate, in care.
- Arrange for child to visit with someone who has a RAC in place if appropriate or possible.

☐ EVALUATION CRITERIA/DESIRED OUTCOMES

The child
- Identifies ways of adapting to changed body image

The child/parents
- Express concerns about physical appearance with catheter in place
- View insertion site
- Participate in catheter care

NURSING DIAGNOSIS #5

Knowledge deficit regarding catheter maintenance and use at home

> **Rationale:** The child/parents must have sufficient knowledge base to manage care independently. Planned instruction and return demonstration allow time for learning and reinforcing newly-learned skill.

☐ GOAL

The child/parents will independently demonstrate correct procedure for catheter care and dressing changes; will state emergency actions to take for a damaged or dislodged catheter; will state troubleshooting and safety measures.

☐ IMPLEMENTATION

- Teach the signs of site infection (e.g., redness, warmth, inflammation, tenderness).
- Teach emergency actions for damaged catheter, dislodged injection cap, or accidental IV disconnection.
- Instruct to contact physician when the catheter becomes clotted or dislodged; provide telephone number of nurse/physician for assistance when problems with the catheter occur at home.
- Have child/parents explain and demonstrate site care and irrigation procedure.
- Have child/parents demonstrate operation of flow control device if appropriate.
- Have child/parents administer prescribed medication or TPN; monitor performance; provide appropriate positive feedback; correct improper technique; explain reasons for specific procedures.
- Ensure that school nurse and teacher know emergency/safety measures for care of catheter if appropriate; encourage parents to assist teacher in preparing for child's return.
- Refer to home health agency for follow-up care.
- Provide the child/parents with a referral number and name if any questions arise.

☐ EVALUATION CRITERIA/DESIRED OUTCOMES

The child/parents

- State emergency actions to take for damaged catheter, dislodged injection cap, or accidental IV disconnection
- Demonstrate correct dressing change/irrigation procedure
- Change injection cap correctly
- List signs of a catheter infection
- Administer prescribed medication/TPN accurately
- Identify appropriate safety/troubleshooting measures

The Child with Scoliosis

Definition/Discussion

Scoliosis is an abnormal lateral curvature of the spine; the condition sometimes includes secondary compensatory curves and rotation of vertebral bodies; occasionally the child will also have *hyperlordosis* (excessive swayback) or *kyphosis* (excessively rounded upper back). The medical treatment of scoliosis involves early detection of scoliosis and prevention of severe deformities by long-term use of orthotic devices.

Surgical correction of scoliosis is usually done with Luque or Harrington rods. Luque rods apply a transverse force on each vertebra to internally stabilize the spine. No casting or bracing is necessary; ambulation begins in 3-4 days and the child is discharged in 7-10 days. Complications include nerve damage due to threading the wire around the nerve column. Harrington rods apply a longitudinal force on the involved vertebrae via a long, rigid rod. A longer hospitalization is required. The child must usually wear a Risser body cast for 6-8 months after surgery to stabilize spine throughout the healing period. Bracing and physical therapy is used to regain lost muscle strength and limb function.

Nursing Assessment

☐ **PERTINENT HISTORY**

Birth injuries, skeletal dysplasia/age, myelomeningocele, metabolic bone disease, neurocutaneous syndrome, connective tissue disorders, developmental delays, neuromuscular disorders (e.g., muscular dystrophy), trauma, infection, radiation to spinal area, family history of scoliosis, postural habits, menarche, previous attempts to correct scoliosis

☐ **PHYSICAL FINDINGS**

Degree of curvature from front, side, back while standing erect and bending forward about 60° with arms extended and hands touching; asymmetric chest or shoulder height, prominent scapula or thoracic rib "hump," uneven hips, or sideways deviation of the spine (one hip touching the arm while the other arm hangs free); pain during undressing and examination; vital signs, respiratory status, weight, condition of skin, neurologic status/strength of lower extremities

☐ **PSYCHOSOCIAL CONCERNS/ DEVELOPMENTAL FACTORS**

Developmental level, fear, anxiety, coping mechanisms, routines/habits, relationships of child with family and peers, impact of body-image changes

☐ **PATIENT AND FAMILY KNOWLEDGE**

Previous experience with scoliosis, including bracing or surgical treatment; pre-/post-op routine, cast care; ability to understand problem; level of knowledge, readiness and willingness to learn

Nursing Care

☐ **LONG-TERM GOAL**

The child will achieve a normal life with a straight, healthy back via the least restrictive means necessary to achieve correction of curvature; the child will express a feeling of independence and responsibility for self-care and successful treatment.

NURSING DIAGNOSIS #1
a. **Ineffective individual/family coping** related to developmental age, altered body image, chronicity, complexity of treatment regimen
b. **Noncompliance** related to developmental age, altered body image, chronicity and complexity of treatment regimen

Rationale: Peer relationships are extremely important to the late school-age child and early adolescent who do not want to appear different from their peers. Visual differences such as a body cast/brace may contribute to low self-esteem, and late school-age children/early adolescents may not comply with treatments if they do not see immediate results. Caring for a child in a body cast at home takes time/energy. Family routines may be disrupted.

GOAL

The child/parents will express fears of the unknown and concerns over treatment restrictions; will express a feeling that they are not alone in facing consequences of diagnosis and treatment; will comply with the treatment plan.

IMPLEMENTATION

- Introduce to the orthotic device (e.g., allow child to touch/explore the device, show pictures of others wearing them while participating in various sports and recreational activities).
- Relate instances of successful treatment so that youth can identify with others in similar circumstances.
- Explain the importance of careful monitoring every 3-6 months; share progress as shown on periodic x-rays.
- Provide child with control by giving realistic decision-making opportunities.
- Establish trusting relationship; assist to explore feelings and to accept responsibility for cooperation with treatment plan; encourage expression of anxiety about condition and concerns (e.g., embarrassment, peer rejection, abnormal body image for the youth, fears for well-being, expense and discomfort of medical visits and surgery, guilt over not noticing something abnormal sooner).
- Offer to provide explanations to absent family members or friends whose opinions and attitudes will significantly affect the success of treatment; rehearse with the child/adolescent if they choose to share the information with others.
- Ensure understanding of all treatment regimens prior to implementation, especially length of time required to wear brace/body cast.
- Discuss clothing that will be most flattering; have some clothes brought from home to be worn after surgery or with brace.
- Assist with the application of body cast; calm child by explaining sensations to be expected.
- Help to deal with realities of limitation of body cast; explore feelings of claustrophobia and depression; teach safe methods of movement; assist with first attempts.
- Reassure female adolescents that body cast has no effect on breast development or menstrual periods; reaffirm that cast will be changed as body grows; review *The Child Experiencing a Body-Image Disturbance*, page 30.
- Provide radio, TV, telephone, social interaction with staff and other youths; encourage visitors; place necessary items within reach; encourage decorating the room with favorite posters/objects from home.
- Encourage to do as much for self as able; assist to resume as many normal activities as possible.
- Tell family members that child's feelings of anger, depression, apathy, and dependence are normal

and expected; help them to look at ways they can respond and cope to reduce tensions and to improve relationships.
- Allow time for questions; provide a written summary of what physician has said about condition and recommended plan of treatment; reinforce or repeat initial explanation as needed.

EVALUATION CRITERIA/DESIRED OUTCOMES

The child
- Adapts to changes in body image
- Develops effective coping mechanisms
- Complies with medical regimen
- Maintains normal contact with peers

The child/parents
- Express concerns and fears
- Participate in planning treatment

NURSING DIAGNOSIS #2
a. **Impaired physical mobility** related to restriction of movement/activities, altered body image
b. **Impairment of skin integrity** related to cast/brace, surgical procedure
c. **Potential for infection** related to surgical incision

Rationale: Restricted movement caused by cast/brace and restriction of some activities might discourage or limit participation in beneficial physical activities. A poorly fitting cast/brace may rub against the skin causing breakdown. Surgical procedures and breaks in the skin provide a potential for infection.

GOAL

The child will comply with activity restrictions; will participate in accepted activities; will be free from skin breakdown and infection.

IMPLEMENTATION

- Teach correct posture (e.g., sit up straight, stand erect with weight equally distributed on both feet).
- Teach that brace or jacket must be worn 23 hours a day with 30 minutes off morning and evening for exercises and general hygiene; explain that time in the brace may be gradually decreased over a 1- to 2-year period but brace must be worn at night until spine is completely mature.
- Check brace for proper fit; massage pressure areas/bony prominences at least 2 times a day
- Demonstrate abdominal and back exercises designed to strengthen muscles and to improve posture

- tilt the pelvis so the small of the back is against the floor while in supine position
- tilt pelvis so the small of the back is against the wall while standing
- tighten buttock and abdominal muscles
- do controlled deep breathing
- do push-ups with pelvic tilt
- Encourage to perform each exercise 10-25 times, twice daily, or as prescribed; praise correct performance of exercises and positive attitudes; schedule range-of-motion (ROM) exercises as necessary for the child who is immobile or has had surgery; refer to *The Child Requiring Range-of-Motion Exercises*, page 237.

Clean traction-pin sites of child in halofemoral skeletal traction with antiseptic solution (e.g., hydrogen peroxide, povidone-iodine) twice daily; gently remove crusts and exudate.

- Change position or logroll every 2 hours after surgery or when on bedrest; check for correct position of feet and forehead when in prone position.
- Keep skin clean, dry, and free from irritants; massage buttocks and bony prominences with every turn.
- Observe for skin redness and irritation caused by diminished circulation and pressure every 2 hours; ensure that stockinette, foam pads, and sheepskin pads are properly placed at pressure points.
- Check incision site every 2 hours for increased tenderness, odor, or excessive drainage.
- Provide a list of restricted activities (e.g., body-contact sports, weight lifing, horseback riding, gymnastics, trampoline, diving).
- Review practical changes for school (e.g., substitute for physical education class, adjust desk-top height, plan school seating).

☐ EVALUATION CRITERIA/DESIRED OUTCOMES

The child
- Performs exercises as prescribed
- Demonstrates correct posture
- Wears properly fitting brace as prescribed
- Has no reddened areas
- Is free from infection
- Maintains firm muscle tone

NURSING DIAGNOSIS #3
a. **Alteration in cardiac output: decreased** related to blood and fluid loss associated with surgery
b. **Impaired gas exchange** related to pre-op pulmonary compromise, surgery, 7-10 days of immobilization prior to casting and ambulation

---

Rationale: *Excessive bleeding/fluid loss without replacement causes cardiovascular compromise. Children with scoliosis often have some pulmonary compromise before surgery as the curve may cause reduced lung expansion/tidal volume. Extended immobilization after surgery may be necessary, further compromising thoracic expansion.*

☐ GOAL

The child will be free from hemorrhage; will maintain effective cardiac function; will have adequate gas exchange.

☐ IMPLEMENTATION

- Monitor and record vital signs, intake and output; color, appearance, and specific gravity of urine; skin color, tissue perfusion, capillary refill, warmth of extremities; peripheral pulses every hour until stable, then according to hospital routine.
- Observe dressing sites for bleeding; record amount of Hemovac drainage.
- Monitor breath sounds and respiratory status (e.g., rate, depth, and equality of expansion, use of accessory muscles, nasal flaring, and color) every hour until stable, then according to hospital routine.
- Encourage coughing and deep-breathing exercises every 2 hours; provide comfort measures (e.g., positioning, pain medication) prior to deep breathing; play games with child to accomplish deep breathing; associate deep-breathing schedule with something familiar to child (e.g., with every commercial, 5-10 breaths with every new TV program or after each chapter read).
- Monitor hematocrit and hemoglobin; report significant changes.
- Maintain patency and proper operation of central venous pressure line, nasogastric tube, and Foley catheter.
- Monitor IV administration every hour and as necessary; refer to *The Child with an Intravenous Catheter*, page 174.

☐ EVALUATION CRITERIA/DESIRED OUTCOMES

The child
- Maintains normal vital signs, balanced intake and output, adequate urine output, good skin color
- Maintains pre-op hematocrit and hemoglobin
- Takes 10 deep breaths and coughs every 2 hours
- Has clear and equal breath sounds with good aeration

NURSING DIAGNOSIS #4
Sensory-perceptual alteration: tactile, visual related to extensive spinal surgery, positioning

Rationale: Spinal fusion surgery carries the risk of spinal nerve damage. If the child is immobilized after surgery in a Stryker frame or CircOlectric bed, the visual range is limited.

☐ GOAL

The child will be free from neurologic/visual impairment.

☐ IMPLEMENTATION

- Monitor nerve and circulatory status of all extremities (e.g., pulses, sensation, movement, complaints of pain, color) at least every 4 hours.
- Observe and report any signs of neurologic problems (e.g., diminished swallow, loss of lateral gaze and ability to follow a moving finger, decreased cranial and spinal cord responses), headache, weakness, pain, incontinence, hyperreflexia of lower extremities, or dysesthesia (impairment of sensitivity, "pins and needles" sensation) of hands or feet.
- Stand in line of vision when talking with child, instruct others to do the same; provide prism glasses for reading or watching television when appropriate.

☐ EVALUATION CRITERIA/DESIRED OUTCOMES

The child
- Is free from neurologic impairment
- Has no tingling or feelings of heaviness in limbs
- Has full range of motion and feeling in lower extremities

NURSING DIAGNOSIS #5

Alteration in comfort: pain related to surgery, spinal fusion, iliac graft, muscle spasms

Rationale: Pain following spinal fusion surgery is significant for 3-4 days postoperatively.

☐ GOAL

The child will be as pain free as possible.

☐ IMPLEMENTATION

- Refer to *The Child Experiencing Pain*, page 216.
- Observe and investigate all complaints promptly (e.g., anorexia, nausea/vomiting, pain in chest, shortness of breath, rapid breathing or heartbeat, pain in legs, abdomen); report promptly.
- Ascertain and correct cause of pain if possible before administering analgesics/sedatives; monitor effectiveness of analgesics.

- Provide age-appropriate diversional activities and comfort measures.

☐ EVALUATION CRITERIA/DESIRED OUTCOMES

The child
- Has no verbal complaints of pain
- Is free from behaviors indicating pain
- Participates in conversation, diversional activities

NURSING DIAGNOSIS #6
a. **Alteration in bowel elimination: constipation** related to poor dietary intake, immobility
b. **Alteration in patterns of urinary elimination** related to immobility, positioning

Rationale: Constipation may result from decreased metabolic needs and the child's exerting control over the environment by refusing to eat. Inability to sit makes defecation more difficult. Embarrassment in using the bedpan may cause the child to ignore the urge to defecate causing constipation.

Urinary tract infections (UTI) are hazards of immobility because a recumbent position may cause urinary stasis in the renal pelvis. Increased calcium excretion from inactivity causes alkaline urine, which promotes bacterial growth.

☐ GOAL

The child will maintain normal elimination patterns postoperatively and while mobility is restricted.

☐ IMPLEMENTATION

- Monitor bowel and bladder function daily; give laxatives or suppositories PRN; record effectiveness.
- Observe for signs of bladder retention or infection (e.g., voiding small amounts, dysuria, frequency, fever).
- Explain the necessity of high fluid intake and high-fiber diet.
- Encourage a high-protein, low-calorie, high-fiber diet with small, frequent feedings.
- Encourage fluids (2,000-3,000 cc/day) to reduce the likelihood of UTI/constipation.

☐ EVALUATION CRITERIA/DESIRED OUTCOMES

The child
- Has soft bowel movement at least every other day
- Has adequate urine output without signs of retention or infection

NURSING DIAGNOSIS #7

Knowledge deficit regarding condition, treatment, exercises, care of appliances, follow-up care

Rationale: *If knowledge deficit exists, child/parents cannot appropriately adhere to treatment, manage appliance, or detect signs of complications.*

☐ GOAL

The child/parents will verbalize an understanding of scoliosis, treatment aims, and anticipated outcomes of selected therapeutic regimen; the child will be free from complications of treatment.

☐ IMPLEMENTATION

- Schedule a team conference with parents, child, teachers, school nurse, and friends to provide information, explore feelings and attitudes; encourage child to take part in the selection of conference participants.
- Instruct regarding exercises, restriction of activities, frequency of follow-up appointments.
- Provide verbal and written instructions regarding proper application of brace (e.g., over a T-shirt, but under pants) and brace care (e.g., mild soap and water cleansing, saddle soap to leather parts, tightening screws).
- Suggest that parent take child to orthodontist for assessment of jaw alignment because of pressure from chin rest on brace (not needed for underarm jacket type).
- Stress importance of regular, frequent follow-up appointments to ensure proper brace/jacket fit and effective wear.
- Reinforce purpose of surgery if appropriate; review hospital equipment (e.g., fracture bedpan, Stryker frame, CircOlectric bed, prism glasses for reading or watching TV, pedestal mirror, absorbent pads or disposable diapers).

- Give suggestions for rental of hospital bed or safe elevation of standard bed prior to discharge; suggest use of bedboard, firm mattress, foot board, trapeze, or rope pull.
- Teach appropriate diet to provide high fiber and prevent weight gain while meeting age/activity needs; weigh weekly on the same scale, at the same time, in the same clothes.
- Describe skin care and prevention of pressure sores; reinforce positioning, turning, deep breathing, exercises.
- Teach care of body cast; refer to *The Child with a Cast*, page 48.
- Explain that with Luque rods activities will gradually be increased to full tolerance except for contact sports, diving, trampoline, and gymnastics; teach that only sponge baths are permitted for the first 2 weeks, then showers are allowed.
- Arrange for child/parents to meet others who have had similar experiences and successfully managed.
- Arrange clinic appointments and make appropriate referrals to community service agencies (e.g., home health, physical therapy, education, mental health counseling) as needed.
- Instruct when pregnant to tell obstetrician about scoliosis correction 5°-8° shifts in curvature can occur.
- Promote community awareness by participating in inservice training sessions with school nurses, physical education teachers, public health nurses, parents, volunteers, physicians, and school administrators; discuss the scope of the program and procedure for examination and referral.

☐ EVALUATION CRITERIA/DESIRED OUTCOMES

The child/parents

- Discuss suitable plan to meet psychosocial and physical needs of child
- Comply with treatment plan
- Keep appointments as ordered for continuing medical observation and x-rays

The Child Experiencing Separation Anxiety

Definition/Discussion

Separation anxiety refers to the anticipation of danger or uncertainty that is generated by separating a child from significant others (usually parents). It occurs in older infants, toddlers, and in the early preschool years. The behaviors that accompany it can be divided into 3 recognizable stages or phases

- *protest*: begins with hospitalization or mother's absence and lasts from a few hours to 3 or 4 days; common protest behaviors (see Nursing Assessment) occur if another adult approaches child when the parents are absent
- *despair*: frequently called the mourning state or "settling in" stage, begins from 1 hour to several days following separation and lasts 1-2 days, or until discharge
- *detachment (or denial)*: period of seeming acceptance or adjustment as the child returns to normal patterns of behavior; has detached self from parents to cope with the emotional pain of wanting them, and easily goes from person to person forming superficial relationships

If the child has had an emergency admission or is placed in a pediatric intensive care unit (PICU), both child and family will encounter a varying combination of additional stressors that can potentiate the separation anxiety, such as

- nature and severity of child's illness
- restrictions and fright caused by necessary treatment (e.g., restraints, intrusive procedures, machines)
- sleep deprivation
- unfamiliar surroundings compounded by altered states of consciousness related to disease, fever, drugs
- imposed separation of family related to space limitations or unit policy
- the emotional impact of critically ill child on the parent (e.g., grief, shock, guilt)
- overwhelming sensory stimuli (e.g., noxious odors, noises)
- imposed bedrest
- threats to infant's/toddler's trust, security, and autonomy/initiative
- threats to older child's body image, integrity, control of functions, pain or fear of pain

Nursing Assessment

☐ **PERTINENT HISTORY**

Number of other siblings, birth order, experiences outside the home, other traumatic separations, previous reactions to separations

☐ **PHYSICAL FINDINGS**

Protest stage: puffy eyes, red face, restlessness and crying, crying out for and demanding presence of primary caretaker; listening for step and looking for approach of primary caretaker; intensified crying when parents leave and when demands are not met; refusal to go to sleep; refusal to cooperate with care or treatment procedures; fighting, struggling, resisting, or pushing caretakers away

Despair stage: regressive behavior (e.g., thumbsucking, holding blanket or toy, incontinence, whining, clinging, use of baby talk); apathy and withdrawal; sometimes hyperactive or overtly aggressive; no eye contact; staying in crib in a fetal position, pretending to be asleep; showing no pleasure when parents are present, crying when they appear, rejection of parents or clinging to them; demanding to be taken home; accepting nursing care passively; allowing staff to handle and touch him/her

Detachment stage: showing an interest in surroundings and others; accepting care and love from almost anyone; complacency; no acting-out behavior or frequent bursts of anger; playing well by self or with others; responding to parents no differently from anyone else

☐ **PSYCHOSOCIAL CONCERNS/ DEVELOPMENTAL FACTORS**

Rituals of child, time of awakening, feeding times and methods, naptimes and bedtime rituals; other significant behavioral patterns

☐ **PATIENT AND FAMILY KNOWLEDGE**

Understanding of behavior, developmental aspects of child care, concept of separation anxiety, level of knowledge, readiness and willingness to learn

Nursing Care

☐ **LONG-TERM GOAL**

The child will experience separation from caretaker during hospitalization with minimal traumatic/residual effects; the child will feel secure and trust others.

NURSING DIAGNOSIS #1

Ineffective individual coping related to separation, hospitalization

Rationale: Learning to separate from parents is normally a gradual process achieved by the child as s/he comes to appreciate own separate individuality; it cannot be forced abruptly. The separation involved in hospitalization, coupled with the stress of illness, is usually beyond the normal adaptive capacity of a child aged 8 months to 6 years.

☐ **GOAL**

The child will experience minimal effects of separation; will not injure self or others; will maintain a secure and trusting relationship with parents; will interact normally and effectively with peers and adults.

☐ **IMPLEMENTATION**

Protest stage
- Review *Normal Growth and Development*, pages 300–314, for age-appropriate needs.
- Provide one consistent care giver for child; have nurse meet child in presence of parent.
- Accept crying and anger; reassure child that parent will return.
- Use language appropriate for child's age and stage of development.
- Allow for safe areas like crib, playroom where no procedures are done.
- Delay intrusive procedures when possible if child is very upset or parents are absent.
- Stay visible but do not force contact with child; respond physically when child initiates contact, then cuddle and comfort as needed.
- Be warm, firm, and reassuring to child.
- Gently restrain if child attempts to escape or injure self or others; use crib nets or high-top cribs when necessary.
- Provide with familiar and cherished objects, if possible.
- Encourage one parent to room in if feasible.
- Encourage parents to visit often, participate in care whenever possible.
- Have parent leave something personal behind (e.g., purse or gloves) so child knows parent will return; have bedside pictures of family, pet, or best friend.
- Encourage visiting of siblings if hospital rules allow.
- Read to preschool child *Curious George Goes to the Hospital* or other appropriate books about hospitalization.
- Use puppets, comedy to attract child's attention and cooperation.
- Arrange for preschooler or older child to visit hospital (e.g., tour and preadmission party) if possible, to alleviate fears and reduce incidence of anxiety.
- Assess the actual effects of additional stressors and plan care according to individual needs of child/family; provide additional explanations, encouragement, touching/stroking, talking/soothing, environmental manipulation as indicated.
- Allow child to make some simple decisions, if able.

Despair stage
- Continue previous successful nursing actions.
- Allow, but do not foster or encourage regressive behavior.
- Provide for physical comfort and closeness; hold and rock child, establish trust.
- Attempt to maintain skills achieved at home (e.g., talking, toilet training); know that the last skill learned will be the first to disappear when child is stressed.
- Allow expression of anger through play with active toys (e.g., play clay, bang toys, balls) or dramatic play with puppets, dolls; refer to *The Child Requiring Play Therapy*, page 226.
- Use games like peek-a-boo or hide-and-seek to desensitize child (especially infant) to separation and to encourage the development of object permanence; tell stories in which people are reunited or brought together.
- Keep track of child's possessions and do not lose them; allow child to wear own clothes; have shoes at bedside so child can see that they are there when s/he needs them to go home.

Detachment stage
- Continue previous successful nursing actions.
- Talk about home, what the people are doing there now, about when child will be going home to room/school/brother/sister, and what s/he will do.
- Continue use of physical contact; explain to parents child's need to be held even if it appears that s/he rejects them.
- Help parents continue nurturing role (they may resent child's acceptance of the nurse and feel nurse is stealing child's love; if parents pull back from child, child may feel s/he is being abandoned).
- Allow child to have some control over own life and any procedures; encourage involvement with other children.

EVALUATION CRITERIA/DESIRED OUTCOMES

The child

- Is allowed to protest within limits
- Accepts care of nursing staff
- Accepts parents when they return
- Uses play activities to express fears
- Talks about home/family
- Interacts effectively with peers/adults
- Returns to previous level of social/interactive behavior

NURSING DIAGNOSIS #2

Knowledge deficit regarding child development, child-rearing practices

Rationale: If a knowledge deficit exists, parents can become overwhelmed by child's behavior and fear the child is acting abnormally or not responding appropriately.

GOAL

The parents will verbalize an understanding of separation anxiety; will anticipate child's behavior and provide appropriate interventions.

IMPLEMENTATION

- Explain the concept of separation anxiety and why the child is acting in certain ways.
- Encourage to verbalize feelings (e.g., confusion, sadness, anxiety).
- Encourage to visit even if child cries more at their appearance; explain this is child's way of coping and is a positive behavior.
- Discourage from "sneaking" away from child; encourage them always to say goodbye.
- Support in efforts at intervention; provide parents with general ideas for interventions but allow them to make the major decisions.

EVALUATION CRITERIA/DESIRED OUTCOMES

The parents

- Describe separation anxiety
- Express feelings toward child having separation anxiety
- Provide interventions for child to prevent separation anxiety

Siblings of the Ill Child

Definition/Discussion

Siblings of an ill child are healthy brothers or sisters of the child who is ill with either an acute episode requiring hospitalization or a chronic condition that may require recurrent hospitalization as well as continuing care at home.

Nursing Assessment

☐ **PERTINENT HISTORY**

Ill child's condition, impact of the illness on the family, general health of siblings, previous experiences with illness

☐ **PHYSICAL FINDINGS**

Observed interactions between ill child and parents/sibling, sibling and parents

☐ **PSYCHOSOCIAL CONCERNS/ DEVELOPMENTAL FACTORS**

Developmental level of sibling and ill child, school performance, involvement in group activities, usual coping mechanisms, usual daily routines of sibling, sibling's experience with hospitals/illness

☐ **PATIENT AND FAMILY KNOWLEDGE**

Sibling's understanding of ill child's condition, parents' understanding of sibling's reactions to the ill child's condition

☐ **LONG-TERM GOAL**

The sibling will make successful adjustment to the changes in family routines necessitated by the ill child's condition; the experiences will be a positive factor in the sibling's development.

NURSING DIAGNOSIS #1
a. **Ineffective individual/family coping** related to inability to handle the stress of the sibling's illness
b. **Alteration in parenting** related to family stress involved with caring for ill child
c. **Altered growth and development** related to parents spending increased time with ill child

---

Rationale: Time and energy demands required by the ill child may leave parents without enough time to meet their individual needs nor the needs of the family. Parents may be so focused on ill child that they may not be aware of the sibling's basic needs. The sibling may experience overwhelming stress and may use ineffective methods for handling the situation.

☐ **GOAL**

The sibling will discuss feelings and fears freely; will develop positive coping strategies; the parents will recognize when the sibling is in crisis and provide support; will develop strategies to assist them with parenting responsibilities.

☐ **IMPLEMENTATION**

• Establish rapport with sibling; encourage expression of feelings and fears by providing a caring atmosphere; utilize methods to assist the sibling to express self (e.g., toys, puppets, role playing, drawing pictures, telling stories); refer to *The Child Requiring Play Therapy*, page 226.
• Discuss specific ways child reacts to various situations.
• Help parents to recognize when sibling is in crisis (e.g., moody, acting-out behaviors, not doing well in school, not participating in activities).
• Cooperate with siblings/parents; develop strategies for sibling to deal with crisis (e.g., special time with parent, outlets to divert energy such as sports, music, crafts).
• Assist parents to discuss the sibling's coping abilities with other adults with whom the child has frequent contact (e.g., teacher, scout leader, coach, clergy, parents of peers); encourage to develop strategies to enable others to report lack of coping or to intervene in sibling's self-destructive behaviors.
• Assist parents to schedule time with sibling; review sibling's developmental level and appropriate activities.
• Encourage parents to express feelings of needing

help; assist to identify support systems/resources available (e.g., help with child care from relatives and friends, respite programs for the chronically ill child and family, day care for sibling, mental health counseling to gain insight into own feelings and needs).
- Refer family to "The Sibling Project," a program that addresses concerns of those who have siblings with disabling conditions.

☐ EVALUATION CRITERIA/DESIRED OUTCOMES

The sibling
- Expresses feelings
- Copes with stress

The parents
- Verbalize signs sibling may exhibit when not coping effectively
- Develop effective strategies to help sibling deal with stress
- Recognize own needs
- Identify support systems/resources available

NURSING DIAGNOSIS #2
a. **Fear** of child's illness related to sibling's knowledge deficit
b. **Knowledge deficit** regarding ill child's condition

Rationale: Children are frightened by things they do not understand or cannot control. Depending on the sibling's developmental level, s/he may not be able to understand pertinent facts about the child's illness and therefore be frightened by it.

☐ GOAL

The sibling will have an age-appropriate understanding of the basic facts of the child's illness, capabilities; the parents will understand how children view illness at different developmental stages.

☐ IMPLEMENTATION

- Teach siblings about the child's illness using age-appropriate terms.
- Explore the sibling's understanding about the illness so that misconceptions can be corrected.
- Encourage sibling visitation with ill child in the hospital, if appropriate; make sure sibling is prepared for what may be seen and answer any questions honestly.
- Instruct parents about responses to illness at the various developmental levels so that they can understand the sibling's behaviors and assist him/her.

☐ EVALUATION CRITERIA/DESIRED OUTCOMES

The sibling
- States basic, correct information about the child's illness

The parents
- Verbalize how the sibling might view the illness according to developmental level

The Child with Sickle Cell Anemia

Definition/Discussion

Sickle cell anemia is a severe, chronic, inherited disorder of hemoglobin formation characterized by the presence of crescent-shaped red blood cells in the peripheral blood, increased breakdown of red blood cells, and increased formation of new cells. It is a genetically transmitted disorder more prevalent in individuals of African or Mediterranean descent.

The young child with sickle cell anemia is often small and gains weight poorly; the older child usually has a short trunk, long extremities, narrow hips and shoulders. Teenagers and adults with sickle cell anemia have a "spider-body" stature with narrow shoulders and hips, kyphosis of upper and lower back, tower-shaped skull, and an increased anterior-posterior diameter of the chest.

Nursing Assessment

☐ PERTINENT HISTORY

Birth history; any other family members with disease; immunizations; previous illnesses, transfusions, surgeries

☐ PHYSICAL FINDINGS

Size for age; energy level; presence/location/characteristics of pain; skin ulceration, especially on legs; diaphoresis; pale or grey skin, mucous membranes, conjunctiva; scleral icterus, vision, level of consciousness, speech, seizures, murmurs, cardiac enlargement, dyspnea, breath sounds, bowel sounds, abdominal distension, hepato/splenomegaly, urine specific gravity, hematuria, enuresis, secondary sex characteristics; age at onset of puberty, menarche; priapism, movement of extremities, limping, frontal bossing, inflammation of the fingers, swelling, pain, redness, warmth in bones or joints

☐ PSYCHOSOCIAL CONCERNS/ DEVELOPMENTAL FACTORS

Developmental level, planning for future, child/parental response to chronic illness, stage of loss and coping, habits (e.g., what comforts child, feeding/bedtime routines, favored objects)

☐ PATIENT AND FAMILY KNOWLEDGE

Pathology, genetic transmission, measures to prevent crisis/infections, preventive care, acceptance of condition and treatment regimen, level of knowledge, readiness and willingness to learn

Nursing Care

☐ LONG-TERM GOAL

The child will live as long as possible with minimum necessary limitations and restrictions; the family will support the child and accept limitations placed on the child during growth and development; the family will adjust to the potential loss of the child.

NURSING DIAGNOSIS #1

Grieving related to the transmission of hereditary, chronic, potentially fatal disease

Rationale: *Both child and parents go through the grieving process as they realize the impact that sickle cell disease may have on the quality and longevity of the child's life.*

☐ GOAL

The parents will work through grief and mourning over transmitting disease to child; the child/parents will work through the stages of loss and deal adaptively with the illness.

☐ IMPLEMENTATION

- Encourage parents to talk about their feelings and fears; set aside private time to focus and listen to concerns/feelings; refer to *The Parent Experiencing Grief and Loss*, page 139.
- Observe for guilt feelings; reinforce that parents are not to blame.
- Inform parents that there is a risk of having other children with trait or disease; refer to genetic counseling or for contraceptive information as needed.

- Offer self as active listener; accept feelings and give support; let child know it is all right to be angry, sad, depressed, just as it is all right to be happy.
- Explain disease and treatment to child in age-appropriate terms; use role playing and play therapy to explore feelings; refer to *The Child Requiring Play Therapy*, page 226; teach parents to assess for fear/anxiety and to practice using role playing as a way to alleviate child's fear and anxieties.

☐ **EVALUATION CRITERIA/DESIRED OUTCOMES**

The child/parents
- Progress through the grief process
- Make realistic plans for the future
- Exhibit no destructive behaviors
- Describe correctly the genetic transmission of the disease
- Do not place blame

NURSING DIAGNOSIS #2

Alteration in tissue perfusion: cardiopulmonary, cerebral related to obstruction of blood vessels by sickled cells, decreased oxygen-carrying capacity of blood

Rationale: As the hemoglobin in the anemic child drops, the body tries to compensate with an increased heart rate and cardiac output. Compensatory mechanisms work for a time; but when the body can no longer maintain cardiac output at needed levels, the cardiac output decreases. Sickling may cause ischemia and infarction (e.g., heart, lungs, and brain). There is a high recurrence rate following cerebral infarction. Blood transfusions every 3-4 weeks may maintain low HgbS levels and prevent further cerebral infarctions. Oxygen may prevent further sickling but usually does not reverse sickling that has already occurred. A vaso-occlusive crisis impedes blood flow and thus perfusion. A splenic sequestration crisis causes blood to pool in the spleen and can lead to shock.

☐ **GOAL**

The child will be free from impaired cardiopulmonary and cerebral perfusion.

☐ **IMPLEMENTATION**
- Monitor blood pressure, pulses, capillary refill, every 4 hours or as necessary; be alert for signs of shock (e.g., restlessness, changes in level of consciousness and orthostatic vital signs); report changes.
- Be alert to complaints of pain, weakness, dizzi-

ness, changes in mobility, signs of cerebral vascular accident.
- Maintain bedrest; limit activities as needed.
- Monitor effect of oxygen administration; report response to oxygen therapy.
- Monitor effect of blood transfusions; be alert for transfusion reactions, hepatitis, and iron overload if receiving multiple transfusions; refer to *The Child Receiving Blood and Blood-Product Transfusions*, page 24.

☐ **EVALUATION CRITERIA/DESIRED OUTCOMES**

The child
- Is free from signs of shock
- Maintains blood pressure, pulse within normal range for age
- Has no orthostatic hypotension
- Is alert

NURSING DIAGNOSIS #3

Impaired gas exchange related to increased secretions

Rationale: The lungs are damaged by occlusion of pulmonary arterioles by sickled cells and repeated pulmonary infections to which the child with sickle cell anemia is susceptible. Repeated assaults on the lung tissue impairs gas exchange, increasing the risk of further sickling.

☐ **GOAL**

The child will be free from pulmonary complications.

☐ **IMPLEMENTATION**
- Report signs of infection immediately (e.g., fever, lethargy, pallor, tachycardia, tachypnea, use of accessory muscles to breath).
- Check immunization status; note if pneumococcal vaccine was given if child is over 2 years of age.
- Keep child away from others with respiratory infection.
- Obtain culture and sensitivity of sputum; monitor response to ordered antibiotics.
- Maintain bedrest to limit oxygen requirements.
- Assist child to plan day so that activity periods are followed by rest periods; plan treatments and activities of daily living (ADL) around rest periods.
- Encourage deep breathing and and coughing to clear secretions.
- Monitor effects of oxygen administration; report improvement (e.g., decreased pain, increased stamina) or lack of therapeutic benefit (e.g., continued pain, increased pallor, restlessness).

☐ **EVALUATION CRITERIA/DESIRED OUTCOMES**

The child

- Is not exposed to anyone with cold/respiratory infections
- Has no fever, tachycardia, tachypnea, retractions
- Has reduced respiratory secretions

NURSING DIAGNOSIS #4

Fluid volume deficit related to inadequate fluid intake, excessive urinary loss

Rationale: The microcirculation of the renal bed is sensitive to the effects of sickling. Kidneys may not concentrate urine well and fluid is readily lost. Sickled cells cause increased viscosity in the capillary bed, which further compounds the problem.

☐ **GOAL**

The child will remain normovolemic and well hydrated.

☐ **IMPLEMENTATION**

- Monitor hydration status (e.g., vital signs, skin turgor, mucous membranes) every 4 hours and as necessary.
- Maintain accurate intake and output.
- Weigh daily at the same time, in same clothes, on same scale.
- Calculate maintenance fluid requirements for child.
- Monitor electrolyte status/IV infusion if ordered; refer to *The Child with an Intravenous Catheter*, page 174.
- Offer oral fluids frequently (every 30-60 minutes); have specific plan for child to follow (e.g., drink 3,000 cc/24 hours; take 250 cc/hour while awake); offer a variety of colorful fluids (e.g., juices, Jell-O, Popsicles).
- Motivate the child to drink (e.g., assess for favorite fluids, play a game, have a tea party, use special cups/straws, place sticker on bottom of clear glass, draw empty glasses on paper and have child color in glass after one is consumed [orange for orange juice, purple for grape]).

☐ **EVALUATION CRITERIA/DESIRED OUTCOMES**

The child

- Maintains weight
- Has moist mucous membranes, flat fontanel (in infant), good skin turgor
- Ingests 1½–2 times fluid maintenance requirements

NURSING DIAGNOSIS #5

Alteration in comfort: pain related to infarctions

Rationale: The child with sickle cell anemia may experience vaso-occlusive crises where the red blood cells sickle, clump together, and block small blood vessels. The tissue beyond these blocked vessels becomes ischemic and infarctions may occur causing pain in the involved area.

☐ **GOAL**

The child will cope effectively with pain; will experience relief of pain.

☐ **IMPLEMENTATION**

- Monitor baseline vital signs.
- Assess for verbal and nonverbal indications of pain at least every 2 hours; determine location, intensity, characteristics of pain.
- Encourage child to evaluate level of pain; refer to *The Child Experiencing Pain*, page 216.
- Discuss previously successful pain-relief methods.
- Administer analgesics as ordered; monitor effects.
- Apply local heat to area as ordered; massage area gently; position for comfort.
- Assess and provide diversional activities.
- Report priapism immediately if it occurs; treat quickly with warm baths, hypotonic fluids, transfusions as ordered.

☐ **EVALUATION CRITERIA/DESIRED OUTCOMES**

The child

- Verbalizes relief of pain, talks, laughs, has good eye contact
- Displays no nonverbal behaviors indicating pain

NURSING DIAGNOSIS #6

Impairment of skin integrity related to altered peripheral circulation

Rationale: The skin, particularly of the lower leg, is susceptible to the effects of decreased peripheral circulation, that may include tissue ischemia, infarction, and subsequent necrosis.

☐ **GOAL**

The child will not experience skin breakdown; the child/parents will report signs of skin breakdown/complications.

☐ IMPLEMENTATION

- Observe for reddened areas, breaks in skin integrity at least every 8 hours.
- Teach child/parents to observe for and report immediately any reddened areas, breaks in skin, or burning sensations.
- Change child's position frequently (e.g., every 2 hours, when sensing pressure) if on bedrest.
- Treat breaks in skin integrity immediately, avoid contamination of site, report to physician.
- Treat leg ulcers promptly (e.g., elevate legs, change dressings frequently); know that grafting may be required.
- Monitor effects of transfusions/therapy (e.g., oral zinc) as ordered.

☐ EVALUATION CRITERIA/DESIRED OUTCOMES

The child
- Has intact skin with no areas of breakdown
- Has diminished wound size with no signs of secondary infection if ulceration has occurred
- Has no complaints of painful areas on skin

NURSING DIAGNOSIS #7

a. **Disturbance in self-concept** related to frequent illnesses, perceived stigma of disease characteristics
b. **Altered growth and development** related to frequent illnesses

Rationale: Many of the effects of sickle cell anemia (e.g., frequent illnesses with the possibility of hospitalization, dependency on others, restrictions on activities, small stature, delayed acquisition of secondary sex characteristics) prevent the child, particularly the adolescent, from developing a positive self-concept.

☐ GOAL

The child will develop a positive self-concept; will accomplish age-appropriate developmental activities; the parents will supply love and set limits needed by child without overprotecting; will understand that the child with sickle cell anemia has the same developmental needs as a healthy child.

☐ IMPLEMENTATION

- Encourage participation in school and social activities between episodes of crisis.
- Reinforce developmentally appropriate activities and skills; refer to *Normal Growth and Development*, pages 300–314; provide positive reinforcement for hobbies and schoolwork.
- Counsel parents to discuss treatment plan with siblings and extended family; encourage family to

set limits and not overprotect or give all their attention to sick child; refer to *Siblings and the Ill Child*, page 261.
- Discuss concerns and feelings regarding developing body.
- Trust the adolescent's ability to assume responsibility for self; prepare for self-care activities.
- Reinforce involvement with peer group and independence.
- Encourage parents to bring child's books, games, hobbies, homework, radio, or tape recorder to hospital; use these activities to help the child focus on health and away from the pain and discomfort; assist child to stay in touch with friends by telephone, letters, and visiting.
- Assess adolescent's need for sex and birth control information; teach as needed; explain that pregnancy is dangerous for the developing female adolescent with sickling; explain to both sexes the chance of passing on the disease to offspring; refer for genetic counseling or birth control as desired and needed; encourage any questions the adolescent has about dating, sex, or birth control.
- Assess the need for vocational counseling; make referrals as needed.

☐ EVALUATION CRITERIA/DESIRED OUTCOMES

The child/adolescent
- Verbalizes positive self-regard
- Accomplishes age-appropriate developmental tasks
- Presents a clean, well-groomed appearance
- Shows no signs of depression, self-derogatory behavior

The parents
- Establish behavioral limits

NURSING DIAGNOSIS #8

Activity intolerance related to pain, fatigue, dyspnea

Rationale: The child with anemia has fewer red blood cells to carry oxygen so the body may have insufficient oxygen to meet normal or exertional oxygen requirements. Pain also limits the activity level.

☐ GOAL

The child will perform ADL; will balance activity with rest.

☐ IMPLEMENTATION

- Evaluate child's activity level (e.g., needs/desires).
- Make plan for day with child scheduling rest and activity periods.

- Encourage child to limit activities when fatigue occurs.
- Provide quiet diversional activities to encourage rest.
- Schedule ADL with rest periods.
- Increase activities as tolerated; work with child to schedule appropriate exercises.

☐ EVALUATION CRITERIA/DESIRED OUTCOMES

The child
- Plans day so activities are spread out and child does not become overly tired
- Performs own ADL

NURSING DIAGNOSIS #9

Sensory-perceptual alteration: visual related to sickling within vasculature of eye

Rationale: The eye has an extensive microvasculature that is sensitive to the effects of sickling resulting in decreased vision. With early detection, therapy may prevent progression of visual deterioration.

☐ GOAL

The child will maintain vision; the child/parents will report early signs of retinopathy to the health team.

☐ IMPLEMENTATION

- Check vision with standard tests and questions (e.g., "Can you see the blackboard from your seat at school?" "Do you have trouble reading traffic signs/billboards?").
- Note complaints of visual disturbances.
- Discuss signs of retinopathy; stress the importance of annual eye exams.

☐ EVALUATION CRITERIA/DESIRED OUTCOMES

The child
- Has eye exam at least yearly and more frequently if indicated
- Maintains visual acuity

NURSING DIAGNOSIS #10

Knowledge deficit regarding pathology, effects of disease, prevention, precipitating factors of crisis, well-child care

Rationale: The child/parents with sickle cell anemia can avoid situations that may precipitate a crisis and can implement wellness behaviors that permit the child to achieve maximum potential with good

---

care at home. Sickle cell anemia affects multiple body systems and child/family education must be adequate to ensure optimal understanding and care.

☐ GOAL

The child/parents will understand genetic transmission and pathology/effects of sickle cell anemia; will avoid situations that may precipitate a crisis; will practice health maintenance behaviors.

☐ IMPLEMENTATION

- Reinforce understanding of the genetic transmission and pathology of sickle cell anemia.
- Prepare parents that child may grow/develop more slowly than unaffected child, may weigh less than peers.
- Teach to avoid exposure to extreme cold, persons with infection, exercise beyond endurance, activities resulting in trauma/bruising, dehydration, high altitudes, and emotional stress.
- Emphasize importance of pacing self according to stamina; encourage rest/periods of quiet activity.
- Teach child to use caution in order not to cut/bump self.
- Discuss the importance of eating a well-balanced diet high in folic acid (e.g., meat, green leafy vegetables and fresh fruit, dairy products, whole grains).
- Give specific amounts for fluid intake (e.g., 12 glasses/day; a glass every 30-60 minutes); teach child/parents to calculate intake and output at home.
- Instruct to increase fluids during hot weather or strenuous exercise.
- Explain to parents that because of the high fluid intake, toddlers may have difficulty toilet training, and bed wetting is very common; encourage parents to continue high fluid intake; elicit their concerns; suggest to parents to have child void frequently during the day, and take child to bathroom when they go to bed and once during the night if it does not disrupt child's sleep; discuss with parents negative effects of limiting fluids or shaming child.
- Allow parents sufficient time to adjust to a diagnosis that requires life-long therapy and medical attention; refer to *The Child/Family Adapting to Chronic Illness*, page 62.
- Discuss importance of regular health maintenance care (e.g., physicals every 1-2 months during first year of life, immunizations, dental care, eye examinations).
- Encourage child to wear Medic-Alert tag; inform significant others of disease (e.g., teachers, babysitters, employers).
- Teach to promptly report any signs of illness

(e.g., vomiting, diarrhea, pain, fever, breaks in skin integrity).
- Caution parents about being overprotective.
- Encourage participation in age-appropriate activities as tolerated.
- List resources available in the community to assist the family (e.g., information, support/counsel).
- Provide written materials to support verbal instructions.

☐ EVALUATION CRITERIA/DESIRED OUTCOMES

The child/parents
- Keep appointments for follow-up with physician/clinic
- Describe factors that contribute to sickle cell crisis and methods to avoid or minimize them
- Contact physician/clinic at first signs of pallor, jaundice, lethargy, fever, pain
- State importance of regular immunizations and immunization against pneumococcus
- Keep record of intake and output

The child
- Ingests nutritional meals
- Exercises within own limits
- Obtains adequate sleep
- Has needed referrals for counseling (e.g., genetic, sex education, birth control, support groups).

The Adolescent who Attempts Suicide

Definition/Discussion

Adolescence is a time of mood swings, depression, loneliness, anger, and other negative feelings balanced by positive new independence, sensations, experiences and relationships, achievements, and pleasures. These rapid changes may elicit a sense of loss of control over one's life—a sense of desperation that may lead to a functional fixedness through which the teen sees no other alternative but to end life. Feelings/motives that precipitate/precede a suicide attempt may include acting out (cry for help), impulsive acts, true death wish, desire to punish others or self, release from despair, or avoiding risk of rejection. An ongoing depressive process is usually present prior to suicide.

Nursing Assessment

☐ PERTINENT HISTORY

Precipitating factors, losses, past patterns of managing stress, chronic or terminal illness, school functioning, physical/sexual abuse, peer/family relations, alcohol/chemical abuse, promiscuity

☐ PHYSICAL FINDINGS

Hygiene, eating, sleeping, and elimination patterns; change in usual motor activity, nervous habits; scratches, bite marks, bruises, lacerations, or burns; orientation to person, time, place

☐ PSYCHOSOCIAL CONCERNS/ DEVELOPMENTAL FACTORS

Developmental level; interactional patterns; expression of affect; self-destructive behavior, rebellion, withdrawal, running away, social isolation, change in behavior, giving away possessions, irritability, low frustration level, restlessness, anger; sexuality, peer relationships, independence, school functioning; unusual sensations or thoughts; feelings of sadness, worthlessness, apprehension, fear of harm from others, inability to cope, difficulty concentrating; problem-solving skills

☐ PATIENT AND FAMILY KNOWLEDGE

Self-evaluation, parental perception of adolescent's behavior, patient and family's awareness of existence of a problem and willingness to work toward resolving issues; level of knowledge, readiness and willingness to learn

Nursing Care

☐ LONG-TERM GOAL

The adolescent will realize that life's frustrations and challenges do have possible solutions and will not attempt to end life; the adolescent will learn effective methods of communicating needs and feelings (e.g., loss, anger, guilt, failure, inadequacy, loneliness).

NURSING DIAGNOSIS #1

Potential for injury related to suicidal gestures/attempts

Rationale: *Depending on the plan, the adolescent is at risk from self-harm. The more definitive the plan, the greater the risk. Suicidal gestures/attempts may include accidents as well as self-inflicted injuries.*

☐ GOAL

The adolescent will not injure self.

☐ IMPLEMENTATION

- Take any comment or mention of death and suicide seriously.
- Do not promise to keep suicidal gesture a secret from individuals who can help.
- Discuss the suicidal ideation with the teen; assess lethality of comment (e.g., Does teen have a plan?, What is it?, Is it feasible?, Does teen have access to methodology?, What is the time frame?).
- Stay with adolescent at all times if lethality is moderate or high (e.g., plans to give overdose of

insulin, is diabetic, has access to materials needed—insulin, syringes).

- Remove potentially lethal objects from the environment.
- Place on one-to-one observation; make statements that indicate caring (e.g., "Staff care and are here to protect you and keep you safe until you are able to do that yourself.").
- Report findings to health care provider/mental health professional.
- Express "I care . . ." statements; articulate your concern for teen's safety and that you will protect him/her from harming self, even if that means informing others.
- Remain calm; be accepting and supportive; do not act shocked, make judgments, or instill guilt.

☐ **EVALUATION CRITERIA/DESIRED OUTCOMES**

The adolescent

- Does not injure self
- Recognizes that someone cares enough to prevent the lethal behavior
- Participates in therapy

NURSING DIAGNOSIS #2

Potential for violence: self-directed related to anxiety, fear, dysfunctional grieving

Rationale: As teens progress through adolescence, they experience a variety of biopsychosocial changes. These may be perceived as threats to self-concept and create anxiety for the teen. Many events may precipitate fear in the adolescent (e.g., peer pressure, diagnosis of chronic illness, loss of a significant other, parental divorce, school failure, sexual development/activity, lack of knowledge about the biopsychosocial changes). The move to adolescence produces actual losses (e.g., childhood, identity, role) that must be grieved. In addition, the usual developmental changes of adolescence and the resulting confusion may cause the teen to experience an otherwise innocuous loss with increased intensity, or to experience disproportional and prolonged grief with a truly significant loss.

☐ **GOAL**

The adolescent will recognize own anxiety and coping patterns; will experience an increase in psychologic comfort; will develop/utilize effective coping skills.

☐ **IMPLEMENTATION**

- Encourage expression of feelings; refer to table 9 *Guidelines for Working with Adolescents.*

- Assess physical and psychologic symptoms that may accompany fear/anxiety/grief.
- Determine actual/perceived stressors/losses; define the significance; assist adolescent to define precipitating factor(s), real or imagined.
- Discuss past and present coping mechanisms; assist to identify effective and ineffective coping mechanisms.
- Assist to identify alternatives to suicide rather than merely postponing it; help find reason to live, something to look forward to.
- Assist to recognize behaviors indicating increased anxiety (e.g., increased restlessness, mood swings, apathy, poor concentration) and to develop mechanisms to manage behaviors (e.g., engage in physical activity, practice relaxation techniques, identify factors that can be controlled, make decisions when realistic, seek professional counseling); refer to *The Child Experiencing Anxiety,* page 11.
- Instruct in use of relaxation techniques (e.g., deep breathing, meditation).
- Role play adaptive coping skills with teen; support and reinforce use.

☐ **EVALUATION CRITERIA/DESIRED OUTCOMES**

The adolescent

- Expresses feelings
- Identifies stressors/losses
- Develops successful coping mechanisms
- Role plays new skills

NURSING DIAGNOSIS #3

Disturbance in self-concept related to distorted body image, decreased self-esteem

Rationale: One of the main developmental tasks of adolescence is to maintain a sameness with one's peers—not to be different. The suicidal adolescent often has a distorted view of self in relation to physical/social/emotional environment. Comparison of the self with a distorted environment can result in an altered sense of self and subsequent decreased self-esteem.

☐ **GOAL**

The adolescent will develop a realistic body image; will increase self-esteem.

☐ **IMPLEMENTATION**

- Note manner of dress and state of hygiene and grooming (e.g., disheveled, unkempt appearance).
- Engage in dialogue regarding feelings/opinions about self and personal appearance (e.g., likes/dislikes, strengths/weaknesses).

- Explore feelings surrounding changes in body with onset of puberty.
- Encourage and reinforce any positive self statements; discuss ways to highlight good feelings about self (e.g., improving grooming/hygiene).
- Assist with hygiene and grooming as needed; reinforce any attempts toward improvement in hygiene/grooming.

☐ EVALUATION CRITERIA/DESIRED OUTCOMES

The adolescent
- Participates in grooming and hygiene
- Makes positive statements about self

NURSING DIAGNOSIS #4

Alteration in family process related to suicidal ideation, gestures

Rationale: The normal supportive environment of the family is altered when an adolescent contemplates/attempts suicide. Members may become overly protective or ignore/deny the issue out of discomfort with the topic.

☐ GOAL

The family will achieve a productive functional state; will be supportive of the adolescent.

☐ IMPLEMENTATION

- Determine level of disruption in family functions and interactions.
- Provide opportunities for members to verbalize feelings (e.g., anger, disbelief) to nurse and one another.
- Assist adolescent/family to listen, hear, and acknowledge one another.
- Be accepting; both the adolescent and the family are feeling very vulnerable.
- Assist the family to identify and use supportive behaviors with one another through role play.
- Collaborate with the family to establish/facilitate goals and treatments.
- Encourage family to seek professional therapy; provide a list of community resources (e.g., mental health clinics, Survivors of Suicide support group, clergy).

☐ EVALUATION CRITERIA/DESIRED OUTCOMES

The family
- Participates in goal-setting and treatment
- Supports one another
- Participates in family/individual counseling

NURSING DIAGNOSIS #5

Knowledge deficit regarding adolescent suicide, early symptoms of suicidal behavior

Rationale: Many teens are unaware that many other "normal" teenagers also think about suicide; the adolescent is not different from the peer group in this respect. Teens who recognize problems, utilize coping skills and support systems are less likely to feel so hopeless. Parents often deny or ignore warning signs.

☐ GOAL

The adolescent/parents will recognize the scope of adolescent suicide; will know warning signs; will seek professional help if these signs appear.

☐ IMPLEMENTATION

- Discuss warning signs (e.g., behavior changes, mood swings, change in peer group or loss of peer group, school failure or absorption, decreased communication, expressing bad feelings about self, verbalizing suicidal ideation, making suicidal gestures/attempts).
- Give resource list of therapists proficient in adolescent and family therapy.
- Educate regarding the scope and seriousness of adolescent suicide.
- Identify community resources with counseling/information available to those contemplating suicide and their families (e.g., Suicide Hotline).

☐ EVALUATION CRITERIA/DESIRED OUTCOMES

The adolescent/parents
- Identify warning signs of suicide
- Verbalize the scope of the problem
- List community resources available

Table 9
Guidelines for Working with Adolescents

- Approach with respect; avoid authoritarian attitudes.
- Let the adolescent be the expert about him/herself.
- Use open-ended questions and be nonjudgmental.
- Avoid use of "why" questions.
- Do not try to be "hip" or use adolescent jargon (it changes almost daily and adults who try to be "one-of-the-gang" create distance and distrust).
- Ask for clarification if adolescent uses jargon or is unclear about situations or events.
- Assess and praise adolescent's strengths.
- Assist to clarify values.
- Avoid giving advice.
- Tell the adolescent "It's okay to feel . . ."; validate feelings.

- Teach assertive communication skills; help adolescent complete "I" statements (e.g., "I feel," "I want," "I don't want," "I like," "I don't like," "I am willing to"); avoid "you" statements (e.g., "You make me mad," "You are sloppy"); instead say "I'm mad at you," "I am upset with the way this room is messed up."
- Role play assertive communication by using simple, nonthreatening situations, with characters (participants) from the individual's or group's everyday life.
- Use role playing and problem solving with guided imagery to explore new behaviors, possible choices, and consequences of behaviors.

- Use positive affirmations to increase adaptive risk taking; offer opportunities to learn risk taking with support of nurse.
- Enable the adolescent to withdraw, plan adaptive coping methods, and try again.
- Reinforce the need for consistency and limit setting to provide stability.
- Reinforce the use of positive coping strategies; give feedback as the adolescent learns to cope adaptively with difficult situations and threatening people.

The Child with a Tonsillectomy and Adenoidectomy

Definition/Discussion

Tonsillectomy (T) is the surgical excision of both tonsils; adenoidectomy (A) is the surgical excision of adenoid tissue. A child who has frequent episodes of sore throat will be treated surgically if medical intervention is not effective.

Nursing Assessment

☐ **PERTINENT HISTORY**

Course of illness (number of sore throats in past year, treatment), last sore throat (onset, duration, treatment); difficulty swallowing or airway obstruction, allergies and treatment

☐ **PHYSICAL FINDINGS**

Vital signs, signs of current tonsilar infection, complaints of pain/discomfort

☐ **PSYCHOSOCIAL CONCERNS/ DEVELOPMENTAL FACTORS**

Developmental level, coping mechanisms, normal routines, previous experience with hospitalization

☐ **PATIENT AND FAMILY KNOWLEDGE**

Indications for surgery, surgical procedure, post-op treatment plan, level of knowledge, readiness and willingness to learn

Nursing Care

☐ **LONG-TERM GOAL**

The child will return to home and family following safe, successful surgery; the child will integrate this experience into self-concept; the child will maintain the ongoing processes of growth and development; the child will resume normal life functioning within the family.

NURSING DIAGNOSIS #1

Ineffective airway clearance related to inability to handle excess secretions

Rationale: Postoperatively, the child may have difficulty handling secretions because of sleepiness, fear of swallowing or spitting out secretions resulting in an accumulation of secretions at back of the mouth that causes obstruction.

☐ **GOAL**

The child will maintain a clear airway.

☐ **IMPLEMENTATION**

- Monitor rate and quality of respirations every hour and as needed; note frequency of swallowing; assess breath sounds; document findings.
- Observe and report respiratory distress (e.g., "crowing," retraction of chest muscles).
- Record presence or absence of tonsillar packing.
- Position prone or lying on side.
- Encourage child to gently spit up mucus secretions.
- Turn and deep breathe every 2 hours.

☐ **EVALUATION CRITERIA/DESIRED OUTCOMES**

The child
- Has normal respiratory pattern and rate
- Is free from respiratory distress
- Produces thin, easily handled secretions

NURSING DIAGNOSIS #2

Alteration in cardiac output: decreased related to post-op hemorrhage

Rationale: A major post-op complication can be excessive bleeding, which leads to decreased cardiac output.

☐ **GOAL**

The child will have a stable post-op course with minimal bleeding; will not develop complications.

☐ **IMPLEMENTATION**

- Observe for signs of bleeding (e.g., increased pulse rate, decreased blood pressure, restlessness, skin color changes); monitor vital signs every hour for the first 4 hours, then every 2 hours or as necessary; document findings; inspect throat when checking vital signs.
- Assess lab values (e.g., hematocrit, hemoglobin) as available.
- Observe for increased frequency of swallowing; note any vomiting of bright red blood.
- Avoid red colored fluids to make it easier to detect bleeding.
- Avoid use of aspirin for pain management (increases possibility of bleeding).
- Remind child to avoid coughing or clearing throat as much as possible.
- Maintain bedrest with bathroom privileges in quiet environment.
- Avoid putting sharp objects (e.g., forks, straws, pointed toys) in mouth.

☐ **EVALUATION CRITERIA/DESIRED OUTCOMES**

The child
- Bleeds minimally postoperatively
- Maintains lab values within normal limits
- Has normal vital signs

NURSING DIAGNOSIS #3

Fluid volume deficit related to decreased intake of fluids, excessive fluid loss

Rationale: Postoperatively, the child may be afraid to swallow fluids due to sore throat or fear of vomiting. Decreased intake of fluids, combined with excessive loss of fluid (e.g., vomiting, increased secretions) leads to fluid deficit.

☐ **GOAL**

The child will have adequate fluid intake; will experience minimal fluid losses.

☐ **IMPLEMENTATION**

- Monitor rectal temperatures, mucous membranes, and skin turgor every 4 hours.

- Chart accurate intake and output; record urine specific gravity every 8 hours.
- Monitor IV (if present) hourly; refer to *The Child with an Intravenous Catheter*, page 174.
- Give medication to control nausea/vomiting if needed; monitor for effectiveness.
- Encourage frequent sips of cool, clear liquids (e.g., ice chips, Popsicles) initially; advance diet (e.g., full liquid, soft, regular) as tolerated.

☐ **EVALUATION CRITERIA/DESIRED OUTCOMES**

The child
- Voids at least 1 cc/kg/hour
- Experiences minimal nausea/vomiting
- Has moist mucous membranes, good skin turgor

NURSING DIAGNOSIS #4

Alteration in comfort: pain related to surgical procedure

Rationale: Surgical removal of the tonsils and adenoids produces swelling and pain in the back of the mouth and throat.

☐ **GOAL**

The child will be comfortable; will obtain adequate rest.

☐ **IMPLEMENTATION**

- Assess for verbal and nonverbal behaviors indicating pain; allow child to express feelings of fear and pain; refer to *The Child Experiencing Pain*, page 216.
- Monitor effectiveness of ordered analgesics.
- Provide mouth care; rinse with cold water every 1-2 hours or as needed; instruct child not to gargle.
- Encourage use of ice collar as tolerated.
- Provide uninterrupted periods for sleep/rest.
- Encourage parents to participate in care to extent they feel comfortable.

☐ **EVALUATION CRITERIA/DESIRED OUTCOMES**

The child
- Does not cry excessively or display other signs of pain
- Has periods of restful sleep

NURSING DIAGNOSIS #5

Knowledge deficit regarding signs and symptoms of post-op complications

> *Rationale:* Parents cannot appropriately manage post-op treatment or detect early signs of complications if knowledge deficit exists.

☐ GOAL

The parents will describe treatments and early signs of post-op complications.

☐ IMPLEMENTATION

- Explain all procedures; instruct regarding medications (e.g., schedule, side effects, necessity of taking ordered).
- Caution about potential for bleeding for 5-10 days postoperatively.
- Teach symptoms (e.g., persistent earache, coughing, swallowing, vomiting blood, fever) that require a physician's attention.
- Instruct to keep child quiet for a few days; to continue soft foods for 7-10 days; to encourage 1-1½ quarts of fluids/day; and to protect child from contact with infection, especially upper respiratory infections.
- Emphasize importance of and schedule follow-up appointment.
- Provide written materials to support verbal teaching.

☐ EVALUATION CRITERIA/DESIRED OUTCOMES

The parents
- Describe necessary post-op home care
- List signs/symptoms of potential complications and necessity of notifying health care provider
- Keep follow-up appointment

The Child Receiving Total Parenteral Nutrition

Definition/Discussion

Total parenteral nutrition (TPN), sometimes called hyperalimentation, is the infusion directly into the blood of solutions containing dextrose, amino acids, lipids, and additives (e.g., vitamins, minerals, electrolytes, essential trace elements) to restore/maintain normal body composition and nutrition in individuals who are unable to meet their needs via the gastrointestinal (GI) tract. TPN is usually administered via an established central venous line or a right atrial catheter. Hypertonic solutions need to be infused directly into a central vein with high blood flow. Less concentrated solutions may be given via a peripheral vein.

Nursing Assessment

☐ **PERTINENT HISTORY**

Health problem that interferes with normal nutrition (e.g., congenital defect, chemotherapy, surgical manipulation of GI tract, bronchopulmonary dysplasia, cystic fibrosis, Crohn's disease); anticipated duration of treatment; previous parenteral nutrition experiences; other chronic illnesses that may affect treatment (e.g., diabetes mellitus, renal disease, cardiac disease)

☐ **PHYSICAL FINDINGS**

Height, weight, and head circumference (in infants); muscle mass; serum proteins, electrolytes, minerals; fluid status (e.g., skin turgor, edema, diaphoresis); ability to ingest oral foods; method of elimination (e.g., usual urinary and GI patterns, ostomies, abnormal losses via vomiting or diarrhea); presence of wounds or fistulas; anticipated caloric and nitrogen needs; established venous access

☐ **PSYCHOSOCIAL CONCERNS/ DEVELOPMENTAL FACTORS**

Age, developmental level, usual coping mechanisms/ habits (e.g., what comforts child, bedtime routine, favored objects), stage of grief response to loss of normal body functioning, family dynamics, daily activities, resources to perform home parenteral nutrition

☐ **PATIENT AND FAMILY KNOWLEDGE**

Level of knowledge, child/family acceptance of health problem necessitating parenteral nutrition, understanding of purpose and mechanics of parenteral nutrition and problems to report, readiness and willingness to learn

Nursing Care

☐ **LONG-TERM GOAL**

The child will receive total parenteral nutrition infusion free from preventable complications.

NURSING DIAGNOSIS #1

Alteration in nutrition: less than body requirements related to inability to absorb nutrients via GI tract, inability to ingest sufficient nutrients

Rationale: Pathophysiology making GI absorption of nutrients a problem for the child will vary depending on specific health problem. Regardless of the specific situation, a child needs enough protein for tissue repair, enough calories for energy (both carbohydrate and fat sources), and enough electrolyte, vitamins, minerals, and trace elements for normal body functioning. Children experience growth spurts which require an increase in required nutrients. The specific health problem and the child's growth pattern determine the exact amount of nutrients needed. General guidelines for daily parenteral nutrition for children vary with age but include: amino acids—1.5-3.0 gm/kg, glucose and lipids—50-120 cal/kg of ideal body weight, sodium—3-8 mEq/kg, potassium—2-4 mEq/kg.

☐ **GOAL**

The child will receive adequate nutrition to restore/ maintain health and growth.

IMPLEMENTATION

- Measure height, daily weight, head circumference (in infants), and periodically plot on growth chart.
- Record oral intake accurately; monitor intake and output; note unusual losses (e.g., vomiting, diarrhea, ostomies, and wounds).
- Collect ordered laboratory studies.
- Assess fluid balance at least every 8 hours.
- Administer solutions using an electronic infusion pump to accurately control rate.
- Calculate caloric intake.

EVALUATION CRITERIA/DESIRED OUTCOMES

The child

- Is free from side effects
- Grows along own growth curve

NURSING DIAGNOSIS #2

a. **Potential for injury** (air embolism, electrolyte and glucose imbalance, impaired catheter integrity) related to infusion of TPN via a central line

b. **Potential for infection** related to central line, TPN

Rationale: Children receiving TPN may be initially malnourished and at risk for infection. Hypertonic glucose solution is an excellent culture medium for bacteria and yeast. Poor aseptic technique may result in contamination of catheter or solution. In addition, TPN bypasses the normal defenses of the GI tract. Disconnection of IV tubing attached to a central line without proper clamping may result in air embolism, clot formation, and a break in integrity. TPN can be infused via a peripheral line but the dextrose concentration must not exceed 12.5% since this is very irritating to the veins. Infiltration of the infusate, since it is hyperosmolar and contains additives (e.g. potassium, calcium), can cause serious tissue necrosis. Because TPN contains high glucose concentrations, insulin production is increased; if TPN is slowed or stopped, the blood sugar may drop rapidly. Inconsistent rate of infusion and inadequate or overdosage of insulin to cover glucose load may lead to hyper/hypoglycemia. Any of these problems may result in breaks and interruption of needed nutrition and can cause serious, even life-threatening problems for the child.

GOAL

The child will be free from injury associated with TPN; will be free from infection.

IMPLEMENTATION

- Use strict aseptic technique when handling catheter; follow established hospital protocol; refer to *The Child with a Right Atrial Catheter*, page 248, and *The Child with an Intravenous Catheter*, page 174.
- Check temperature every 4-6 hours and report elevations above 100°F (37.8°C).
- Culture any purulent drainage from any part of body; perform routine blood and urine cultures as ordered.
- Refrigerate TPN solution until 1 hour before administration; inspect solution for turbidity, precipitates, or cracks in the bottle before administration.
- Administer solution via IV tubing with 0.22 micron in-line filter to remove impurities; do not allow solution to hang for more than 24 hours.
- Monitor hourly for signs of phlebitis and infiltration; discontinue IV infusion and follow hospital protocol for TPN infiltration (applicable for both peripheral and central infusions).
- Tape all catheter connections securely to avoid inadvertent disconnections; change position of tape tag on a central catheter during dressing change to prevent repeated stress on same area; keep specially designed toothless nontraumatic clamp in close proximity to child (e.g., on IV pole, at bedside).
- Clamp catheter at tape tag when changing IV tubing to avoid air embolism; if child becomes short of breath, has chest pain, coughing, or cyanosis, clamp catheter and position on left side to keep air from going into pulmonary circulation, left heart, and into arterial circulation; report immediately.
- Do not increase rate to catch up if solution infuses too slowly; if solution infuses ahead of schedule, infuse 10% dextrose in water (or as per hospital protocol) to keep system open until time to resume TPN.
- Administer intralipids as ordered using an electronic infusion pump
  - given via a peripheral vein because these solutions are isotonic
  - may be given piggyback into TPN infusion to decrease the osmolarity and make the solution less irritating to the veins
  - do not use an IV filter because particles are too large to pass through filter
  - take baseline vital signs and repeat every 10 minutes during first 30 minutes of infusion to monitor for side effects (chills, fever, flushing, diaphoresis, allergic reactions, chest and back pain, nausea and vomiting, headache, vertigo, pressure over the eyes)
  - discontinue infusion if side effects occur
- Check blood sugar or urine sugar/acetone every 4 hours during therapy; administer insulin coverage as ordered; observe for manifestations of hypogly-

cemia (e.g., sweating, pallor, palpitations, nausea, headache, hunger, shakiness, blurred vision) or hyperglycemia (e.g., nausea, weakness, thirst, headache, polyuria).
- Flush catheter with heparin solution between infusions if treatment is intermittent rather than continuous.

☐ EVALUATION CRITERIA/DESIRED OUTCOMES

The child
- Is afebrile
- Has no redness, swelling, or discharge at catheter insertion site
- Maintains negative urine and blood cultures
- Is free from shortness of breath, chest pain
- Maintains serum glucose between 80-120 mg%; urine sugar less than 3+

NURSING DIAGNOSIS #3

Alteration in oral mucous membranes related to prolonged fasting

Rationale: TPN infusate is hyperosmolar and may cause dehydration thus drying mucous membranes. Children receiving TPN are frequently NPO and thus receive no oral stimulation from eating. Salivation is often decreased (increases with the thought/ sight/smell of food). Additionally, the presence of oral ulceration may make the child unwilling to cooperate with routine oral hygiene. Brushing the teeth/rinsing the mouth stimulates gingival health by increasing local circulation.

☐ GOAL

The child will maintain oral mucous membrane integrity.

☐ IMPLEMENTATION

- Inspect oral mucous membranes every 8 hours and record.
- Provide oral hygiene every 2-4 hours; massage gums, wipe new teeth for infants; brush teeth in older children and rinse mouth as able.

☐ EVALUATION CRITERIA/DESIRED OUTCOMES

The child
- Has intact oral mucous membranes

NURSING DIAGNOSIS #4
a. **Alteration in health maintenance** related to digestive dysfunction
b. **Social isolation** related to fear of being different
c. **Grieving** related to perceptions of lost body function and inability to eat normally
d. **Ineffective individual/family coping** related to perceptions of altered health status
e. **Altered growth and development** related to lack of oral/motor stimulation, imposed restrictions on movement

Rationale: Eating is both a time to meet the body's need for nutrition and a time for social interaction. The child who is unable to eat normally due to dysfunction of the digestive system, and family may experience a grief process over the loss. This may progress normally with development of alternative behaviors to deal with the loss or may develop into ineffective coping behaviors. The child may avoid social contact with others. Infants need oral stimulation to meet sucking needs and develop positive feeding behaviors. The catheter and IV tubing put restrictions on movement that limit the active exploration of the environment necessary to foster attainment of developmental milestones/tasks.

☐ GOAL

The child/parents will develop effective coping behaviors to deal with a socially different method of nutritional support.

☐ IMPLEMENTATION

- Be an empathic and supportive listener; use open-ended, leading statements to facilitate expressions of feelings; refer to *The Parent Experiencing Grief and Loss,* page 139.
- Monitor for signs of depression and hopelessness; provide support and clarify facts as needed.
- Educate child/family regarding the treatments and long-term needs; assist in the resumption of normal social contacts; teach others beside parents/ primary caretaker (e.g., relative, neighbor) child's routine and care needs to provide needed respite for caretaker; encourage parents to leave child with this individual and take time for themselves.
- Work with overprotective family members to encourage child to be as independent as possible.
- Encourage child to participate in family meals; the child may tolerate small amounts of clear liquids or elemental formula, and can schedule this during usual mealtimes; offer infant/toddler pacifier.
- Encourage resumption of normal schedule of activities

- children/families infuse solutions at night; conceal catheter beneath clothing during the day
- avoid contact sports
- cover dressing with plastic wrap if swimming and change dressing immediately when finished
- plan travel
- Refer to *The Child Experiencing a Body-Image Disturbance*, page 30.
• Ensure parents have address of a national organization such as Lifeline Foundation, Inc. (2 Osprey Rd., Sharon, Maine 02067).

☐ EVALUATION CRITERIA/DESIRED OUTCOMES

The child/parents
• Progress through grief response
• Utilize effective coping behaviors to deal with alteration in diet
• Participate in family meals and social situations that include food
• Resume preillness schedule of activities, making changes as needed to protect catheter
• Express feelings to staff and supportive others

NURSING DIAGNOSIS #5

Knowledge deficit regarding new method of nutritional support

Rationale: The child/parents who understand health problems and treatment will be better able to participate in therapy. They will be willing to ask questions, avoid many problems (e.g., sleep pattern disturbances, high levels of anxiety, noncompliance with treatment), and know how to recognize and deal with complications.

☐ GOAL

The child/parents will verbalize need for parenteral nutrition; will cooperate with treatment.

☐ IMPLEMENTATION

• Explain treatments; keep explanations brief; reassure that TPN is a method of supplying complete nutritional need.
• Teach those who will administer TPN at home
  - rationale for TPN
  - dressing change technique
  - symptoms to report to physician

- irrigation technique of the catheter with heparinized saline between infusions and how to change catheter cap
- infusion set-up and delivery via an infusion pump
- safety measures (e.g., put pump out of reach of young child to prevent them changing rate/turning pump off, pump alarms on; intercom in child's room to monitor child and quickly respond to alarms; ready access to clamps; catheter tucked under clothing to prevent pulling at catheter and dressing)
- identification of complications and what to do about them
• Teach to monitor intake and output and blood/urine glucose, and administer insulin as needed.
• Teach to weigh every other day on same scale, at same time, in same clothes.
• Teach to infuse solution at night while sleeping; reassure that infusion pump has an alarm if problems with flow occur; instruct to set alarm.
• Demonstrate techniques and obtain a return demonstration.
• Assist to incorporate TPN into usual schedule.
• Include supportive others in the instruction.
• Refer to support groups as necessary.
• Ensure child has an appointment for return visit to physician.

☐ EVALUATION CRITERIA/DESIRED OUTCOMES

The child/parents
• Explain rationale for TPN and how to perform procedure at home
• Demonstrate procedures before discharge including
  - changing the dressing and observing site
  - heparinizing catheter
  - changing catheter cap
  - setting up infusion, including adding vitamins, minerals, and elements to solution
  - testing blood/urine glucose testing
  - administering insulin
• Discuss safety measures and methods of implementation
• List complications that may occur and how to deal with them
• State when and how to notify physician of progress or problems
• List at least one health agency and one support group available for assistance

The Child with a Tracheostomy

Definition/Discussion

A tracheostomy is the surgical creation of an opening (stoma) into the trachea. It is performed to circumvent upper airway obstruction, to facilitate removal of tracheobronchial secretions, to optimize or for prolonged mechanical ventilation, or to enhance ventilation for any child with decreased chest muscle capability. The tracheostomy may be temporary or permanent.

Nursing Assessment

☐ **PERTINENT HISTORY**

Reason for tracheostomy, date of procedure, temporary or permanent; size/type of tracheostomy tube in place; oral fluids/foods status

☐ **PHYSICAL FINDINGS**

Color; vital signs with emphasis on respirations, breath sounds; color, consistency, amount of secretions; condition of skin around stoma; presence/absence of cuff (inflated/deflated)

☐ **PSYCHOSOCIAL CONCERNS/ DEVELOPMENTAL FACTORS**

Age, developmental level, inability to communicate verbally, fear of asphyxia, change in body image, habits (e.g., what comforts child, bedtime/feeding routines, favored objects)

☐ **PATIENT AND FAMILY KNOWLEDGE**

Purpose of tracheostomy, permanent or temporary; understanding of anatomy, especially the difference between the trachea and esophagus and how child can still eat after tracheostomy placement; hygiene regimen to be followed after discharge; indications for contacting physician after discharge; level of knowledge; readiness and willingness to learn

Nursing Care

☐ **LONG-TERM GOAL**

The child will maintain optimum ventilation; the child/family will care for stoma, incorporating changes necessary to accommodate this alteration in life-style.

NURSING DIAGNOSIS #1

Ineffective airway clearance related to inability to expel excess secretions

Rationale: This artificial opening into the tracheobronchial tree bypasses the glottis and the expulsive forcefulness of the cough is reduced. The upper airway passages are also bypassed so that humidification, warming, and filtering of air are decreased. Children often have plastic or silastic tracheostomy tubes (as opposed to metal). These materials allow the tube to have a more acute angle to accommodate a child's airway. They also resist crust formation and thus do not have to have an inner cannula. The child must still be watched closely to prevent occlusion of the tube by secretions or small objects.

☐ **GOAL**

The child will maintain a patent airway.

☐ **IMPLEMENTATION**

- Auscultate chest, record respiratory rate and characteristics every 4 hours; assess for tactile fremitus.
- Suction every 2-4 hours or as needed; choose appropriate sized catheter; with suction off, insert the length of the tube (may be only 2-3 inches in young child); apply suction and withdraw using a twisting motion; limit insertion and suctioning time to 5 seconds in infants and 15 seconds for older children; allow at least 30 seconds for reoxygenation and recovery between suction passes; record color, consistency, and amount of secretions.
- Observe for restlessness, anxiety, nasal flaring, stridor, tachycardia, cyanosis, trouble sucking/eating; monitor blood gases if ordered, especially pCO_2; ascertain that monitor, if used, is working properly and alarms are on.
- Turn and deep breathe every 2 hours; encourage activity.
- Provide humidification using humidity collar in

hospital or a cool, mist humidifier in child's room at home; change water daily, clean unit weekly according to manufacturer's recommendations.
- Ensure fluid intake of at least maintenance requirement/day unless contraindicated.
- Perform percussion and postural drainage to maximize airway clearance.
- Elevate head of bed or place in semi-Fowler's position; place small rolled blanket under shoulders to gently extend neck.
- Keep obstructive materials such as sheets, cotton, hair from pets, or stuffed animals away from stoma; if dressing is desired, use clean 4 × 4s without cotton filling and fold, do not cut, to fit, or use presplit gauze; use nonplastic bibs to keep food and fluids out of tracheostomy; check toys for small parts that can be inserted into tracheostomy.
- Tape obturator to head of bed; maintain an extra, appropriate-size tracheostomy tube/hemostat at bedside.
- Change tracheostomy tube every 7-10 days or as ordered
  - schedule 2-3 hours after meals to prevent vomiting
  - have second person assist
  - position child supine with small roll under shoulders or on assistant's lap
  - have all equipment ready at hand
  - suction child
  - cut old tracheostomy ties, remove old tracheostomy tube
  - in one fluid movement, quickly insert new tube with obturator, hold tube in place at flange with other hand, and remove obturator
  - observe for correct placement (e.g., chest moving with respiration, color)
  - securely knot tracheostomy ties on side of neck snug enough to just fit one finger under them

☐ **EVALUATION CRITERIA/DESIRED OUTCOMES**

The child
- Breathes easily with respiration rate within normal limits for age
- Demonstrates clear breath sounds upon auscultation
- Takes food and fluids without choking

NURSING DIAGNOSIS #2
a. **Potential for infection** related to altered pattern of ventilation, ineffective airway clearance
b. **Impairment of skin integrity** related to presence of secretions on skin

Rationale: With the body's first line of defense (an intact skin as a protective barrier) compromised

---

and the upper airway passages no longer functional, there is an access route for infectious organisms to enter the respiratory tract. If the child is unable to expel excess secretions, the likelihood of infection increases as the accumulated secretions provide a medium for the growth of organisms. Infants also have short, fat necks, which makes keeping them clean and dry difficult while predisposing them to skin maceration.

☐ **GOAL**

The child will remain free from infection; will maintain intact skin.

☐ **IMPLEMENTATION**

- Assess for signs of infection (e.g., temperature above 100.5°F [38.0°C], increased amounts of or change in smell or color [yellow-green] of mucus) every 4 hours.
- Inspect skin around stoma for signs of inflammation (e.g., redness, swelling, warmth, increased tenderness) every 2-4 hours during first few days postoperatively, then at least every 8-12 hours; recognize that some incisional inflammation is expected during the early post-op period; report unexpected changes in appearance (e.g., exacerbation of signs of inflammation or drainage around stoma).
- Use sterile technique when suctioning and performing tracheostomy care; use half-strength hydrogen peroxide and cotton-tipped applicators to clean around stoma every 4-8 hours and as necessary.
- Change external dressing and ties when wet or soiled; never remove old ties until new ones are in place or unless a second person holds the flange in place.
- Administer prophylactic antibiotics if prescribed, carefully monitoring for effectiveness (e.g., afebrile, normal pulse and respiratory rate, white blood count within normal limits, negative sputum cultures) and toxicity (e.g., abnormal hematologic, renal, liver function studies).
- Assess for other etiologic factors (e.g., impaired nutritional status, immunosuppression, environment, existing disease processes) that might contribute to the development of infection; initiate measures to modify these factors.

☐ **EVALUATION CRITERIA/DESIRED OUTCOMES**

The child
- Has clean, dry skin around the stoma
- Maintains temperature within normal limits
- Expectorates clear respiratory secretions
- Has normal laboratory values

NURSING DIAGNOSIS #3

a. **Impaired communication: verbal** related to effects of tracheostomy
b. **Altered growth and development** related to others' perceptions of the child being an invalid, lack of opportunity for communication

Rationale: *The artificially created opening bypasses the larynx, making phonation impossible and interfering with achievement of developmental milestones. Individuals may respond to the tracheostomy instead of to the child with normal developmental needs and a tracheostomy.*

☐ GOAL

The child will establish an effective method of communication and achieve developmental milestones.

☐ IMPLEMENTATION

- Explain to child/parents that child will not be able to vocalize (e.g., cry, speak) after the tracheostomy is placed, and reassure child someone is always nearby; reassure that voice will return after tracheostomy is taken out.
- Provide pad/pencil or erasable slate for writing, picture board for pointing to desired objects; work out an alternative method of communication for common needs (e.g., tongue clicks, eye blinks, finger taps).
- Arrange signals for bells or buzzer; suggest ways parents can monitor young child (e.g., make anklet with bells, use intercom).
- Always have caretaker in close proximity to young child; leave apnea monitor on while child is sleeping and turn monitor off while awake to help normalize environment.
- Talk to child frequently; point out objects in environment, provide tactile stimuli (e.g., hold, cuddle).
- Encourage parents to let child explore/achieve as developmentally appropriate; remind them that child needs discipline and limits, and parents should not be lenient because they feel sorry or guilty for child's condition; refer to *Normal Growth and Development*, pages 300–314.
- Teach, when condition permits, to occlude tracheostomy and phonate.

☐ EVALUATION CRITERIA/DESIRED OUTCOMES

The child
- Communicates needs and wants effectively with minimal frustration
- Achieves developmental landmarks appropriate for age

NURSING DIAGNOSIS #4

Ineffective family coping related to needs/demands of caring for child with a tracheostomy

Rationale: *The presence of a technologically dependent child in a family places great demands on family members both for care-giving requirements and sacrifice in terms of time and ability to meet own needs. These demands may strain family relationships and coping abilities.*

☐ GOAL

The family will cope with caring for/meeting the needs of all family members.

☐ IMPLEMENTATION

- Teach another caretaker child's routine, care demands, and CPR to give parents respite from the demands of care; encourage/give permission to parents to take time for themselves and not feel guilty; reinforce that they should feel fresher and better able to cope with the constant demands of care after a break.
- Encourage both parents (when appropriate) to share care demands, not leaving care responsibilities totally up to one.
- Help explain tracheostomy to siblings and gently remind parents not to overlook needs of siblings in order to concentrate on ill child; refer to *Siblings and the Ill Child*, page 261.
- Encourage parents to verbalize concerns, be an empathic listener; refer to *The Parent Experiencing Grief and Loss*, page 139.
- Arrange for parents to meet others who have a child with a tracheostomy and cope successfully; refer to community health agency for follow-up of teaching and reinforcement of home care, counseling as necessary.

☐ EVALUATION CRITERIA/DESIRED OUTCOMES

The parents
- Verbalize comfort in caring for child and meeting needs of all family members
- Have person(s) they trust with whom to safely leave child

NURSING DIAGNOSIS #5

Anxiety related to weaning process

Rationale: *Some children will need a tracheostomy for a limited period of time. It is likely that the child/parents will display some anxiety about the child getting enough air when the decision is made* *to start weaning. In addition, the child with a chronic respiratory condition and parents may be concerned that the weaning will be unsuccessful. The return to normal ventilation pathways can be achieved by a planned progressive set of actions.*

☐ GOAL

The child will ventilate through the nose, pharynx, larynx, and trachea; the child/parents will express decreased anxiety.

☐ IMPLEMENTATION

- Explain weaning process carefully (varies according to surgeon preference and the reason the tracheostomy was done; possibilities include gradually decreasing tracheostomy tube sizes, doing a bronchoscopy in the OR, then decannulating and suturing the stoma followed by close observation in the ICU, occasionally plugging the tube).
- Stay with child, monitor respiratory status closely.
- Reassure child/parents of progress.
- Refer to *The Child Experiencing Anxiety*, page 11.

☐ EVALUATION CRITERIA/DESIRED OUTCOMES

The child
- Demonstrates normal respiratory effort without tachycardia, stridor, retractions
- Breathes through normal passages

The child/parents
- Express decreased anxiety about weaning process

NURSING DIAGNOSIS #6

Knowledge deficit related to tracheostomy care

Rationale: The tracheostomy requires constant care in order to provide the child with adequate ventilation.

☐ GOAL

The child/parents will suction the airway and provide routine trach care; will know how to proceed if the tracheostomy should become displaced; will take caution with environmental and safety factors that might lead to aspiration of foreign particles and to prevent complications.

☐ IMPLEMENTATION

- Implement teaching plan for tracheostomy care and CPR with adequate time for practice and mastery of skill before discharge; include
  - routine tracheostomy tube changes
  - changing tracheostomy ties
  - skin care of stoma and neck
  - assessing need for suctioning appropriately (e.g., when child sounds coarse)
  - caring for equipment
- Encourage the child/parents to provide total independent care while still in the hospital.
- Review physician's instructions as to what to do should the tracheostomy become displaced and collaboratively plan with physician for parents to demonstrate tracheostomy tube change prior to discharge.
- Advise to avoid swimming, sandboxes; baths may be taken/wading pools used with careful adult supervision.
- Suggest using a porous covering for the stoma to filter out dust/foreign objects when playing outdoors or in very windy/cold conditions; avoid smokers, using aerosol sprays/powder/cleaning solutions around child.
- Encourage wearing a Medic-Alert bracelet.
- Teach parents to prepare and plan for excursions away from home (e.g., always have extra tracheostomy tubes and ties, battery-operated portable suction, and catheters).
- Have parents post list of emergency numbers in home; notify the telephone and electric companies of presence of child with a tracheostomy in the home.

☐ EVALUATION CRITERIA/DESIRED OUTCOMES

The child
- Wears a Medic-Alert bracelet upon discharge

The child/parents
- Demonstrate procedure for routine changing of tracheostomy tube and ties, skin care, caring for equipment, and appropriately assessing need for suctioning with minimal anxiety
- Demonstrate appropriate CPR techniques
- Describe process for reinserting the tracheostomy tube and avoiding aspiration

The Child in Traction

Definition/Discussion

Traction is the application of force through a system of ropes, pulleys, and weights to an injured or diseased body part in order to maintain it in a correct position. Traction may be applied to the skin with tape, bandages, halters; or it may be applied directly to the skeletal system with wires, pins, or tongs. Types of traction include: *running traction* (pull is exerted in one plane) and *balanced suspension traction* (produced by a counterforce other than the person's body weight; the affected part "floats" in the traction apparatus).

Nursing Assessment

☐ **PERTINENT HISTORY**

Onset of symptoms, mechanism of injury (if appropriate), previous musculoskeletal history, medication history, allergies

☐ **PHYSICAL FINDINGS**

Muscle spasms, bone fractures, x-ray studies, pain, decreased mobility, range of motion (ROM), skin condition

☐ **PSYCHOSOCIAL CONCERNS/ DEVELOPMENTAL FACTORS**

Age, developmental level, usual interaction patterns, habits (e.g., what comforts child, bedtime routine, favored objects), living situation, usual coping mechanisms

☐ **PATIENT AND FAMILY KNOWLEDGE**

Understanding of purposes of traction and how it works, potential complications related to traction and preventive measures, readiness and willingness to learn

Nursing Care

☐ **LONG-TERM GOAL**

The child will maintain proper alignment of the affected body part; the child will be free from complications related to circulation, nerve function, and immobility.

NURSING DIAGNOSIS #1

Alteration in comfort: pain related to condition requiring traction

Rationale: There are a variety of conditions and situations that require a child to be in traction (e.g., fracture, spinal curvature, dislocation). Children are often in acute pain; the traction will maintain alignment of the extremity and decrease pain.

☐ **GOAL**

The child will maintain an adequate level of comfort with minimal side effects.

☐ **IMPLEMENTATION**

- Ask verbal child to describe level of discomfort using a 0-10 self-rating scale; monitor preverbal child continuously for signs of pain (e.g., change in behavior, refusing to move/sleep).
- Determine preferred route of administration and administer analgesics PRN as ordered to reduce sensation of pain.
- Return 30 minutes after administering the analgesics to evaluate effectiveness of the medication; chart effect.
- Refer to *The Child Experiencing Pain*, page 216.

☐ **EVALUATION CRITERIA/DESIRED OUTCOMES**

The child
- Verbalizes decreased pain; appears comfortable if nonverbal
- Participates in self-care as age-appropriate

NURSING DIAGNOSIS #2

Fear/anxiety related to perceptions of equipment/procedures and being in traction

Rationale: Many children placed in traction experience anxiety and fear about unfamiliar procedures/

---

equipment and how successful the traction will be. Parents have many of the same feelings which the child may sense, thus intensifying the child's reaction. All the fears and anxieties need to be explored and instruction given to help alleviate some of these feelings.

☐ GOAL

The child/parents will verbalize feelings; will cope with the traction.

☐ IMPLEMENTATION

- Identify child/parent anxieties/fears related to traction.
- Orient to environment using simple explanations; explain traction set-up and equipment to be used (will vary depending on the type of traction)
  - usually consists of weights, ropes, and pulleys
  - may include an overbed frame with a trapeze
- Explain the type of traction that will be used
  - *skeletal:* pins, tongs, or wires directly connected to the bone with ropes connected to the pins
  - *skin:* traction straps (adhesive or nonadhesive) are placed on the skin and wrapped with elastic bandages, then are attached to ropes
- Explain which activities are permitted
  - *suspension traction:* child may sit, turn slightly, and move head as desired
  - *running traction:* the head of bed may be elevated to the point of countertraction
  - child may not turn from side to side because twisting will cause the bony fragments to move against each other
- Discuss with child/parents how they can help with care.
- Teach child how to call for assistance; ensure that someone is always close by to help; answer calls for assistance promptly.

☐ EVALUATION CRITERIA/DESIRED OUTCOMES

The child/parents
- Verbalize decreased feelings of fear and anxiety or demonstrate less fearful behaviors (e.g., calm readily, do not fight equipment)
- Verbalize an understanding of specific type of traction used and the activities permitted
- Adapt positively to limitations imposed by the traction

NURSING DIAGNOSIS #3

Potential for injury related to improper alignment

Rationale: *If alignment of the affected extremity is not properly maintained, injury resulting in perma-*

---

nent misalignment and decreased ROM of the affected extremity may occur. When immobilized, musculoskeletal structures must be maintained in an anatomically correct position to prevent this type of injury.

☐ GOAL

The child will maintain correct alignment of the affected extremity; will be free from injury.

☐ IMPLEMENTATION

- Verify desired position of the ropes, pulleys, supports, and amount of weight to be used; verify activities and movement permitted (will differ depending on purpose and desired outcome of the traction for each specific child).
- Maintain proper alignment; place on a firm mattress with a bedboard, footboard, and overhead frame and trapeze (dependent on type of traction).
- Ensure that ropes and pulleys are in straight lines, at correct angles, and unobstructed (e.g., not resting on the bed, floor, or any other object to prevent the ropes from hanging freely); ensure ropes are well knotted and not frayed, and weights are allowed to hang freely.
- Keep slings clean, dry, and secure.
- Do not remove skeletal or adhesive skin traction straps; when nonadhesive skin traction straps are used, traction may be removed as designated by physician.
- Ensure that child in Bryant's traction has buttocks slightly elevated off bed (child's weight supplies the counter traction).
- Check sandbags, pillows, restraints (e.g., jacket, pelvic sling), and other supports every 1-2 hours.
- Keep child centered in the bed with head elevated at the proper level; instruct as to why positioning is so important; help child know proper position by putting sticker on trapeze in appropriate position and tell to keep his/her nose under it.
- Place toys, call light, phone, bedside table, and necessary items within easy reach.

☐ EVALUATION CRITERIA/DESIRED OUTCOMES

The child
- Maintains proper position while lying in bed
- Verbalizes importance of positioning to maintain alignment and prevent permanent injury
- Maintains traction in a freely hanging position
- Is free from injury

NURSING DIAGNOSIS #4

Potential for infection related to skeletal traction

Rationale: With skeletal traction, pins, wires, and tongs are surgically placed directly on the skeletal structures. In this invasive procedure, there is the risk of introducing pathogens through the pin sites and there is, therefore, potential for developing an infection locally or in the skeletal structures.

☐ **GOAL**

The child will be free from infection at wound sites.

☐ **IMPLEMENTATION**

- Monitor for signs/symptoms of infection (e.g., inflammation, edema, hematoma, wound drainage, elevated leukocyte count, elevated temperature).
- Provide pin care according to hospital protocol using strict sterile technique.
- Use strict sterile technique when changing the dressings.
- Administer antibiotics as ordered and observe child's response.

☐ **EVALUATION CRITERIA/DESIRED OUTCOMES**

The child
- Has no drainage or odor from pin sites or other wounds
- Maintains temperature and leukocyte count within normal limits

---

NURSING DIAGNOSIS #5
a. **Alteration in tissue perfusion: peripheral** related to compromised circulation
b. **Impairment of skin integrity** related to immobility

Rationale: When the blood supply to an area falls below that required for survival, the skin and the underlying tissues are destroyed. Cellular nutrition and respiration are dependent on adequate blood flow through the microcirculation. There is often pressure upon the vessels and the nerves during immobilization via traction. The pressure on the vessels compromises the circulation to the area and causes decreased perfusion to the surrounding tissues; the pressure on the nerves can cause decreased sensation and palsy of various nerves. A complication of overhead traction (e.g., Dunlop and particularly Bryant's) is Volkmann's syndrome. This is an ischemic process that progresses from arterial occlusion to muscle anoxia and vasospasms. The resulting lack of blood supply leads to muscle necrosis, paralysis, and contractures.

☐ **GOAL**

The child will exhibit adequate peripheral circulation; will be free from thromboembolus and impaired nerve function; will maintain intact skin.

☐ **IMPLEMENTATION**

- Carefully assess back and other bony prominences (especially the heels) every 2 hours for signs of impaired circulation (e.g., reddened areas of the skin, broken skin).
- Use appropriate decubitus-prevention measures and devices; refer to *The Child at Risk for Hazards of Immobility*, page 156.
- Check splints, bandages, and elastic wraps for tightness and bunching with every contact; remove/replace elastic wraps as ordered.
- Check skin and affected extremity for temperature, color, sensation, and movement every hour to assess neurovascular functioning; monitor for signs of Volkmann's syndrome (e.g., severe pain, absent pulses in affected extremity, pallor or cyanosis, paresthesia, paralysis); report immediately.
- Avoid pillows and pads under the knees or calves; monitor for signs/symptoms of thromboembolus (e.g., pain in leg or chest, calf tenderness, shortness of breath, coughing up blood) and report any findings.
- Instruct in ROM exercises (often not needed in active child) for unaffected body parts to prevent contractures and increase circulation; refer to *The Child Requiring Range-of-Motion Exercises*, page 237.

☐ **EVALUATION CRITERIA/DESIRED OUTCOMES**

The child
- Has normal neurovascular checks
- Performs ROM exercises if needed on a regular basis with minimal prompting
- Exhibits normal peripheral pulses
- Is free from signs and symptoms of thromboembolus
- Is free from signs and symptoms of pressure sores
- Participates as able in preventive care of decubitus ulcers

---

NURSING DIAGNOSIS #6
a. **Diversional activity deficit** related to imposed prolonged immobilization
b. **Altered growth and development** related to lack of stimulation, inability to perform age-appropriate activities
c. **Alteration in self-concept: body image** related to perceptions of immobility, traction apparatus, injury

Rationale: The nursing challenge in caring for a child in traction is keeping the child involved in

---

enough activities/providing diversion so s/he will tolerate the immobility needed to maintain traction. Children may perceive the traction apparatus as an extension of self or may have distorted perceptions of the body part because of the imposed immobility.

☐ **GOAL**

The child will participate in age-appropriate activities; will have appropriate body-image perception.

☐ **IMPLEMENTATION**

- Provide age-appropriate toys/activities; refer to *Normal Growth and Development*, pages 300–314.
  - *infant/toddler:* mobile, busy box, music box, rattles, squeak toys, stuffed animals; audiotape of parents reading; talk to, stroke, play "peek-a-boo", "this little piggy"; look at books, name body parts, have parents bring in favorite objects
  - *preschool:* watch children's video programs then discuss them, color, Play-doh, blunt scissors, medical kits, puppets, stories
  - *school-age:* discuss friends, have classmates send cards/visit/call; books, puzzles, arrange for visiting teacher, hang "punching bag" from overhead frame, play basketball (e.g., attach string to ball so can retrieve it by self).
  - *all ages:* push bed into hallway/playroom, arrange to eat meals with family/other children, use volunteers to play with child, decorate room
  - Refer also to *The Child Requiring Play Therapy*, page 226, and *The Child Experiencing a Body-Image Disturbance*, page 30.

☐ **EVALUATION CRITERIA/DESIRED OUTCOMES**

The child
- Does not complain of boredom
- Performs age-appropriate tasks as allowed/able
- Verbalizes positive body image/draws self-portrait with all body parts present and to scale (as age appropriate)

NURSING DIAGNOSIS #7

Knowledge deficit regarding condition requiring traction, care at home

---

Rationale: The child and parents will need instruction about activity restrictions, mobility, safety, pain management, and any further rehabilitation that may be necessary for complete recovery.

☐ **GOAL**

The child/parents will verbalize an understanding of the discharge rehabilitation plan including pain management, return to school and activities, exercise, mobility, and safety.

☐ **IMPLEMENTATION**

- Assess need for referral to a home health agency for physical therapist to instruct child in progressive ambulation program and to assess the home for equipment necessary to ensure safety and complete healing without complications.
- Instruct about use of pain medications and possible side effects of prescribed medications; teach noninvasive measures.
- Give written instructions for progressive, active exercises as appropriate.
- Instruct in care of incisions/wound sites per hospital protocol until all open areas are completely healed.
- Teach signs/symptoms of infection (e.g., painful swelling in affected extremity or pin sites; redness, drainage, odor from pin sites/incisions; elevated temperature) and appropriate action to take.
- Review activity restrictions (this will vary depending on type of injury and the success of traction); suggest appropriate diversional activities.
- Counsel regarding safety measures to prevent accidents.

☐ **EVALUATION CRITERIA/DESIRED OUTCOMES**

The child/parents
- Verbalize understanding of the need for continued rehabilitation at home
- State approved exercises/activities that may be performed

The parents
- Demonstrate care of incisions and/or pin sites
- Identify correctly signs/symptoms of infection and when to call physician
- Describe activity restrictions
- Verbalize correct usage of pain medications and demonstrate the use of noninvasive measures to relieve pain and discomfort

The Child Requiring Tube Feedings

Definition/Discussion

Nutrition and medications are administered through a nasogastric (NG) tube or a gastrostomy tube (GT) to meet the basic daily metabolic requirements for those children who are unwilling or unable to take nutrition orally.

Nursing Assessment

☐ **PERTINENT HISTORY**

Previous medical/surgical diagnoses, congenital defects, gastrointestinal (GI) disorders; prior diet history (e.g., breast, bottle, solids), onset of symptoms, medications

☐ **PHYSICAL FINDINGS**

Weight, height, head circumference (in infants) plotted on standardized growth chart, nutritional status, elimination patterns, level of consciousness, status of oral and pharyngeal mucosa, placement of tube; color and amount of gastric secretions, tolerance of nutritional formulas, ability to suck/swallow

☐ **PSYCHOSOCIAL CONCERNS/ DEVELOPMENTAL FACTORS**

Age, developmental level, previous experience with NG/gastrostomy tube, usual coping mechanisms, available support systems, habits/rituals (e.g., what comforts child, bedtime activities, favored objects)

☐ **PATIENT AND FAMILY KNOWLEDGE**

Purpose, side effects, potential complications, level of knowledge, readiness and willingness to learn

Nursing Care

☐ **LONG-TERM GOAL**

The child will maintain adequate nutrition via NG or gastrostomy tube with safety and reasonable comfort.

NURSING DIAGNOSIS #1
a. **Self-care deficit: feeding** related to medical condition
b. **Fluid volume deficit** related to condition, inadequate intake
c. **Alteration in nutrition: less than body requirements** related to condition

Rationale: Various conditions and situations such as chemotherapy, respiratory distress, neurologic impairment, trauma or surgery to the head, neck, mouth, or esophagus, and eating disorders, all preclude children from being willing or able to swallow, thus necessitating tube feedings.

☐ **GOAL**

The child will maintain optimal nutrition via tube feedings with minimal discomfort and complications.

☐ **IMPLEMENTATION**

* Obtain baseline weight/height/head circumference and plot on growth curves so that progress of nutritional status can be monitored.
* Weigh every day on the same scale, at the same time, in the same clothes.
* Check orders to determine the strength of the formula to be administered; formulas are usually given at quarter to half strength initially to determine child's tolerance for the feedings.
* Wash hands and arrange all necessary equipment
  - formula/enteral feeding solution at room temperature
  - enteral feeding administration set and solution container
  - 10-60 cc syringe (depending on child's size)
  - water for irrigation
* Explain procedure and position upright/on right side with head of bed elevated.
* For feedings, unclamp the tube, attach the syringe, and aspirate gastric residual (NOTE: do not aspirate GT postfundoplication; allow residual to drain by gravity).
  - measure and record gastric residual; if less than

half of previous feeding, return gastric aspirate to stomach and proceed with tube feeding; subtract residual from amount to be fed (e.g., if feeding is 50 cc and residual refed was 5 cc, then only give 45 cc this feed); if more than 50% of previous feeding, assess for abdominal distension, notify physician, and postpone tube feeding until instructed further
  - verify placement of NG tube after checking residual by auscultating with a stethoscope before each feeding (place stethoscope over the gastric region and introduce 1-10 cc air quickly into tube with a syringe; listen for the crackling or gurgling as the air exits tube into the stomach)
- Flush the tube with 3-10 cc water (depending on size of child) to clear and assess for patency; pinch the tube before the water completely runs out to avoid instilling air.
- Add formula to syringe gradually for *intermittent bolus feedings*; it may be necessary to gently push plunger to start feeding flowing, then remove plunger and allow feeding to flow by gravity; raise and lower the tube as needed to regulate the flow so that the total feeding takes approximately 20 minutes; avoid instilling air; do not use force to administer feeding.
- Follow the prescribed amount of formula with 3-10 cc water; clamp tube before the water empties and plug with a clean catheter plug.
- Leave head of bed elevated for at least an hour after feeding to prevent aspiration; have child lie on right side or ambulate if possible.
- Use enteral infusion pump for *continuous feedings*, hang 4 hours of formula supply at a time; check NG placement every 2 hours and check for residual every 2-4 hours; with gastrostomy, vent stomach every 4 hours or as necessary; stop continuous feedings for at least 30 minutes before and during treatments such as physical, pulmonary, or x-ray therapy; check infusion rate hourly to ensure an appropriate rate.
- Record tolerance of the feeding, amount of formula infused, and length of time bolus feeding administered.
- Assess for signs and symptoms of dehydration (e.g., inelastic skin turgor, dry mucous membranes, sunken fontanel/eyeballs, fever, low urine output with high specific gravity) at least every 4 hours.
- Monitor urine/blood glucose 4 times a day; monitor serum electrolytes as ordered to ensure that nutritional formulas are appropriate for the child's metabolic requirements.
- Refer to dietician as appropriate.

☐ EVALUATION CRITERIA/DESIRED OUTCOMES

The child
- Maintains fluid balance, is free from signs and symptoms of dehydration

- Demonstrates weight gain
- Has normal urine specific gravity, blood sugars, electrolytes

---

NURSING DIAGNOSIS #2
a. **Alteration in oral mucous membranes** related to prolonged tube feedings/NPO status
b. **Impaired gas exchange** related to aspiration of tube feeding
c. **Alteration in comfort: pain** related to prolonged placement of NG tube
d. **Altered growth and development** related to lack of stimulation during feeding, restrictions on movement

Rationale: These are all conditions or side effects that may occur as a result of tube feedings and having an NG tube in place. The tube can cause laryngitis, esophagitis, or pharyngitis when left in place for several days. Oral mucous membranes can become dry and ulcerated. Dehydration and osmolar overload can occur with children who receive too high a concentration of formula in too short a period of time. Tube feedings administered too rapidly or in high volume may cause abdominal distension, which may precipitate aspiration. If a child does not associate sucking with feeding and a feeling of fullness or feeding as a pleasurable experience, s/he may not gain weight as rapidly or may refuse to eat orally when physically able to do so.

☐ GOAL

The child will experience minimal side effects/complications of the tube feedings.

☐ IMPLEMENTATION

- Refer to *The Child Requiring Nasogastric Intubation*, page 194, and *The Child with a Gastrostomy*, page 135.
- Provide mouth care at least every 4 hours to preserve oral mucosa and provide comfort, or have child gargle and rinse mouth 3 times a day to keep the oral mucosa cleansed.
- Have child brush teeth (if present) and massage gums to stimulate oral tissues, prevent ulceration, and to provide oral-motor stimulation.
- Suggest sucking on hard candies, if permitted and if child is old enough, to coat throat and provide a pleasant taste in the mouth.
- Apply cream/ointment to lips and nose to counteract dryness and irritation.
- Monitor for signs/symptoms of aspiration (e.g., coughing substance that looks like feeding, change in breathing pattern or behavior) continuously.

- Administer non-narcotic analgesics as ordered to decrease discomfort; evaluate effectiveness.
- Monitor child's emotional reaction to tube feeding; always hold/cuddle/talk to infant during feeding; offer pacifier and have infant suck during feeding; make it a pleasant experience.

☐ **EVALUATION CRITERIA/DESIRED OUTCOMES**

The child
- Maintains intact nasal and oral mucosa
- Has decreased verbalizations/appearance of side effects or complications

---

NURSING DIAGNOSIS #3

Knowledge deficit regarding maintenance and care of feeding tube and tube feedings

Rationale: If child is discharged on tube feedings, the child/parents need instructions on total management of the feedings at home, including type and preparation of the formula, method of tube feeding, care of NG or gastrostomy tube, equipment required for the feedings, and signs/symptoms of complications/side effects from the feedings with appropriate action.

☐ **GOAL**

The child/parents will verbalize and demonstrate understanding of tube feedings, potential complications/side effects of the feedings, and maintenance of the tube and equipment at home.

☐ **IMPLEMENTATION**
- Refer to *The Child Requiring Nasogastric Intubation*, page 194, and *The Child with a Gastrostomy*, page 135.
- Instruct in principles of tube feedings as outlined above.
- Teach about potential complications and side effects (e.g., signs and symptoms of aspiration of formula, feeding intolerance, potential mechanical

problems) and appropriate action to take for each complication.
- Provide repeated demonstrations and have parents give return demonstrations of the tube feedings (e.g., type, concentration, and preparation of formula to be used; anchoring techniques; verification of tube placement before each feeding; and administration of feeding).
- Teach to administer medications per tube, using similar principles for intermittent tube feedings; reinforce administering medication via gravity and to flush tube well to ensure total dose administration and maintain tube patency.
- Instruct in the use of equipment necessary for the tube feeding; include information about care of the equipment, trouble-shooting measures, and how to obtain supplies.
- Instruct in care of mucous membranes and comfort measures.
- Provide written instructions for parents to take home to ensure proper administration of tube feedings with minimal complications and proper care of the equipment.
- Assess need for referral to home health agency for continuity of care; provide parents with a list of resources.

☐ **EVALUATION CRITERIA/DESIRED OUTCOMES**

The child/parents
- Describe the principles of tube feedings and care of the tube
- List potential complications/side effects of tube feedings
- Identify signs/symptoms of aspiration of tube feeding and appropriate action
- Demonstrate preparation of the correct formula and verification of tube placement
- Administer tube feeding without complications
- Demonstrate correct administration of medications via NG or gastrostomy tube
- List community resources where formula and supplies can be obtained
- Describe techniques to protect mucous membranes and to provide comfort measures

The Child with Ulcerative Colitis

Definition/Discussion

Ulcerative colitis is a chronic mucosal inflammatory disease limited to the colon. It starts in the rectosigmoid colon and spreads upward. The disease is characterized by bloody diarrhea, fluid imbalances, and remissions and exacerbations. The peak age of onset in children is between 10 and 19 years.

Nursing Assessment

☐ **PERTINENT HISTORY**

Medical and surgical history, history of the disease, family history of gastrointestinal (GI) problems, nutritional status, eating patterns, food allergies

☐ **PHYSICAL FINDINGS**

Discomfort/pain: site, frequency, character, rebound tenderness and guarding in the right lower quadrant; weight loss; growth retardation; edema; temperature elevation; signs of dehydration (e.g., decreased skin turgor, dry mucous membranes), nausea and vomiting; bowel sounds; palpable liver; number, character, amount, presence of blood (e.g., overt, positive guaiac test), pus, and mucus in stool; excoriation/erythema of perineal skin from severe diarrhea; nutritional deficiencies; anemia; delayed sexual maturation

☐ **PSYCHOSOCIAL CONCERNS/ DEVELOPMENTAL FACTORS**

Developmental level, usual personal/family coping mechanisms, habits (e.g., what comforts child, bedtime routine, favored objects), roles and responsibilities, age, available support system, apprehension, tenseness, restlessness

☐ **PATIENT AND FAMILY KNOWLEDGE**

Exacerbating/relieving factors; skin care; level of knowledge, ability, readiness and willingness to learn

Nursing Care

☐ **LONG-TERM GOAL**

The child will heal and regain normal bowel function; the child will adhere to medical regimen and required life-style changes to prevent recurrence of symptoms.

NURSING DIAGNOSIS #1
a. **Alteration in comfort: pain** related to abdominal cramping/perineal skin excoriation
b. **Impairment of skin integrity** (perineal) related to diarrhea

Rationale: In ulcerative colitis, lower abdominal cramping is usually present because of the irritable bowel. The cramping pain is followed shortly by urgency and bloody diarrhea. As the bowel becomes scarred, thickened, and shortened, cramping is less marked. An increase in pain and tenderness may indicate impending obstruction from inflammation, edema, and scarring. The constant perineal irritation of severe diarrhea can lead to skin excoriation.

☐ **GOAL**

The child will have decreased/relieved abdominal pain; will maintain/regain perineal skin integrity.

☐ **IMPLEMENTATION**

- Ask child to assess discomfort using a 0-10 self-rating scale or a picture board with unhappy faces as an objective measure of the pain; refer to *The Child Experiencing Pain*, page 216.
- Assess location, duration, pattern, frequency, characteristics, and precipitating factors of pain; determine causative factors (e.g., stressful events, food intolerance); eliminate factors that can be eliminated.
- Monitor for and record abdominal distension, increased temperature, decreased blood pressure, rectal bleeding, characteristics of stool.
- Cleanse perineal area with mild soap and warm water after each bowel movement; apply ointments as necessary.
- Administer analgesics; evaluate effectiveness; administer anticholinergics, steroids to relieve spasm of the GI tract; monitor for desired effects.
- Administer and encourage sitz baths as necessary for local soothing and comfort.

EVALUATION CRITERIA

The child

- Verbalizes lessening or absence of pain
- Has no perineal erythema or excoriation

NURSING DIAGNOSIS #2

Alteration in bowel elimination: diarrhea related to intestinal inflammatory process

Rationale: Frequent watery stools are typical of the disease. The need to defecate may be sudden, painful, and related to ingestion of irritant foods.

GOAL

The child will experience less frequent bowel movements of normal consistency.

IMPLEMENTATION

- Have bedpan/bathroom facilities readily accessible at all times; empty bedpan promptly; use room deodorizer and avoid undue embarrassment for child.
- Observe and record number, characteristics, amount, and precipitating factors of diarrhea.
- Promote intestinal rest by restricting foods and fluids that precipitate diarrhea (e.g., raw vegetables and fruits, whole grain cereals, condiments, carbonated drinks, milk.)
- Promote rest and relaxation to decrease bowel motility.
- Monitor for signs/symptoms of perforation and peritonitis (e.g., fever, tachycardia, lethargy, leukocytosis, decreased serum protein, anxiety, prostration).
- Administer medications to decrease bowel motility and inflammation; evaluate and chart response.
- Observe for long-term side effects of steroids (e.g., growth retardation, GI upset, masking of and lowered resistance to infections, fluid retention).

EVALUATION CRITERIA

The child

- Defecates stools of normal consistency at less frequent intervals than on admission

---

NURSING DIAGNOSIS #3

a. **Fluid volume deficit** related to diarrhea
b. **Alteration in nutrition: less than body requirements** related to dietary restrictions, pain, diarrhea

Rationale: Stools are watery and frequent; the scarred and denuded bowel loses plasma and electrolytes profusely and is unable to absorb nutrients properly. Children with severe diarrhea may lose 500-1,700 cc water and 2-8 gm sodium in 24 hours. Nausea, odor, cramping, and diarrhea decrease the inclination for food. The child with chronic colitis usually manifests growth retardation and delayed sexual maturation. Inadequate diet and decreased absorption may lead to vitamin K deficiency and defects in coagulation.

GOAL

The child will maintain adequate fluid volume and electrolyte balance; will ingest sufficient calories to maintain/gain weight.

IMPLEMENTATION

- Maintain accurate intake and output record; include number, character, and amount of liquid stools; monitor serum electrolytes.
- Weigh child daily on the same scale, at the same time, in the same clothes.
- Observe for indicators of excessive fluid loss (e.g., excessively dry skin and mucous membranes, decreased skin turgor, oliguria, decreased temperature, weakness, increased hematocrit and hemoglobin, elevated BUN and urine specific gravity).
- Encourage bedrest/limited activity during acute phase of illness.
- Administer parenteral fluids and TPN in acute exacerbations; refer to *The Child Receiving Total Parenteral Nutrition*, page 276.
- Resume oral food intake when diarrhea decreases; begin with clear liquids and progress to small, frequent feedings of high-calorie, high-protein, low-residue bland foods; administer elemental diets, blended feedings, and commercial preparations (e.g., Vivonex).
- Discuss limitation of fats, spicy foods, milk products, eggs, potatoes, wheat, and tomatoes.
- Note clotting studies and observe for overt or occult bleeding.
- Allow child to participate in dietary planning.
- Administer iron supplements by deep intramuscular injection using z-track technique; administer vitamin B_{12} (folic acid).
- Administer antiemetics to prevent vomiting and further nutritional losses; evaluate and chart effectiveness.

EVALUATION CRITERIA/DESIRED OUTCOMES

The child

- Stabilizes/gains weight
- Has normal skin turgor, mucous membranes, temperature, BUN, and urine specific gravity
- Excretes at least 0.5-2.0 cc/kg/hour urine

- Maintains hematocrit and hemoglobin within normal limits
- Has normal electrolyte values

NURSING DIAGNOSIS #4

a. **Ineffective individual coping** (depression) related to the chronicity of the condition
b. **Alteration in self-concept: body image** related to perceptions of disease, retarded growth, delayed sexual maturation

Rationale: Recurrent exacerbations often lead to discouragement, anxiety, and preoccupation with the physical self. The child may feel "different" and unable to fit in with peers since s/he is often smaller and has delayed acquisition of secondary sex characteristics. Peers may also tease the child about this.

☐ **GOAL**

The child will cope effectively with the disease and its treatment; will have a positive self-image.

☐ **IMPLEMENTATION**

- Provide an atmosphere of trust and caring; encourage verbalization of fears and concerns.
- Determine ongoing strengths and values; discuss these with child.
- Identify potential solutions to present problems; assist to set realistic goals.
- Assist to identify some new effective coping mechanisms; provide positive reinforcement when they are utilized; role play situations with child.
- Encourage independence; provide opportunities for active participation in self-care to maintain dignity and feelings of self-worth.
- Encourage involvement of family in coping process; this may assist child to cope with stressors.
- Keep informed of physical condition; initiate realistic discussion of disease, diagnostic studies/treatments.
- Refer to pastoral care as desired; obtain social service and home care consults if necessary.
- Refer to *The Child Experiencing Depression*, page 96, *The Child/Family Experiencing Anxiety*, page 11, and *The Child Experiencing a Body-Image Disturbance*, page 30.

☐ **EVALUATION CRITERIA/DESIRED OUTCOMES**

The child

- Verbalizes feelings
- Identifies individual strengths

- Develops at least 1 new effective coping mechanism
- Identifies/uses external resources
- Verbalizes positive self-concept

NURSING DIAGNOSIS #5

Knowledge deficit regarding stress, self-care management of a chronic bowel disorder

Rationale: Stress and emotional tension may precipitate an exacerbation of chronic bowel disease. In addition, a chronic disease requires child/parent knowledge for cooperation to help avoid and minimize symptoms.

☐ **GOAL**

The child/parents will manage stress and deal with the prescribed regimen for chronic illness.

☐ **IMPLEMENTATION**

- Provide with information about disease process, medications, and symptoms of complications.
- Instruct or have dietician instruct regarding high-protein, high-calorie, high-vitamin, and low-fiber diet that avoids milk products.
- Teach about medications that decrease bowel motility and inflammation.
- Instruct to increase fluid intake when diarrhea occurs.
- Teach perineal hygiene, use of analgesic rectal ointment or sitz baths for anal discomfort.
- Instruct on relaxation techniques (e.g., breathing exercises) when emotional tension/stress is present.
- Assist to identify foods/fluids/stressors that may exacerbate symptoms and ways to eliminate or deal constructively with them.
- Advise to maintain a regular sleep schedule and to schedule daily activities to avoid fatigue, taking rest periods as needed.
- Instruct regarding signs indicating possible exacerbations or complications (e.g., abdominal pain, increasing diarrhea, presence of blood or pus in the stool, fever, progressive weight loss).
- Instruct to plan for regular follow-up care; refer to outside resources as indicated.

☐ **EVALUATION CRITERIA/DESIRED OUTCOMES**

The child/parents

- List signs indicating possible exacerbations or complications
- Verbalize and initiate appropriate interventions to deal with prescribed regimen

The Child with a Urethral Catheter

Definition/Discussion

A tube (catheter) is introduced through the urethra into the urinary bladder. The retention catheter encloses a second smaller tube throughout its length. This second inner tube connects to an inflatable balloon near the tip, which, when expanded after insertion, holds the tube in place within the bladder. Surgical procedures on both male and female reproductive structures and urinary systems may call for the use of an indwelling urinary catheter postoperatively. Any critically ill child may require an indwelling catheter for continuous assessment of fluid status. Some children who are post-op or who have congenital defects are discharged home with an indwelling catheter in place or instructions for intermittent catheterization. They require frequent monitoring of their health status in order to prevent complications such as infection.

Nursing Assessment

☐ PERTINENT HISTORY

Congenital defects; incontinence or bladder distension; operative site needing protection from urine; critical condition requiring frequent monitoring of urinary output during treatment

☐ PHYSICAL FINDINGS

Presence of congenital defects; neurogenic bladder, bladder obstruction or overdistension requiring intermittent drainage; incontinence after being toilet trained; daily urine output, specific gravity, gastrointestinal (GI) symptoms

☐ PSYCHOSOCIAL CONCERNS/ DEVELOPMENTAL FACTORS

Developmental level; embarrassment about urine collection receptacles in clear view; body image, dependency, habits/routines (e.g., sleep patterns, what comforts child, favored objects)

☐ PATIENT AND FAMILY KNOWLEDGE

Purpose of intermittent/indwelling catheter; care of the catheter after discharge, prevention of bladder/renal infections, signs and symptoms of urinary tract infection (UTI); frequency of follow-up regimen; level of knowledge, readiness and willingness to learn

Nursing Care

☐ LONG-TERM GOAL

The child will maintain a properly functioning urinary drainage system; the child will be free from cystitis, more serious infections, and complications.

NURSING DIAGNOSIS #1

Potential for infection related to presence of indwelling catheter, interruption of flow of urine from bladder to urinary collection receptacle, technique of self-catheterization

Rationale: *While the bladder is normally a sterile organ resistant to inflammation and infection, a catheter left in for more than a few hours can greatly increase the chances of bacteriuria. Most infections are caused by E. coli, Klebsiella, Aerobacter, Pseudomonas, and Proteus organisms, normally found on the skin or in the hospital. Strict aseptic technique is essential. Stasis of urine in the bladder predisposes the child to development of bladder infection and other complications. If the collection receptacle is positioned higher than the bladder, reflux of old urine into the bladder causes contamination.*

☐ GOAL

The child will be free from bacterial growth and nosocomial infection; will maintain normal urine composition, specific gravity, and pH; will maintain gravity flow drainage without backflow into bladder, blockage of flow, or interruption of closed system.

☐ IMPLEMENTATION

• Observe and record color, odor, amount, and appearance of urine each time collection unit is emptied or intermittent catheterization is done; check

- patency of drainage system every 2 hours; explain the system to child/parents; enlist cooperation of child when possible.
- Determine specific gravity and pH of urine collected 1 hour after collection receptacle has been previously emptied or when catheterization is done; report specific gravity greater than 1.030.
- Record total intake and output at least every 8 hours; monitor critically ill children more frequently; report to physician hourly output of less than 1 cc/kg.
- Be alert to indications of renal calculi (e.g., low abdominal distension or pressure, flank pain), pyelonephritis (e.g., fever, chills, vomiting, lower back pain), or urinary tract infection (UTI)
    - infants: signs of sepsis (e.g., poor sucking and feeding, vomiting, lethargy or irritability, fever, jaundice, abdominal distension, failure to thrive)
    - toddler, preschooler: GI symptoms (e.g., lower abdominal pain, anorexia, vomiting, diarrhea), urgency, frequency, dysuria, regression to bed-wetting
    - older children: frequency, urgency, dysuria, lower abdominal pain
- Note sediment buildup, mucus threads, blood clots, or stones that impede flow; use sterile equipment and technique to irrigate and clear blockage if "milking tube" does not work; slowly, gently infuse room-temperature solution to reduce likelihood of bladder spasms and discomfort.
- Explain procedure when inserting the indwelling catheter verbally, through drawings, or using doll play; refer to *The Child Requiring Play Therapy*, page 226; enlist the aid of another nurse to help restrain/comfort child as needed.
- Use only sealed, sterile units (e.g., catheter, drainage tube, and collection container); choose catheter of appropriate size for child (often 8-10 French or a smaller soft, flexible feeding tube if these are too large).
- Employ strict aseptic technique; cleanse perineum with solution, designated by hospital protocol; use antibacterial lubricant on catheter tip and meatus before insertion.
- Secure catheter with nonirritating tape; place drainage tube between or under legs and secure it to linens at side of bed to allow child freedom of movement.
- Keep drainage tube descending directly to collection unit without any dependent loops that could cause urine to move uphill slowly before flowing into container.
- Keep collection unit and tubing covered by sheets (ease of visibility to a passing nurse is less important than preventing the older child's embarrassment); leave infant's tube uncovered so passing nurse can ascertain that unit is intact.
- Change catheter and complete unit only when necessary for accumulated sediment or leakage (average every 1-4 weeks) and per hospital protocol.
- Cleanse perineum at least twice daily with mild soap and water; rinse and dry thoroughly; apply ointment around meatus per hospital protocol.
- Obtain urine specimens with a sterile 25-gauge needle and 5 cc syringe; after cleansing rubber port with antiseptic swab, insert at an angle into the flared or distal end of catheter or specially designed port; send specimen to lab in sterile container.
- Clamp tubing whenever collection unit is lifted to the height of the mattress, such as when turning child or moving by gurney; keep collection unit below bladder level at all times; hang bag at the correct level attached to the gurney or back of wheelchair when transporting child; instruct child/parents in prevention of reflux.
- Never disconnect catheter from drainage unit unless absolutely necessary; transport or ambulate child with closed unit intact; when disconnection is unavoidable, use sterile catheter plug and discard after single use; before emptying drainage bag, wipe spigot with alcohol sponge; do not let the spigot touch anything else.
- Use a three-way catheter or connecting Y-tube when irrigations are needed more than once daily.
- Explain procedure as developmentally appropriate when performing intermittent catheterization; choose appropriate sized catheter for child; use sterile technique as described above or use clean technique if child will be discharged requiring intermittent catheterization and will be using clean technique at home; assemble equipment, keeping catheter in its container until needed; wash hands (health care personnel should also use gloves to further decrease the chance of nosocomial infection); insert catheter until urine starts to drain; when it stops, tell child to squeeze tummy (as with bowel movement), slowly remove catheter; if urine begins to drain again, stop and allow bladder to empty; remove catheter and wash it and hands with soap and water, rinse through with clear water, dry and store in clean, dry container (e.g., margarine container, plastic bag).
- Ensure a fluid intake of 1,500 cc/m^2/24 hours (unless contraindicated).
- Give cranberry or prune juice to promote a slightly acid urine; provide acid-ash foods (e.g., eggs, meat, poultry, cereal, corn, prunes, plums).
- Give orange juice, citrus fruits, vegetables if child is on streptomycin or sulfonamide therapy to promote alkaline urine; reduce intake of acid-ash foods previously listed.
- Instruct child/parents in purpose and rationale of catheter, catheter care, hand washing, and prevention of contamination.
- Discuss with child/parents the signs/symptoms of urinary infection and when to contact physician/clinic/visiting nurse.

☐ EVALUATION CRITERIA/DESIRED OUTCOMES

The child

- Maintains an appropriate fluid balance for each 24 hours
- Excretes urine free of bacteria and with normal specific gravity and pH
- Is free from bladder infection, renal calculi

NURSING DIAGNOSIS #2

a. **Urinary retention** related to catheter removal

b. **Functional incontinence** related to catheter removal

c. **Anxiety** related to fear that control will not be achieved

Rationale: Children who have had indwelling urinary catheters for long periods of time may experience difficulty in regaining bladder control after the catheter has been discontinued because of decreased muscle tone. It may be necessary to institute bladder training measures to facilitate achieving independence and to maintain positive self-esteem. The child may be anxious about regaining normal urinary patterns and may express concerns that something is wrong if immediate control is not present.

☐ GOAL

The child will regain and maintain normal muscle tone and function of the bladder to the extent possible; the child/parents will express decreased feelings of anxiety about voiding pattern.

☐ IMPLEMENTATION

- Clamp catheter for 2- to 3-hour intervals prior to draining for at least 2 days before removing catheter (for those who have had indwelling catheters for long periods).
- Encourage an increased fluid intake (unless contraindicated) if child has had catheter removed after a period of days or after pelvic surgery; offer bedpan/urinal or assist to bathroom every 2 hours.
- Catheterize for residual urine as ordered; if unable to void within 6 hours of catheter removal, it may be necessary to recatheterize for a period of time.
- Maintain calm manner while assuring child that these measures will promote bladder control.
- Explain that it may take some time for normal functioning to be restored; listen to expressed concerns; validate that others have expressed similar feelings.
- Point out positive achievements (e.g., if catheterization for residual ordered, tell child when residual amount minimal or absent).
- Know that anxiety tends to interfere with normal urinary elimination; work with child to decrease

anxiety prior to removing catheter and as necessary afterwards; refer to *The Child Experiencing Anxiety*, page 11.

☐ EVALUATION CRITERIA/DESIRED OUTCOMES

The child

- Is prepared for catheter removal
- Regains normal bladder function after catheter removal

The child/parents

- Express decreased feelings of anxiety regarding return of bladder control

---

NURSING DIAGNOSIS #3

Knowledge deficit regarding necessary care at home

Rationale: If the child is to be discharged with an indwelling catheter or needing intermittent catheterization, child/parents will need instruction to ensure adequate catheter care.

☐ GOAL

The child/parents will properly manage the care of the indwelling catheter, or to perform intermittent catheterization.

☐ IMPLEMENTATION

- Demonstrate intermittent catheterization/routine catheter care to the child/parents; provide time for practice and return demonstrations; reinforce appropriate behaviors and correct mistakes.
- Review the signs/symptoms of urinary infection and renal calculi and provide a written list; instruct to contact physician should symptoms develop.
- Reassure that the inability to void or control voiding is not uncommon and may be directly related to neurologic changes as a result of medical/surgical condition; encourage discussion with physician if this is a problem area.
- Initiate referrals for home health care as needed.
- Ensure that written instructions are provided at time of discharge if bladder training is to be done at home.

☐ EVALUATION CRITERIA/DESIRED OUTCOMES

The child/parents

- Verbalize understanding of the purpose and rationale of the indwelling catheter/intermittent catheterization
- Demonstrate correct daily care of catheter/intermittent catheterization
- List early signs and symptoms of urinary infection; know to call physician/clinic/nurse

The Child with Wilms' Tumor

Definition/Discussion

Wilms' tumor is the second most commonly occurring pediatric solid tumor and is most frequently found in toddlers. The etiology is unknown but is often associated with certain congenital anomalies such as hemihypertrophy, cryptorchidism, and hypospadias. Treatment involves surgical removal of the tumor, followed by radiation and combination chemotherapy. Wilms' tumor is classified according to the following staging system.

- *Stage I*: tumor confined to the kidney and completely removed surgically
- *Stage II*: tumor extending beyond the kidney but completely removed surgically
- *Stage III*: regional spread of disease beyond kidney with residual abdominal disease postoperatively
- *Stage IV*: metastatic disease to lung, liver, bone, distant lymph nodes, or other distant sites
- *Stage V*: bilateral disease

Nursing Assessment

☐ **PERTINENT HISTORY**

Medical (e.g., vague abdominal pain, malaise, anorexia) and surgical history, congenital anomalies, date discovered/diagnosed, metastatic disease, family history, life-style

☐ **PHYSICAL FINDINGS**

General health status, height, weight, nutritional status, fever, enlarged abdomen, abdominal mass, hypertension, hematuria, renal function, pain, staging of tumor

☐ **PSYCHOSOCIAL CONCERNS/ DEVELOPMENTAL FACTORS**

Age, developmental level/tasks, sex, child's/family's available coping mechanisms, roles and responsibilities, experience with cancer/cancer treatment, family structure, cultural/religious beliefs, routines (e.g., sleep patterns, favored objects, what comforts child)

☐ **PATIENT AND FAMILY KNOWLEDGE**

Type of cancer, prognosis, course of treatment, level of knowledge, readiness and willingness to learn

Nursing Care

☐ **LONG-TERM GOAL**

The child will adapt effectively to the diagnosis and treatment of Wilms' tumor as well as the biopsychosocial changes that will occur; the child will return to previous roles in the family and community after a reasonable period.

NURSING DIAGNOSIS #1

Anxiety related to perception of the diagnosis of Wilms' tumor, treatment regimen

Rationale: The diagnosis of cancer will evoke anxiety in the child/parents due to its potentially fatal outcome and aggressive treatment. The possibility of several different stages of Wilms' tumor is frightening as diagnosis is sometimes delayed because of vague presenting symptoms. Surgical removal of the involved kidney (treatment of choice) may cause fear for the remaining kidney.

☐ **GOAL**

The child/parents will express fears, anxieties, feelings, and questions associated with the diagnosis/ treatment of Wilms' tumor; will use appropriate coping mechanisms to manage anxiety.

☐ **IMPLEMENTATION**

- Know what the physician has told the child/parents regarding diagnosis, treatment, and prognosis; clear up any misconceptions, answer questions.
- Be honest; keep information/communication continuous and current.
- Allow time for parents to express emotions and concerns without child present.
- Allow child (if appropriate) to express emotions and concerns without parents present.
- Encourage continued expression of concerns and questions.

- Assess previous coping mechanisms and support systems and encourage child/parents to utilize them; introduce new coping mechanisms (e.g., methods of information seeking, clergy, active participation in care) as necessary.
- Arrange a meeting with another child with a similar diagnosis if possible.
- Refer to *The Child Receiving Chemotherapy*, page 57, and *The Child Undergoing Radiation Therapy*, page 234.

☐ EVALUATION CRITERIA/DESIRED OUTCOMES

The child/parents
- Express relief of/reduction in anxiety
- Identify and utilize effective coping mechanisms/support systems
- Verbalize feelings about Wilms' tumor, life-style and role changes, coping mechanisms

---

NURSING DIAGNOSIS #2

Alteration in comfort: pain related to cancerous invasion of the kidney, surgical removal of kidney

Rationale: Although Wilms' tumor is not likely to cause discomfort prior to diagnosis, pain will occur after surgery is done to remove the tumor and involved kidney.

☐ GOAL

The child will experience relief/control of pain.

☐ IMPLEMENTATION

- Assess the child's level of pain using a developmentally appropriate scale to obtain an objective measure of the pain (e.g., color scale, 1-10 scale); refer to *The Child Experiencing Pain*, page 216.
- Assess for nonverbal cues of pain (e.g., flat affect, grimacing, not moving in bed, guarding).
- Administer analgesics as ordered; assess and chart their effectiveness frequently.
- Teach muscle and total-body relaxation techniques as developmentally able; assist child to use newly learned skills.
- Provide diversional activities to enhance relief of pain (e.g., coloring, games, reading).
- Utilize effective nonmedication pain-relief techniques (e.g., massage, heat, cold).

☐ EVALUATION CRITERIA/DESIRED OUTCOMES

The child
- Expresses/demonstrates relief/control of pain

NURSING DIAGNOSIS #3

Grieving related to perceptions of the loss of kidney and kidney function

Rationale: The kidneys provide a vital physiologic function. A diagnosis of Wilms' tumor necessitates the removal of the affected kidney. The child's/parents' grieving process for this kidney begins when the diagnosis is made and the treatment alternatives are made known.

☐ GOAL

The child/parents will express grief and the meaning of the loss as developmentally appropriate.

☐ IMPLEMENTATION

- Assess the stage in the grieving process; be aware of the usual stages including denial; assist to progress through the grieving process.
- Recognize and help to see that feelings of depression, hostility, resentment, frustration, helplessness, and hopelessness are normal.
- Provide time to verbalize feelings; ask questions and express concerns; be an empathic listener; do not challenge/discourage any expressions; assist to focus on adaptive feelings after adequate time for grieving.
- Arrange for another with similar disease to talk with child/parents and share experiences, present life-style changes, and coping strategies.
- Be honest and open regarding expected outcome of treatment; be realistic about impairments to expect while offering alternatives to deal with loss.
- Initiate referral for psychologic counseling if requested/assessed that grieving is interfering with normal functioning.

☐ EVALUATION CRITERIA/DESIRED OUTCOMES

The child/parents
- Express grief and move toward resolution
- Identify effective coping patterns/appropriate support systems for continued resolution of loss

---

NURSING DIAGNOSIS #4

Knowledge deficit regrading diagnosis of Wilms' tumor, treatment regimen

Rationale: Wilms' tumor is a complex and unfamiliar disease. The child/parents must understand the disease, treatment regimen, and follow-up care to accomplish biopsychosocial adaptation.

☐ GOAL

The child/parents will understand the disease process, treatment regimen, and follow-up care for Wilms' tumor.

☐ IMPLEMENTATION

- Assess level at which to direct education.
- Arrange scheduled, uninterrupted sessions with the child/parents.
- Provide written material to enhance/review verbal instructions (e.g., signs to watch for and report, medications to be given, appointments to be made, appropriate activity).
- Give instructions at developmentally appropriate level, in terms of what the child will see, hear, feel, taste, smell.
- Provide with names and phone numbers of physicians/appropriate individuals to contact for follow-up and emergency care.
- Refer to community support group/home health service as appropriate.

☐ EVALUATION CRITERIA/DESIRED OUTCOMES

The child/parents
- Comply with instructions
- Verbalize an understanding of Wilms' tumor and its treatment
- Know when and how to contact appropriate person(s) for follow-up or emergency care
- List support groups/home health services available

APPENDIX 1
Normal Growth and Development: Infant

Definition/Discussion

Infancy is the initial period of an individual baby's life cycle, generally spanning from 4 weeks to 18 months.

- Childhood is sequentially divided into stages or critical periods to denote a specific span of time that is maximally favorable for the accomplishment of a new developmental process or task.
- Developmental task (Erikson's central problem) to be resolved in infancy is the development of a sense of trust versus mistrust.
- Overall nursing responsibilities during infancy include meeting the infant's needs for nutrition, warmth, sucking, comfort, sensory stimulation, security, and love; supporting and guiding the parents to a responsible, nurturing, and understanding relationship with their child; observing, assessing, and recording normal and abnormal patterns of infant growth and development.
- The common parameters of physical development and behaviors for the infant are outlined below; corresponding nursing implications and parental teaching or guidance suggestions follow in *italics*.

☐ AGE 1 TO 6 MONTHS

Weight: gains 5–8 oz/week (14–22 gm); average American baby now doubles birth weight by 4⅔ months.
- *Review with parents the accuracy of their knowledge on formula or breast-feeding techniques. Reinforce that baby does not need solid foods until 4–6 months.*

Height: grows approximately 1 in/month (2.5 cm).
- *Teach normal growth, development, and safety needs to parents, repeating as necessary.*

Posterior fontanel: closes by about 2 months.
- *Show parents how to handle head gently while fontanels remain open, but not to be afraid to wash scalp.*

Skin: diaper rashes common; infantile acne on face at about 4–5 weeks is common; lasts 4–6 weeks, disappears without treatment; is thought to be associated with disappearance of mother's hormones and the activation of baby's oil and sweat glands.
- *Wash baby clothes prior to use in mild detergent (not soap as it decreases flame retardancy) and rinse well.*
- *Remind parents to keep diaper area clean, dry, and aerated; change diapers frequently washing area with warm water, mild soap after bowel movements; avoid perfumed soaps, bubble bath products, and overuse of commercial diaper wipes (contain alcohol, fragrance, and other additives); protect skin with a thin layer of water-barrier ointment (e.g., zinc oxide, Desitin, A&D), not petroleum jelly, which predisposes to yeast infections; lay infant on pad without diaper and leave area open to air for short periods; teach that using powder is not necessary but if parents insist, then to apply small amount to their hand away from baby's face and then put on baby; do not let baby play with powder container.*

Immunity: passive immunity received from mother is lost unless infant is breast-feeding; then immunity to some diseases remains through breast-feeding period.
- *Encourage parents to seek health care at recommended intervals, usually 2 weeks, 2, 4, 6, 9, 12, 15, and 18 months. Ascertain that parents have a health care provider who is available, accessible, and within transportation and financial means.*
- *Remind parents of need to have immunizations at recommended visits (see table 5); inform of risks/benefits of immunizations so they can make an informed choice*
- *Review common signs of illness and importance of early medical attention.*

Teething: begins at approximately 5–6 months; salivation increases at 3 months when salivary glands mature; drooling, which occurs as infant has not yet learned to swallow saliva effectively, is not a sign of teething though may become more evident when teething begins.
- *Suggest a bib to absorb saliva. Teach that prior to eruption, baby's gums are swollen and tender, baby is irritable and restless, may have slight fever or change in bowel habits. Rubbing gums with finger, a cold spoon, or chilled teething rings may ease discomfort. Sometimes the dentist will prescribe a medication to numb the gums. Symptoms subside when teeth erupt.*
- *Teach parents that high fever, diarrhea, or upper respiratory symptoms are not teething symptoms; these illnesses should be reported promptly to health care provider.*

Reflexes: sucks reflexively in response to touch; quiets in response to sucking.
- Strong palmar grasp reflex; reaches to mouth; "mouths" objects and fist at 2 months; chews at 4–6 months.
  - *Encourage parents to allow baby to satisfy sucking needs (other than during feeding) by permitting baby to suck fingers or thumb, or by using a pacifier.*
  - *Warn parents to be sure that all objects within baby's reach are too large to be swallowed; provide washable, safe toys.*
- Moro (startle) reflex present from birth to 4 months.
  - *Try to avoid loud noises or startling moves around baby.*

- Tonic neck reflex response reaches peak about 3 months, then gradually disappears.
  - *Tell parents to turn baby's head periodically to prevent unsightly flattening and balding of head from sleeping too much with head turned to preferred side since baby exhibits a definite preference for turning head to one side.*
  - *Suggest reversing crib's position in room or hanging bright objects on the neglected side of the crib to stimulate interest.*

COMMON BEHAVIORS

2 Months

Movement: can move in crib; holds head erect in mid position for a few seconds, but still wobbly.
  - *Be certain crib slats are no greater than 2 3/8 in (6 cm) apart; mattress should fit snugly. Secure infant seat so it cannot tip over with baby's movement. Restrain infant when in seat (a three-point restraint is more effective than a lap belt only).*
  - *Reinforce and emphasize car seat safety; use only approved car seats that meet Federal safety standards; always use car seat and buckle baby in correctly; start early and be consistent and firm in use to make compliance expected and to foster appropriate "car behavior." The safest place in the car is the back seat, optimally the middle. Car seats should be rear facing until the infant can sit and hold head erect (about 6 months), then may be forward facing.*

Play: likes bright, colorful, large toys of varied shapes, configurations, and textures; spongy, squeeze toys that make sounds.
  - *Turn feeding, dressing, bathing, and diapering into pleasurable play.*
  - *Provide washable, durable toys without sharp edges or small, loose pieces; avoid fuzzy toys (present an inhalation danger).*
  - *Use crib gyms with stable items for grabbing (infants get frustrated by items that always swing out of reach when they grab for them); rotate toys in crib or playpen to provide various stimuli.*
  - *Use infant seats and swings for awake baby but caution against excessive use. Sometimes place baby in prone position and surround with toys; other times, use back or chest carrier to keep baby close to mother.*
  - *Hold baby and dance to music while humming or singing along.*

Crying: becomes differentiated as to cause (e.g., pain, cold, offensive odors, loud noises).

Smiling: an open-eyed, alert smile involving whole face, eyes crinkling; responds to another's smile.

Vision: can follow a bright, moving object from outer corner of eye to midline; stares indefinitely at surroundings, fixating on 1 or 2 objects (especially moving objects); prefers person to object; begins to coordinate senses (e.g., sucking at sight of bottle, anticipating or looking for sound of objects); attempts to bat or grab objects; begins to hold objects for a few moments.
  - *Teach parents that there is no really "average" baby; each is unique with its own pattern of eating, sleeping, crying, temperament, and activity.*
  - *Encourage to ward off a deluge of unsolicited advice and to take questions and concerns to someone they trust (e.g., health care provider).*
  - *Urge to interview and train at least 2 or 3 mature, reliable baby sitters, or to use licensed child care persons. Try to have sitter spend time with baby while parent is there. Have parent fully explain and demonstrate details of baby's routine, as well as special likes and dislikes.*
  - *Encourage to employ, when possible, healthy nonsmokers;*

children who are exposed to a lot of second-hand smoke have been shown to have a higher incidence of upper respiratory infections and a possibly higher risk of developing cancer.

Sleep: 18–20 hours/day; may sleep 7 hours at night after a late night feeding; shows a definite preference for sleep position; stays awake longer with social interaction.

Feeding: needs approximately 115 cal/kg/day; eats approximately every 4 hours and anticipates feedings. Breast-feeders may eat more frequently.
  - *Hold baby for feedings, looking down and talking to baby, thus providing both stimulation and positive interactions for both baby and care giver.*

Bathing: enjoys bath, kicking, and splashing; exhibits delight and excitement.
  - *Encourage water play during bath time. Pick up baby's legs and move them in circles while singing a song or saying a rhyme. Baby may like being nude, being stroked, massaged, and tickled slightly.*

3 Months

Movement: moves arms and legs vigorously; begins purposeful movements; when on stomach, raises head and chest, supported by forearms; holds hands in front and stares at them, wiggling fingers; reaches for objects, bringing hands together in front; puts hands and objects in mouth. Coordinates looking/grasping/sucking movements.

Play: similar to that of a 2-month-old.

Crying: less.

Smiling: more spontaneous.

Vocalization: babbles and coos in response to sounds. Begins to localize sounds, voluntarily turning toward them; distinguishes speech sounds from other sounds and responds.
  - *Keep diaper pins and other small, loose objects out of baby's reach.*
  - *Move baby from bassinette to a full-sized crib and from mother's bedroom to another room if this has not yet been done. Establish satisfactory sleep patterns by using crib only for sleep, by avoiding stimulation just before bedtime, by setting a consistent habit of presleep activities, and by putting baby in preferred sleep position.*
  - *Rock, cuddle, hum, or play soft music, but avoid practice of putting baby to bed with a propped bottle, as this will foster dental caries, ear infections, and promote association of feeding with bedtime. "Nursing bottle" decay occurs when naptime or bedtime bottles of sweetened liquids are given; the decay process begins during the sleeping hours.*

Sleep: 16–20 hours/day; may sleep 10 hours at night, although may awaken and fret; will fall back to sleep if left undisturbed.
  - *Babies who sleep on their stomach "nest" down, appearing to burrow into mattress; therefore be sure mattress is firm with no loose plastic sheets or pillows to cause smothering.*

4 Months

Appearance: birth hair is gradually replaced by permanent hair. Eye changes to permanent color (although some babies will retain blue eyes up to 2 years before changing color).

Movement: holds head steady and erect for a short time; lifts head and shoulders off surface at 90° angle when prone; supports body with hands. Rolls from back to abdomen and from stomach to side, gradually able to go from stomach to back. Begins "swimming" motions preliminary to creeping and crawling. Picks up objects with whole hand, or may take small objects between index and second fingers.
  - *Never leave infant alone on bed, table, or sofa; use playpen (those with mesh sides must always have them up; children can roll into the mesh and be smothered), crib with rails up, or an infant seat that is securely anchored.*

Play: likes brightly colored rings, large plastic or wooden beads, spoons, keys, noisemakers. Shows preference for certain toys or blankets.

- *Hold toys within baby's vision so s/he can reach for them, but do not put on string that can strangle a neck or wrist.*
- *Toys should be safe for chewing but not able to be swallowed.*

Smell: distinguishes between and shows interest in different smells.

- *Provide opportunities for baby to smell different foods, fragrances, etc.*

Vision: eyes can focus at different lengths and follow different objects for 180°. Stares at place from which an object drops; discriminates between familiar and strange faces, responding with more pleasure to familiar, smiling faces than strangers.

- *Give brightly colored toys to hold; put brightly colored pictures with simple designs in line of vision; put in front of mirror.*

Socialization: likes attention, having people around to handle, play, and talk to him/her; becomes fussy, demanding, or bored if ignored. Enjoys sitting up and being part of a busy environment. Listens, recognizes voices, turns head toward sounds; is quiet and attentive to music.

- *Keep infant in close proximity to others; smile at/talk to frequently while doing chores, encourage siblings to interact with infant while playing nearby, play various types of music (avoid loud noises that may damage hearing).*

Vocalization: expresses moods of enjoyment or protest; makes sounds, laughs, gurgles, or shrieks; laughs in response to light tickling.

- *Repeat sounds baby makes; call by name; laugh with baby; talk to baby about environment, things that are occurring.*

Sleep: sleeps through nights for up to 10 or 11 hours (although some babies will continue to wake at night and demand a feeding for as long as a year).

Feeding: needs approximately 110 cal/kg/day; learning to eat from a spoon may be possible now.

- *Encourage mother to breast-feed infant as long as desired; formula feeding should continue through the first year. Avoid overfeeding or excessive calories.*
- *Introduce solid foods at 4–6 months depending on health care provider's recommendation, care giver's desire, and baby's readiness. Introduce solid foods, one at a time, each week, watching carefully for allergies or intolerances (e.g., rashes, vomiting, diarrhea). Begin with single-grain enriched cereals: rice, barley, oatmeal (delay offering wheat, corn cereals, or mixed grain cereals for several weeks).*
- *Do not force feed, keep mealtime pleasant, happy; let baby play with spoon, get used to smell and taste of new food as well as feel in mouth.*
- *Give vitamin supplements as directed; fluoride supplements may be needed if water supply for homemade formula is not fluoridated. Breast-fed infants need fluoride supplements.*
- *Encourage parents to let baby meet sucking needs (e.g., bottle of water, fingers, pacifiers); if using pacifier, NEVER put it on a string around baby's neck or attached to gown.*

5 and 6 Months

Movement: sits momentarily without support in forward-leaning position, gradually extending time able to sit. Hitches (moves backward in a sitting position). Begins creeping (moves along with abdomen on floor). Gradually able to roll completely over, from stomach to back to stomach. Touches knees, brings feet to mouth; can be pulled up to standing position easily. Tonic neck reflex disappears. Likes to sit in high chair to watch family activity. Enjoys outings in carriage or stroller.

- *Be sure to strap in seat safely; use harness in carriage or food shopping cart.*
- *Keep floor clear of small and dangerous objects; keep cords out of reach; cap all unused electrical outlets.*
- *Close off open stairwells; block off unsafe step-downs.*

Play: enjoys unrestricted movement, to exercise limbs and to observe environment. Likes to look at self in mirror. Enjoys bath and noisy water toys. Likes large soft balls and musical balls. Has longer attention span; can roll, play with toys for an hour or so. Shows interest in books, pictures, paper; likes being read nursery rhymes. Loves social games.

- *Provide opportunities for baby to have unrestricted movement (e.g., carpeted floor, large playpen); let creep around in front of large mirror; limit walker use. Play social games (e.g., peek-a-boo, pat-a-cake, piggy-went-to-market).*

Socialization: distressed around strangers.

- *Give baby an opportunity to be around strangers before they hold/care for baby.*

Vocalization: utters syllables such as "ma," "ba," "da," adding new ones each week; crows, squeals, grunts, purrs, clicks, coughs, babbles.

Feeding: begins to finger-feed, hold bottle and spoon.

- *Limit formula amounts to approximately 20–24 oz daily, while increasing solids to meet development and weight needs.*
- *Add vegetables and fruits, one new each week, checking for food allergies and intolerances.*
- *Neither approve nor scold the spitting back or blowing of food; be persistent and encouraging, patiently spooning food off face, chin, or bib back into mouth.*
- *Realize that amounts and portions of foods vary depending on the baby's size, activity, health status, and appetite, as well as the number of other foods taken and amount of formula given. Offer bottle after eating solids.*
- *Allow baby to be part of family at mealtime; provide with finger food.*

☐ AGE 7 TO 12 MONTHS

Weight: gain after 6 months slows to approximately 4–5 oz/week (11.4–14 gm).

- *Evaluate child's growth status in terms of self; comparisons with charts or siblings may be inappropriate.*

Height: approximately 26–28 in (65–70 cm) at 6 months; grows ½ in/month (1.25 cm).

- *Arrange for 6-month check-up.*
- *Because of baby's rejection of strangers at this time, try to do as much of the exam as possible while baby is sitting in mother's lap. Proceed with the less distressing tasks first, giving baby something to interest and distract.*
- *Remember to smile and talk to baby while conducting examination.*

Teeth: begin to erupt around 6 months; 2 central lower incisors first, then 2 central upper incisors, then upper and lower lateral incisors.

- *Show mother how to clean newly erupted teeth of placque by using a clean washcloth. "Baby" teeth or primary teeth are important for chewing, for appearance, for proper development of jaws and mouth, and for reserving space for permanent teeth. Placque and decay need prompt care to control.*

COMMON BEHAVIORS
7 to 9 Months

Movement: toe sucking common. Sits alone well by 9 months. Raises self to sitting position. Tries various ways to move body; some may crawl (on all four limbs with abdomen up off floor). May start pulling self to a stand, learning later how to return to floor. Bounces and bears some weight in standing position.

- *Hand things to baby directly in front of eyes and chest; don't try to change way baby tries to grasp them.*
- *Never leave alone in bathtub; keep electrical appliances (e.g., can openers, hair dryers) out of reach.*
- *Keep wastebaskets hidden and out of reach; avoid pinching baby's fingers when closing doors, cupboards, drawers.*
- *Strap baby safely into strollers, carriages, grocery carts, high chairs. Close off stairs or teach baby how to crawl down them, feet and legs first.*

Play: likes large plastic and wooden blocks, nesting boxes or cups, stacking rings, water toys, paper to crumple, plastic keys, measuring cups and bowls.

- *Use play pen, cushioned furniture to practice standing and improve muscle tone. Play "hide-a-toy" with baby. Continue social games; give toy telephone; play music of many kinds, provide simple rhythm instruments (e.g., drum, bells, xylophone); read rhymes, poems, sing-song stories with repetitive sounds (Dr. Seuss-type) and ABC rhyme books with pictures.*

Socialization: wriggles and giggles in anticipation of play; learns meaning of "no" by voice tone; pats mirror image; resists doing what s/he doesn't want to do. Wants to play in presence of family; perform for audience. Shows open and fond affection for family members; exhibits comfort around children; fear of strangers reaches peak, then starts to lessen. Begins to understand disappearance concept, may look to floor for object dropped in front of him/her. Imitates adult movements such as clapping, swaying, making sounds and noises.

- *Because of stranger anxiety, cost of sitters, and baby's comfort around children, it is tempting and convenient to involve older siblings in a large amount of baby care while mother is otherwise busy; safety of baby and maturity of older child must be prime considerations, as well as possibility of sibling rivalry and the need of older child to have usual routines of afterschool activities.*

Vocalization: loves to imitate; coughs, clicks, buzzes; says syllables like "ma," "da," "ga,"

Sleep: 14–16 hours/day, including 1–2 daytime naps.

Feeding: eats 3 meals/day; holds spoon, drinks from a cup, enjoys finger foods, tastes everything; may or may not show readiness for weaning; still has strong sucking needs and the emotional need to be held even though willing to hold own bottle.

- *Allow longer time for feeding so child can practice new skills.*
- *Show excitement at baby's achievements.*
- *Gradually decrease amount and frequency of formula or breast-feedings, while increasing foods of various kinds and textures; include meat, soft pieces of fruit, cheese, toast.*
- *When eating 3 meals/day, milk intake should be approximately 24 oz/day.*
- *Avoid foods that can cause choking (e.g., raw carrots, nuts, popcorn). Start good nutritional habits by avoiding too many sweet cookies and salty crackers. Do not introduce candy or ice cream.*

10 to 12 Months

Movement: crawls and creeps well; climbs up and down from furniture; climbs up stairs, but needs to be taught how to crawl down backwards. Pulls self to feet; by 12 months, can stand alone for a few minutes and pivot body 90°. "Cruises" or sidesteps along furniture (average 11 months). Begins walking (average 12 months). Stoops, squats, bends, leans, reaches, opens drawers, lifts lids. Begins to help dressing self. Can pick up objects now and can voluntarily release them. Can hold 2 or more objects in hand; can "store" object in mouth or under arm while grabbing another one. Likes to handle, shake, bang, roll, fill, empty, push, spin, drop, and otherwise manipulate all objects.

- *Allow freedom to creep and walk in safe, baby-proof areas; never leave alone in bathtub.*
- *For babies who can climb out of crib, use a net or put crib side down, placing crib next to a bed to cushion descent.*
- *Baby-proof bedroom and be sure baby cannot open door. Close off stairways or teach baby how to crawl down backwards, safely.*
- *Use only toy hampers without lids to prevent pinched fingers.*
- *Assure parents of a "quiet" baby (or one that is "late" developing motor skills) that when baby is ready, learning and practice time is often shorter than for those babies who started to crawl, climb, or walk earlier; some babies show interest in movement, others in vocalization, still others in passive study and observation.*
- *Whether babies should learn to walk in bare feet or soft-or hard-soled shoes is controversial. Consult health care provider and consider own needs and environment. When purchasing shoes, buy them only ½ in longer and ¼ in wider than baby's foot to allow natural spread and growth. Too-large shoes are clumsy, cause blisters, and force unnatural foot position to develop. Too-small shoes also cause problems, so check size and fit at least monthly.*
- *Minor toeing-in is normal for the new walker and can correct itself when baby's balance is better.*
- *Teach baby meaning of "hot" and "don't touch." Set firm, consistent limits. Try to be patient and persevering. Join a parent support group for mutual aid and help.*
- *Show love openly; touch, hold, rock, be active with child.*
- *Supervise older children "sitting" with or playing with baby, so they don't frighten or inadvertently hurt baby; help older children express frustrations at baby's behavior in socially acceptable and safe ways.*
- *Do things as a family, showing love and respect for older child's needs.*

Play: likes rocking horse and riding toys. Likes to play chase. Prefers push toys to pull toys. Likes to rock, sway, keep time and "dance" with someone to music. Actively searches for vanished objects.

- *Provide new and different toys that stimulate curiosity (e.g., milk cartons, fabric or cardboard boxes, containers to fill and spill, pots).*
- *Do not pretend to be something fearful or jump out at baby with loud noises.*
- *Play music in baby's bedroom or playroom.*
- *Play "hide-a-toy"; let baby see the object covered, then search for it.*

Socialization: may begin temper tantrums. Seeks approval but is not always cooperative. Shaking head "no" is easier than nodding "yes." Shows moods.

- *Walk away from baby having a temper tantrum, or place in own room. Reward verbally for cooperative behavior.*

Verbalization: responds to own name. Identifies (by pointing to) objects such as sky, airplane, familiar animals, and people. May be able to say 3 or 4 words (e.g., "ma-ma," "no," "hi," "hot").

- *Be alert to detect early hearing losses. See a pediatric audiologist if baby does not respond to own name, cannot imitate simple sounds, or cannot point to familiar objects.*

Sleeping: some active babies sleep only 11–12 hours at night with 1-hour daytime nap. Some babies still wake at night to stand, to be rocked, to have a bottle.

Feeding: will eat less solid food if formula or breast-feeding not correspondingly reduced; gains less weight as movement increases.

- *Do not force baby to eat more than s/he wants or force foods that baby dislikes. Allow longer mealtime if baby is feeding self. Allow baby to use fingers and do not force spoon usage at all times. Give baby a spillproof plastic cup; a plastic sheet or newspapers on floor during mealtimes will ease cleanup of spills.*

☐ AGE 12 TO 18 MONTHS

Weight: average 20–24 lb (9–11 kg), triples birth weight by 12 months, gaining 2–6 lb in next 6 months.
- *Recommend 1 year physical check-up, with Hgb, Hct, urinalysis, Tb skin test.*

Height: approximately 29 in growing to approximately 33 in by 18 months.

Size: head and chest circumference are about equal at 12 months.

Pulse: 100–140/minute. Respirations: 20–40/minute.
- *Measure vital signs at rest.*

Reflexes: Babinski sign disappears.

Anterior fontanel: closes (average 10–24 months).
- *Evaluate fontanel and cranial configurations.*

Abdomen: protrudes.

Teething: continues with 10–14 primary teeth by 18 months, including lower and upper molars and cuspids. Good chewing, sucking, and swallowing movements.
- *Urge dental hygiene (e.g., brushing, fluoridated drops, encourage weaning from bottle, no candy/raisins).*

COMMON BEHAVIORS

Movement: able to walk alone with a widebased gait. Climbs upstairs, holding onto hand or rail, one step at a time. Throws, turns pages in a book, builds a tower of three objects/blocks. Helps in dressing self with hat, shoes, lifting arms or legs appropriately.
- *Protect child from kitchen accidents (e.g., hot liquids, overhanging handles, cords on appliances, long table cloths).*
- *Reinforce importance of earlier safety teaching. If not done earlier, lock up all medicines, poisons, gasoline, fertilizers, cleaning agents.*
- *Check all houseplants, keeping them out of reach; discard poisonous varieties.*
- *Keep matches out of reach.*
- *Put safety plugs in electrical outlets.*
- *Supervise yard play.*
- *Never leave alone in bath water, wading or other pools.*

- *Always use seat belts and approved car seats.*
- *Use safety devices on cabinet drawers and all doors.*

Play: Likes large cars and trucks, dolls, mops, brooms, kitchen utensils, stuffed animals, 2- to 10-piece puzzles, balls, picture books. Loves to throw and retrieve objects. Delights in pushing, pulling, or riding toys; climbing up, down, and through indoor gym/slide combinations. Enjoys solitary play or watching others.

Socialization: explores everything with rapid attention shifts. Curious; trial and error behavior teaches s/he can control some things around self; enjoys new skills; shows pride in achievements. Imitates and mimics household chores. Security is focused on one object (e.g., doll, blanket, stuffed animal, thumb, diaper).
- *Know that the parents' reaction to child's failure or accomplishment affects the child's self-concept. Showing anxiety over minor injuries, anger at childish carelessness, or ignoring accomplishments can have an unhealthful effect on child's self-esteem. Try to treat minor injuries, failures, with casual acceptance.*
- *Show pleasure at new social or physical skills. Set firm, safe limits.*

Verbalization: can point to parts of body when asked; can say 3 to 12 meaningful single words (e.g., "ma-ma," "da-da," "no," "hi," "hot," "bye-bye," "go," "baby," "wa-wa" [water]). Begins to follow a few simple commands (e.g., "Give it to me," "Show me the _____ ").

Elimination: may be able to control bowel movements or void at will on potty chair, but usually not interested.
- *Delay bowel/bladder training until baby's readiness is evident (e.g., shows interest and cooperation, able to express needs, walk to bathroom).*

Feeding: feeds self with spoon and drinks from cup by 18 months; appetite decreases with decreasing growth rate. Needs 100 cal/kg or approximately 1,300 cal/day (range: 900–1,800 cal).
- *Do not force feed, coax, wheedle, bribe, threaten, or punish poor appetite or feeding if growth rate is proceeding normally.*
- *Give regular table foods in a 3-meal-a-day pattern with nutritious between-meal or bedtime snacks. Give very small helpings. Keep child at table only as long as interested in eating. Do not give snacks as an alternative to mealtime eating.*
- *Do not appease a fussy or crying baby with a cookie or sweets. Do not use food as a reward, as a comfort for small hurts, or as a substitute for love and attention.*

Normal Growth and Development: Toddler and Preschooler

Definition/Discussion

Toddlerhood is the developmental period in a child's life between 18 months and 3 years. Preschool covers from 3 to 6 years of age.
- Rate of growth and development as well as task mastery varies with each individual child. Parental and environmental influences may stimulate and nurture or retard development, but innate differences and individual readiness will strongly affect level and rate of achievement.
- Developmental task (Erikson's central problem) to be resolved during toddlerhood is *autonomy or independence ver-*

sus *shame or doubt,* and during the preschool period it is *initiative versus guilt.* Successfully achieved, the youngster develops pride, high self-esteem, and good will to self and others.
- Special fears of toddlers and preschoolers are of abandonment and separation from parents. Learning to separate from parents and to cope effectively is an important task of the young child. Success can be achieved when the child experiences positive periods of short separation and feels trust and security with those who care for him. Coping skills begin to include modes of self-expression and elementary self-

reliance. Familiar surroundings and care giver's presence are no longer always necessary for the child to feel secure.

- Cognitive abilities develop rapidly in the preschool years and the child learns many things. The toddler has a concept of time limited to the present experience, focuses on only one aspect of objects, problem solves through trial and error, imitates language heard, and perceives through senses. Piaget calls this the "sensorimotor" stage of cognitive development. The preschooler's thinking, termed "preoperational," is literal, concrete, and absolute (e.g., good/bad, right/wrong, hurt/doesn't hurt). S/he views the world and people's actions in terms of own self and consequences to self, refusing others' viewpoints. The preschooler asks "why" and "how" frequently, extends concept of time to include past as well as present, and has a longer memory span than toddlers.
- Imagination is heightened in the preschooler; fantasy and reality are often interchangeable. Imaginary companions people this fantasy world, are often blamed for the youngster's own misbehavior, and serve as coping mechanisms for controlling situations, especially stressful ones.
- Play in the toddler period is active, informal, spontaneous, and often centered around motor activity. Characteristically, toddler play is singular and referred to as "parallel play" (when two children play alongside but not with each other). When the child learns to give in order to receive, s/he makes the transition into the preschool type of play known as cooperative or associative play.
- Ritualism is a common behavioral pattern of these two periods; activities of daily living are best scheduled and performed precisely and regularly in order to provide security and stability for the child in a rapidly changing period of growth and development.
- Negativism and the consistent use of the word "no" for everything is characteristic of this period. It is the toddlers' way of controlling people and events, acting on their own terms, doing things by themselves ("Me do it myself!"); the negative response becomes quite an automatic one.
- Temper tantrums are the young child's way of expressing frustration and releasing anger at people, things, and self in an effort to gain control. An angry, kicking toddler in the midst of a tantrum cannot be effectively dealt with by threats or reasoning for s/he is oblivious to reality. Walk away from a child having a tantrum; do not be a sympathetic or angry bystander; reward verbally for cooperative, socially acceptable behavior.
- The common parameters of physical development and behaviors for the toddler and preschool child are outlined below; corresponding nursing implications and parental teaching or guidance suggestions follow in italics.

☐ **AGE 18 MONTHS TO 3 YEARS (Toddler)**

Weight: average 28–30 lb (13 kg) (birth weight quadruples by 2½ years).

Height: average 33–37 in (82.5–92.5 cm) (approximately 50% of eventual adult height at 2 years).
- *Caution parents that appetite and weight gain level off during this period; thus child can eat less and still maintain activity levels. Recommended daily dietary intake is about 41–45 cal/lb (90–100 cal/kg).*
- *Provide appropriate counseling for children above 95th percentile or below 5th percentile for height or weight. Any child whose pattern has changed markedly (e.g., from 50th to 10th percentile or vice versa) also should be further evaluated.*
- *Check all measurements and ascertain that they are accurate.*

Norms are based on children being weighed with no clothing except light undergarments.

Pulse: 90–120/minute; respirations: 20–35/minute.
- *Count for 1 full minute.*

Teeth: 16 at 2 years, acquiring a full set of 20 primary teeth by 3 years.
- *Establish nutritious, noncariogenic dietary and snacking habits for proper tooth formation and bone development. Offer pretzels, fruits, fruit juice, and raw vegetables. Avoid carrot sticks, popcorn, and nuts because of possible choking. Keep candy, cookies, raisins, pastries, sweetened soft drinks and gum to a minimum.*
- *Encourage parents to take child for first dental visit by age 2 or before all 20 primary teeth have erupted. Take to dentist immediately for any cavities noticed or for injuries to teeth. Make first dental visit a pleasant, friendly one, preparing child with a positive, matter-of-fact explanation. Read child a book about visiting the dentist. Remember that parental attitudes and examples can mold a child's feelings about dental care for many years.*
- *Teach, demonstrate, and supervise cleaning (brushing and flossing) of teeth.*
- *Apply topical fluoridation treatments for additional decay protection. Continue fluoride supplements for children who do not live in community with fluoridated water supply.*

Vision: visual acuity is approximately 20/70 in the 2-year-old. Depth perception remains poor (cerebral rather than visual developmental function) increasing development of the neurovisual pathways leaves most 3-year-olds with good ability to assess size and location of objects.
- *Recommend a complete eye exam by a specialist for every child between 1 and 3 years of age.*
- *Provide address for free brochure on children's vision (The Children's Eyesight Society, 7420 Westlake Terrace, Suite 1509, Bethesda, MD 20034).*

Body proportions: changing, with abdomen protruding, arms and legs lengthening rapidly, and trunk and head growing slowly. Falls and stumbling may increase during this period due to changing body proportions and rapidly increasing motor skills. In addition, toddlers assert autonomy and overestimate physical capabilities.
- *Supervise constantly and initiate precautions necessary to minimize accidents.*
- *Install stairway rails, sturdy high fences; remove loose throw rugs, tables with sharp edges, glass objects that can topple over.*

Immunization: refer to table 5 for immunization indications and side effects. Current CDC guidelines suggest that *H. influenzae* type B (HIB) vaccine be given to all children 24 months and older. Toddlers 18–24 months old in daycare centers should also receive the vaccine but need to be revaccinated when they reach 24 months.
- *Reinforce need for well child check-ups at 18 and 24 months.*

COMMON BEHAVIORS
2-Year-Old

Movement: gait is steady; walks, runs, jumps with both feet. Climbs stairs one at a time with both feet on each step, holding rail. Can open doors and turn knobs. Can kick a ball without falling, even when running. By 2½ can ride a "kiddy" car and tricycle. Can throw objects overhead, string large beads, and begin to use scissors. Can scribble and copy vertical and straight lines. Assists with dressing and undressing self. Washes and dries hands. Uses toothbrush, but not skillfully.
- *Supervise carefully all outdoor and indoor play.*
- *Teach child street and traffic safety.*

- Use fire-retardant night clothes.
- Lock up all dangerous products.
- Lock doors or put plastic holders over doorknobs to prevent toddler usage.
- Use car seats for every car ride.
- Post a poison chart with poison control center phone number.

Play: has short attention span; needs combination of motor activities with quiet play. Enjoys stories, music, TV, sandbox with toys, Play-Doh, clay, mud, and finger paints. Likes construction toys, cars, trucks, pull toys, wagons, doll buggies, and riding toys like fire engines, tricycles, kiddy cars. Enjoys climbing and swinging playground apparatus, puzzles with large pieces, drawing paper, musical and rhythm instruments, dolls, stuffed animals, and toy household items for imitative play (e.g., brooms, lawnmowers). Parallel play predominates.

- Supervise water play constantly.
- Encourage swim lessons to begin if pool is present and accessible, even if only occasionally.
- Make sure riding toys are in good working order.
- Provide opportunities to practice and develop skills.

Socialization: is egocentric, the center of own world, viewing all in relationship to self. Treats other children almost as if they were objects. May bite in anger or frustration or just to use teeth. Other frequently observed behaviors include self-stimulation (e.g., rocking, masturbation), thumbsucking, ritualism, and negativism.

- Do not expect child to do more than s/he is able to do. Child has a need for peer companionship, even if unable to share.
- Teach parents that biting back, slapping, shouting, or putting something unpleasant in mouth (e.g., soap or hot sauce) usually do not work. Verbal disapproval, removal of child from stressor, or addressing cause (e.g., sibling rivalry) may have some positive effect.
- Accept the normalcy of behavior for this stage. Remain consistent in discipline; provide periods of special quiet time alone with child, reading stories, playing music, cuddling, and providing individual attention.
- Give choices when possible. Do not offer choices where none are present.

Verbalization: has vocabulary of about 200 words, understands more. Begins using phrases of two to four words (e.g., "go bye-bye," "more cookie," "where daddy," "me do it"). Most popular words: "no," "me," "my," "mine."

- Include child in conversations; have child use words to express wants; use concrete examples of words (let child handle object and identify the name for it; look at books, magazines, and identify objects).

Elimination: may gradually become toilet trained at least during daytime.

- Introduce toilet training if child shows signs of readiness (ability to stand and walk well, hold urine for 2 hours at a time, regular schedule of bowel movements, willingness to please care giver, ability to indicate need to eliminate).
- Stress to not start toilet training during stressful periods (birth of a sibling, weaning, moving, family separations, illness).
- Make teaching a positive, pleasant, nonpunitive, nonpressured, and geared to the particular child.
- Expect accidents when child is tired, excited, preoccupied, busy with play, or otherwise in a stressful situation. React casually and noncommittally.
- Keep potty chair accessible or a step stool near a standard toilet fitted with a smaller seat adaptation.
- Be consistent in reinforcements (rewards); use praise, not sweets. Use correct terminology for body parts. Begin foundation for health/sex education; refrain from negative responses for normal curiosity. Child may want to see

elimination products or not want them flushed away immediately; postpone it temporarily.
- Recommend loose-fitting, easily removed outer clothing and training pants that child can manage without help.

Sleeping: 10–14 hours/day, including an afternoon nap. Does not go to sleep immediately, prolongs process of going to bed.
- Monitor TV programs; avoid violent programs.
- Reinforce bedtime ritual; have quiet time at consistent hour; play soothing music, read stories.
- Teach parents not to use going to bed as punishment; use familiar stuffed animal, nightlight if afraid of dark.

Feeding: drinks/feeds self without spilling, plays with food.
- Keep portions small; choose foods from basic 4 food groups; limit milk to 2–3 glasses/day to avoid excessive calories and leave room for nutrients provided by other foods; do not rush child.

☐ AGE 3 YEARS TO 6 YEARS (Preschool)

Weight: approximately 44 lb; 4- to 6-year-olds require approximately 36–41 cal/lb (80–90 cal/kg).

Height: approximately 44 in (100 cm) (about double birth length at 4 years). Height and weight are about even at age 5.

Pulse: 80–120/minute; respirations: 20–30/minute.
- Count for 1 full minute.

Blood pressure: 85–90/60 mm Hg.
- Use child-size blood pressure cuff. Let child handle equipment and listen to own heart beat.

Teeth: begins to lose primary teeth at approximately 5–7 years.

Immunizations: see table 5.

Vision: visual acuity is approximately 20/40 in 3-year-old, 20/30 in 4-year-old, and normal 20/20 by age 6. Depth perception is developing and color vision fully established.
- Evaluate physical condition, immunization, vision, hearing, and kindergarten readiness skills before starting school; provide appropriate corrections and assistance.

Body proportions: loses much of baby fat and protruding abdomen; waist not discernible; legs continue to grow rapidly equaling approximately 44% of total length.

COMMON BEHAVIORS
3-Year-Old

Movement: climbs stairs, alternating feet, but still holding rail. Tries to draw a picture, a mass of lines and circles. Can hit a pegboard with a hammer with more accuracy than before, ride a tricycle. Dresses self with help on grippers, zippers, buttons, and shoe tying. Can help with minor tasks such as drying dishes, emptying waste baskets, getting or putting away items such as cleaning utensils or groceries.
- Continue supervision and safety precautions, even though child shows signs of using more caution and responsibility.
- Teach child what to do if lost while shopping or in new situation. Encourage ID bracelet. Teach child name, age, and phone number, including area code.
- Give small errands or jobs to do around house. Watch and wait before offering help or suggestions.

Play: uses blackboard and chalk, activity related dolls (e.g., can feed, dress, take for stroller rides), housekeeping toys, windup musical toys, child's typewriter, record player, tape player, mechanical games, increasing numbers and varieties of books, puzzles, trucks, building toys.
- Assist parents to expand child's world with same age group play experiences (e.g., babysitting co-ops or playgroups, nursery or Sunday schools, trips to zoo, playgrounds, story hours).

- *Encourage development of cooperative, sharing, or associative play skills.*

Socialization: tolerates short periods of separation, especially if child is in a happy, play-type situation with competent adults.

- *Encourage child to express feelings verbally and accept feelings, while redirecting unacceptable behavior to more acceptable behavior.*

Verbalization: has mastered most vowels, half the consonants; speaks in 3-or-more-word sentences that become more complex. Has a rapidly expanding speaking vocabulary of about 1,000 words. Frequently repeats words and syllables as a means of learning them. 90% of 3-year-olds should be readily understood by others. Knows first and last name, age, and sex. May stutter as attempting to learn complex pronunciation skills. Questions with "what?" "when?" "why?" and "how?" Understands simple explanations of cause and effect.

- *Teach parents to help develop child's language skills by talking aloud about what they are doing, thinking, and feeling; also by "parallel" talk describing what someone else may be doing, thinking, feeling while it happens. Ignore stuttering.*
- *Provide simple but honest explanations, patiently, upon request. Show and describe how things work and why something is dangerous or unwise to handle.*

Elimination: Goes to bathroom with minimal help.

- *Remind child to go before going outside or when playing busily.*

Sleeping and feeding: similar to 2-year-old.

4-Year-Old

Movement: walks with a freeswinging, adultlike stride; walks backwards; can walk upstairs without grasping rail. Can stand on 1 foot for 5 seconds. Runs well. Hops 2 or more times. Throws ball overhead with control and increasing accuracy to someone. Uses scissors to cut out pictures, following outline with increasing accuracy. Can draw a picture of a person with head, eyes, and 2 other parts.

- *Check play areas to remove unsafe hazards. Clear trash heaps; cover holes, ditches, tunnels; lock empty refrigerators or remove doors; properly discard faulty appliances, paint cans, plastic bags, aerosol cans.*

Play: is cooperative; dramatic, imitative play predominates. May have an imaginary companion. Likes jumpropes; play tools; paste and various scraps (e.g., cloth, leaves, paper) to arrange in collage; easels with paints; tires and very large boxes to climb around in; gym sets.

- *Provide dressup clothing for imitative play (e.g., cowboy hats, guns, holster, purses, jewelry, adult clothes).*
- *Take to children's plays, musical performances, puppet shows.*
- *Enroll in dance classes, swim lessons, exercise classes, and other learning opportunities.*

Socialization: brags, shows off, looks for praise, criticizes others, tattles. Developing a conscience that influences behavior. Develops romantic fantasies about parents of opposite sex. Common age for nightmares, castration fears, fears of scary objects and animals. As nightmares are common at this age, child may want to sleep with parent.

- *Invite friends over for parties, play activities, group games.*
- *Start child in own bed, perhaps with light on and relaxing music.*
- *Stress that temporary cuddling in parents' bed for nightmares can be condoned, but when child falls asleep, return to own bed. Patience and persistence, along with growing out of this stage will return the child to a regular, secure sleeping routine.*

Verbalization: has a speaking vocabulary of 1,500 words, expanding approximately 600 words/year depending on stimulation by adults and older siblings. Understands prepositions and opposites. Talks/questions incessantly; knows phone number, and some know address. Begins use of socially unacceptable words for their shock effect. Knows primary colors, some numbers and alphabet letters.

- *Reinforce new knowledge with toys, games, books about numbers, colors, and letters.*

Sleeping: 11–12 hours/day, napping only occasionally when very tired or ill.

Feeding: rarely needs assistance, interested in setting table, pours well from pitcher.

- *Have rules concerning table manners; encourage setting table, serving self; make mealtime a pleasant experience (give everyone a chance to talk about their day).*

5-Year-Old

Movement: can run and play games at same time; hops and skips well; some may attempt to ride a 2-wheel bicycle without training wheels. May be able to swim standard swim strokes a distance of 25 yards. Begins to use fork and knife. May be able to print first name, sometimes a short last name. Some may be able to tie shoelaces, but many are unable to do this until 6–8 years. Draws a recognizable person with body, head, arms, legs, and 4 other parts. Counts to 20 and may recognize coinage of a penny, nickel, dime. Washes self without wetting clothes. Brushes teeth correctly with reminders and some supervision.

- *Teach safe use of toys and riding or moving equipment (e.g., bikes, skates, skateboards).*
- *Teach safe street crossing, obeying traffic lights and crosswalk lines.*
- *Teach how to phone for help (e.g., fire, police, paramedics, emergency 911).*
- *Reinforce how to recite name, age, phone number, and address.*

Play: can use rollerskates, iceskates, sleds, scooters, skateboards, riding toys. Likes building sets, toy soldiers, plastic people, toy animals, doll houses.

- *Add more books, games, puzzles, involving increasing manipulative and cognitive skills. Do not pressure to achieve but let child enjoy the activity.*

Socialization: takes some responsibility for actions, following directions and rules. Increased respect for truth. Growth of modesty and wish for privacy. Able to sit quietly for 10–15 minutes to hear a story or lesson. Interested in meaning of family relationships (e.g., aunts, uncles, cousins, grandparents).

- *Teach personal safety habits (e.g., always tell care giver where they will be, walk with other children in well travelled areas, never talk to strangers or go near strange cars, yell "This isn't my daddy," scream, kick, bite if someone grabs them; don't let anyone do things to their body they shouldn't do; "say no to drugs").*
- *Keep behavior rules simple, enforce consistently; avoid prolonged arguments.*
- *Keep in close touch with kindergarten teacher to learn more about child's progress, abilities, needs, and to get suggestions for helping and guiding child. Help to build child's self-confidence by praising new skills, positive attitudes, and acceptable behavior.*

Verbalization: has a vocabulary of 2,000+ words. Can explain to others how and why of games or activities. Begins sentences with "I" instead of "me," "he" instead of "him." Although child may mispronounce some sounds and make some grammatical errors, most of the time language should closely match that of the family and neighborhood. Stuttering is inappropriate past the sixth birthday.

- *Get further evaluation from health care provider for suspected problems.*

Normal Growth and Development: Midchildhood

Definition/Discussion

The school years are the developmental period in an child's life between 6 and 11 years of age.

- Developmental task (Erikson's central problem) to be resolved during this period is industry versus inferiority. The child moves out into many different social groups and, while the family remains the chief socializing agent, s/he learns new and important skills and attitudes from peers: (1) the art of compromise, cooperation, and persuasion; (2) fair play through competition; (3) increased autonomy from the home; (4) reinforcement of appropriate sex-role behaviors; and (5) an ongoing development of self-concept.
- Cognitive development: time is now well understood and the child can plan ahead. There is a mature concept of causality. Formal logical thinking is present, which is based on perceptually concrete events, not abstractions. Conservation, the ability to see changing states of matter as unchanging, develops during this period. The child expands knowledge rapidly through formal and informal educational means. The child begins to combine others' viewpoints with his own. S/he is capable of prolonged interest and attention span. The memory is good for concrete sequences of numbers and letters and for 2 meaningful and related ideas.
- Special fears of this period are those of bodily injury, concern about death, fear of parental loss, school phobia/failure, fear of the dark, and fear of embarrassment from criticism or ridicule.
- Play is centered around groups of same sex after 6 or 7 years of age; "gang" activities predominate in both school and recreational interests (e.g., clubs, teams, scouts, parties, enrichment classes, neighborhood play groups). Peer-group influence becomes important and peer criticism begins for deviation from sex roles, intellectual or physical skill differences, sociocultural differences, and noncomformity in language, dress, social behaviors. Quarrels are frequent but usually short lived. The school-age child has now learned to share and take turns and can participate in organized games requiring coordinated efforts.
- The common parameters of physical development and behaviors for the school-age child are outlined below; corresponding nursing implications and parental teaching or guidance suggestions follow in italics.

☐ AGE 6 TO 11 YEARS

Weight: 45 lb (20 kg) at 6 years, child gains 5–7 lb/year on average; 62 lb (28 kg) at 7–10 years.

Height: 46 in (117 cm) at 6 years; growth occurs in spurts; overall height increases average approximately 3 in (7 cm)/year to approximately 52 in (132 cm) at 7–10 years.

Pulse: 80–100/minute at 6 years; approximates adult norm at 10–11 years.

- *Refer to growth charts as guidelines, but do not use as rigid criteria.*

Respirations: 18–20/minute at 6 years; approximates adult norms at 10–11 years.

- *Encourage annual well-child check-ups.*

Blood pressure: 95–108/60–68; approximates adult norms at 10–11 years.

- *Verify immunization status complies with state requirements.*

Vision: 20/20 by 7 years.

- *Promote vision testing every 2 years.*
- *Encourage children to sit no closer than 4 ft to TV.*

Nutrition: calorie requirements for 7 to 10-year-old are 32–36 cal/lb (70–80 cal/kg).

- *Assess nutritional status and further evaluate children in the upper or lower percentiles of weight. Have parent keep food diary for 1 week (with child's help). Reinforce basic nutrition ideas and stress healthful eating habits.*

Teeth: first permanent molars come in at 6–7 years; primary teeth are lost in order of eruption; has 10–11 permanent teeth by 10–11 years.

- *Remind parents to schedule twice-yearly dental check-ups and to continue supervision of correct brushing and flossing techniques.*

Sex characteristics: early development may begin in girls as soon as 8 years, and in boys as soon as 10 years. Early developers are often subject to ridicule and embarrassment. Adolescent growth spurt often begins by 10–11 years but may not occur until nearly 14.

- *Provide education and counseling to assist children to understand and accept the changes in their bodies.*
- *Help parents increase their effectiveness in providing sex education for their children.*

COMMON BEHAVIORS
6-Year-Old

Movement: large muscle ability exceeds fine motor coordination. Girls are ahead of boys in fine motor skills, physical development, and achievement. High energy levels; very active, impulsive, and constantly in motion. Balance and rhythm are good. Can hop, skip, run, jump, gallop, and climb. Can kick, throw, and catch a ball well. Can ride a 2-wheel bicycle without training wheels. Able to draw a recognizable human figure, house, flowers. Dresses self with almost no help; can master buttons, grippers, zippers, and shoelaces.

- *Reinforce traffic safety, provide adult supervision of play.*
- *Teach child to avoid strangers, never get in an unknown car, never take candy, food, or pills from strangers.*
- *Provide for a balance of rest and activity.*
- *Teach cold prevention (e.g., separate drinking cups) and good health practices, including reinforcement of dangers of drug abuse and taking medicines or pills not prescribed by a physician.*

Play: plays well alone, but enjoys groups of both sexes in small groups. Likes simple games with basic rules. Likes to make things (starts many, but finishes few). Likes imaginary, dramatic play with real costumes, running games of tag, hide-and-seek, rollerskating, kickball, soccer, jumprope games, hopscotch, iceskating, skiing, and skateboarding. Plays house; builds with plastic blocks. Still plays with dolls, airplanes, cars, and trucks. Enjoys electronic and musical games, puzzles, and books with words as well as pictures. Likes to draw, color, paint, paste, and cut.

- *Give some responsibility for household duties within ability and maturity level.*

Socialization: boisterous, verbally aggressive, assertive, bossy, opinionated, outgoing, active, argumentative, sometimes whiny, and know-it-all. Expresses sense of humor in riddles, practical jokes, and nonsense. Moods and feelings (fear, joy, affection, anger, shyness, jealousy, sadness) expressed in extremes. Can use a telephone. Has a strong need for teacher approval, affection, and acceptance. Very aware of teacher's social attitudes and values as communicated by behavior. Learns concepts of coinage, right and left, morning and afternoon, days of week, months of year, beginning reading and printing. Peer-group influence also becoming important.

- *Assure parents that aggressiveness is normal for age; suggest sidestepping power struggles; offer choices when possible.*
- *Frequently reassure the child of his/her competence, basic worth and lovability.*
- *Encourage parents to visit school, talk with teacher and resolve problems. Successful school experience is critical at this age to establish positive attitudes to learning and later educational experiences.*

Verbalization: has a vocabulary of 2,000–3,000 words. Communicates to share thoughts and ideas with others. Understanding of language greater than ability to use it. Can verbalize similarities.

- *Note any speaking or language difficulties; seek further evaluation and necessary remediation. Confer with school authorities first.*

Nutrition: needs approximately 2,000 cal/day. Eats 3 meals/day plus several snacks.

- *Provide snacks like fruit, raw vegetables, cheese, milk, and juice; have a snack shelf in refrigerator for child to help self.*

7-Year-Old

Movement: motor control has improved, but it is not as important at this age. Capable of fine motor hand movements.

- *Continue to reinforce safety guides.*
- *Assist parents to tolerate "quiet" days and periods of shyness as part of growing up. May be subjected to various fears and nightmares; do not permit child to sleep with parent; reassure, comfort, but do not oversympathize or give undue attention and importance to these unless they increase in severity and frequency (then see counselor).*
- *Stress the importance of teaching and setting examples regarding harmful use of drugs, alcohol, smoking.*

Play: begins to prefer to play with own sex. The importance of the peer group becomes central now. Enjoys games that develop physical and mental skill. Wants more realism in play. Collects things for quantity, not quality (rocks, bottle caps, baseball cards, shells). Enjoys illusion and magic tricks. Likes table and card games, dominoes, checkers. Likes books to read by self; also radio, records, TV; skateboards and bicycles. Girls this age often ready also for lessons in dancing, piano, or gymnastics.

Socialization: is less impulsive and boisterous in activities; quiet and reflective. Begins to deal with the complex organization of concrete concepts; can count by 2s, 5s, and 10s; can add and subtract; can tell time, days, months, and seasons; anticipates things like Christmas, birthdays, holidays. Thinks before acting; thought is more flexible now. Begins to classify and group objects on a general level. Nervous habits are common. Mutilation, body image, and castration fears develop. Wants to be like friends; competition is important. Likes school, considers ideas of teacher important.

- *Help parents form realistic expectations of child's school achievement, development, and behavior. Parents need affirmation that child's unpredictable and changing behavior is normal and expected.*

8-Year-Old

Movement: returns to an active, vigorous phase with fine motor coordination acquired. Movements are more graceful.

- *Teach safety around autos including using seat belts, knowing rules of bike safety.*

Play: enjoys making detailed drawings. Reads comic books, cartoons and books (often adventure stories). Likes board games, electronic games, craft kits, sports of all types.

Socialization: again gregarious, becomes a self-assured and pragmatic character on home ground. Eager to absorb the world around and render opinions on all matters. Curiosity is boundless; able to collect and classify objects in a qualitative manner now. Increasingly modest about own body. Strongly prefers the company of own sex; is selective in choice of company; likes group projects, clubs, and outings. Uses language as a tool; likes riddles, jokes, and word games; has a sense of humor. Art work begins to show new perception of subjects.

- *Reinforce the need to be considered important by adults and given small responsibilities.*
- *Provide simple explanations, honest answers to questions regarding sex.*
- *Avoid negative reinforcement of teasing, nailbiting, enuresis, whining, poor manners, swearing.*

Nutrition: needs approximately 2,100 cal/day.

- *Plan meal and snack times, as child is often too busy to take time for eating proper amounts with good eating habits.*

9-Year-Old

Movement: active, constantly on the go; plays and works hard, often to the point of fatigue. Large group skills and activities predominate (swimming, other sports, dancing). Uses tools fairly well. Uses both hands independently.

- *Have parents teach safety with firearms including storing them away from the bullets, handling them carefully, never referring to them as a toy.*
- *Assess health knowledge and spend time with child discussing health habits.*

Play: peer activities dominate with strong sex differences in play choices; hopscotch, jacks, jumprope, and crafts for girls; war games, fort building, tag, and football for boys. Both sexes like soccer, kickball, and softball. Board games, electronic games, afterschool hobbies, music and dancing lessons popular. Reading still enjoyed by many, but school-age children now thought to watch more than 20 hours TV/week.

Socialization: rules become a guiding force in all aspects of life. Overly concerned with peer-imposed rules. Interested in family life, activities, and vacations, but parents are excluded from a major portion of child's life. Shows a consuming interest in how things are made; how and what makes weather, seasons; outer space, rockets, and science fiction. Much antagonism and rivalry between sexes and between siblings, leading to frequent quarrels and teasing. Lying and stealing to gain recognition or attention may become a problem.

- *Avoid harsh and severe punishment; try to restrict to room or home, cancel treats; try system of rewards with charts or lists of desired behavior. Understand and accept the child as s/he is.*
- *Stress importance of parents knowing playmates and their parents.*

10-Year-Old

Movement: very active with good coordination. Marked differences in motor skills between the sexes appear, with boys surpassing girls in strength, endurance, and agility while girls may exceed in flexibility and graceful movement; training and interests are determining variables.

- *Parental guidance and support are the strongest influence on school achievement.*
- *Competitiveness in school activities may lead to difficulties for the child in handling failure. Low self-esteem is often related to learning difficulties, below average physical skills, family and neighborhood problems.*
- *Assist to seek counseling and help if problems occur.*

Play: likes gangs and clubhouse with secret codes, rules and rituals; experiments in all areas. Enjoys crafts like weaving, jewelry and leather work; singing in choral groups. Likes mystery stories and TV. Interested in hobbies (e.g., collections of stamps, coins, rocks, shells, beer cans, bottle caps, license plates). Parental involvement and commitment are needed to encourage participation of child in organized clubs, sports, and youth groups.

- *Stress importance of serving as "team parent" or helper as most of these activities are organized and conducted by volunteer, interested parents. Parents need to understand that while child needs time alone or with friends, there is still a need to supervise and protect child from harmful companions and influences (e.g., "R" rated movies and some TV programs [including cable TV]).*

Socialization: is happy, cooperative, casual, and relaxed; usually courteous and well-mannered with adults. Has a growing capacity for thought and conceptual organization; is able to discuss problems, see other person's point of view, think about social problems and prejudices. The peak of the gang age; companionship is more important that play activities. Needs occasional privacy; wants independence. Can understand transformations of state in size, shape, weight, and volume. Has the ability to plan ahead.

- *Provide list of organized community programs for "latchkey" children (youngsters under 12 who are on their own and unsupervised after school while both parents are working).*
- *Continue sex education and preparation for adolescent body changes. Since peers share sexual (mis)information, be sure children are given correct facts. Become involved with the health education program at child's school.*

Nutrition: needs approximately 2,400 cal/day.

11-Year-Old

Movement: differences between sexes may become more noticeable, as girls no longer compete on an equal basis with males in some areas of physical strength. Manipulative skills nearly equal to those of adults. May be the start of a stormy, active period of constant activity like finger-tapping, foot-drumming, or restless leg swinging while sitting.

Play: enjoys projects and working with hands in metal craft, ceramics, auto mechanics, bicycle repair, knitting and crocheting. Likes to do jobs and run errands that will earn money (e.g., gardening, babysitting). Very involved in sports, dancing, and talking on telephone. Likes participation in all aspects of drama (e.g., production, stage manager, makeup, props, publicity). May show an interest in golf, tennis, racquetball, jogging/running, water sports, and both street and ice hockey. Indoor games of choice may include arcade games, electronic games, Ping-Pong, pool, volleyball, and basketball. Enjoys listening to popular music; wants

records, tapes of favorite stars and to attend rock concerts or movies.

- *Encourage inactive preteens to engage in some organized, regular play or physical exercise. Establish life-long habits of regular exercise for physical and mental well-being.*

Socialization: rebels at routines, doing homework, or household chores. Has wide mood swings with rapid changes from moodiness to cheerfulness. May cry and lose temper if hair doesn't look "perfect" before going somewhere. Begins to take daily showers, shampoos without urging, especially as s/he begins to take notice of opposite sex. Peers are very significant; "put-downs" and taunting over physical attributes, clothing, or school skills are very common. Participates actively in community, team, and school affairs. Wants unreasonable amounts of freedom to do as s/he wishes. Wants to be trusted and given responsibility; wants to earn extra money over allowance (e.g., washing cars, mowing lawns, babysitting). Boys begin to tease girls to get attention. Hero worship is prevalent. Can be very critical of selves, own work or skills. Interested in whys of health measures; beginning to understand reproduction when accurately taught.

- *Set realistic limits that can be tolerated by both sides. Offer support and give democratic guidance as child works through feelings. Help channel energy in the right direction.*
- *Assist parents to set clear expectations and enforceable limits on preteen behavior.*
- *Help schools arrange for suitable educational materials on smoking and alcoholism by contacting local agencies of PTA and American Cancer Society. Use power of suggestion rather than dictating behavior; set good examples of moderation and moral values for children.*
- *Provide explanations of body changes and special understanding for child that surges ahead or lags behind. Recognize that they may have a need to rebel and deprecate others.*
- *Encourage parents and schools to address sex education (e.g., reproduction, venereal disease, taking responsibility for own actions, the right to say no, birth control) since the time of menarche continues to occur at earlier ages (it is not unusual to see menstruation occur at age 11, also some pregnancies).*
- *Encourage parents to discuss beliefs (e.g., religion and birth control).*

Sleep: needs approximately 8–10 hours/night.

Nutrition: boys need approximately 2,500 cal/day; girls approximately 2,250 cal/day.

- *Discourage excessive sugar snacks and junk foods. Reinforce basics of good nutrition.*

Normal Growth and Development: The Adolescent

Definition/Discussion

Adolescence spans the developmental period terminating childhood, from 12 through 19 years of age.

- Developmental task (Erikson's central problem) to be resolved in adolescence is *identity* versus *identity diffusion* (e.g., Who am I really? Who do I want to be? How am I

different from others?). During this period the adolescent continues to develop a self-concept and identity that is acceptable to him/her and to significant others. To this end s/he "tries on" many different roles in deciding what career, role, and personality characteristics are most desirable.

- Acceptance is a critical element in the adolescent's pursuit for a self-concept; conformity of dress, eating, activities, ap-

310 APPENDIX 1

pearance, and beliefs are all efforts or attempts at acceptance by the peer group.

- The overriding importance of peers of the last period of the middle years of childhood takes on a different character during adolescence as peer groups are no longer restricted exclusively to one sex; the individual has significant peer relationships in groups of both sexes serving different needs.

- The all-consuming importance of rules for the school-age child gives way to a severe criticism of authority and rule and a desire to change the world, making it a better place to live. To this end the adolescent joins activist groups and groups promoting civic change to make a contribution and effort at achieving his high goals for mankind.

- Stress-related disorders in adolescents (e.g., anxiety and phobic reactions, eating disorders, depression, alcohol and drug abuse, suicidal and delinquent behaviors) are more prevalent today than in previous generations due to increased social pressure and expectations of peers versus parents. Teenagers often need help to learn that everyone has problems, conflicts, tensions; that help is available from caring others, that s/he can successfully face own feelings and understand and accept self; and that by developing stress management skills, s/he will be able to cope effectively with own problems.

- More than 12 million teenagers are sexually active (Guttmacher Institute Report, 1982). While use of contraception is increasing, more than one million teenage girls get pregnant each year. About 75% of these pregnancies are unintended. Studies show teenagers to be seriously misinformed on basic sex education facts. More than two-thirds never practice contraception, or do so inconsistently. Nearly 50% of the sexually active teenage females think they can't get pregnant, yet 20% of teenage pregnancies occur within the first month after start of intercourse; half the pregnancies occur within the first 6 months. Studies show that peers and the media (movies, TV) are the primary source of adolescent sex education. Less than 25% of teenage students receive a significant amount of school-based sex education. A heightened awareness and concern among the public, along with a strong commitment, may help correct this growing problem.

- Adolescence is a special period of childhood where the individual undergoes numerous physical and emotional changes to develop into the unique individual s/he has been maturing into throughout childhood. Due to the uniqueness of each individual, it becomes difficult to set rigid standards for patterns of development, yet there is a sequential progression of behaviors during this period.

- The common parameters of physical development and the broad changes in behaviors for the adolescent are outlined below; corresponding nursing implications and parental teaching or guidance suggestions follow in italics.

☐ AGE 12 THROUGH 19 YEARS

Weight and height
- girls
  11–14 years: 101 lb (46 kg); 62 in (157 cm)
  15–19 years: 120 lb (55 kg); 64 in (163 cm)
- boys
  11–14 years: 99 lb (45 kg); 62 in (157 cm)
  15–18 years: 145 lb (66 kg); 69 in (176 cm)
  19 years: 147 lb (67 kg); 70 in (178 cm)
- *Provide information regarding weight gain, growth spurts, and episodes of fatigue that accompany adolescent physiologic changes.*
- *Counsel in a patient, supportive manner to bolster self-confidence; see table 9.*

- *Encourage sound dietary practices and hygiene.*
- *Provide a wide degree of variability based on individual differences.*
- *Screen for scoliosis and refer as needed.*
Pulse: 50–100/minute.
Respirations: 15–24 minute.
Blood pressure: 110–118/65–74.
Teeth: Wisdom teeth usually come in, if at all, by 18–20 years. Caries common during this period.
- *Arrange at least twice yearly dental check-ups; screen for orthodontic problems.*
Female Sex Characteristics
- *primary:* increase in size of internal and external genitalia; changes in endometrial lining and vaginal secretions; ovulation and menarche (average age of onset 12–13 years)
- *secondary:* increase in breast size, bone growth, basal metabolic rate; changes in shape of pelvis, pubic and axillary hair patterns; increased fat deposits in breasts, buttocks, and thighs; increasingly smooth and soft skin
Male Sex Characteristics
- *primary:* growth and development of testes, scrotum, and penis; production of mature sperm
- *secondary:* changes in body hair distribution; increase in size of vocal cords; increased thickness of skin, sebaceous secretions, basal metabolic rate, and bone growth with broadening of shoulders
- *Answer questions regarding the physical changes in their systems in an honest and direct manner to prevent misconceptions and to foster a positive self-image. Listen sympathetically to expression of feelings (e.g., worries, fears) regarding changes; initiate conversation on points the adolescent may be reluctant to discuss (e.g., unequal breast size).*
- *Provide information on antiprostaglandin preparations (Motrin, Ponstel, Anaprox) to help with dysmenorrhea. They should be taken at the onset of menstrual period and stopped as the flow subsides. They are also useful for decreasing heavy bleeding, but not shortening the period. They should be taken with milk or food, but not with aspirin or any other medication. Caution teenagers not to take each others' prescriptions. Each girl should be examined by a competent physician to evaluate whether cause of the dysmenorrhea is primary or secondary to some organic problem, infection, or tumor.*
- *Teach girls to use sanitary pads or tampons (regular-size only), and to change them at least every 4 hours. Caution against use of tampons used when girl is being treated for any pelvic inflammatory disease or vaginal infections.*
- *Have an open discussion about menstruation to encourage sharing of questions, beliefs, and feelings. If girls have been raised in families comfortable with occasional discussions of growth and sex, the beginning of menstruation will be accepted naturally with little embarrassment or tension. Simply dropping a book on the subject in the girl's hands is unwise, unless requested or read together by mother and daughter. The action of giving the child something to read can be interpreted as lack of caring, unwillingness, or inability on the part of the mother to discuss such private subjects.*
- *Provide clear, concise, accurate information about menstruation in a matter-of-fact way to enable the girl to reject inaccurate information shared among her friends.*
- *Assure girls that they can continue with normal activities, that discomfort is often only temporary, and that their periods may be very irregular for a year or more.*
- *Teach youth to cleanse face thoroughly (washing gently, not scrubbing) with a mild, unscented soap; rinse; apply a 5% or*

10% benzyl peroxide gel 1–2 times daily for pimple prevention as well as treatment.

COMMON BEHAVIORS
12 to 15 Years

Movement: often awkward and uncoordinated, as the adolescent adjusts to physical changes in height and size. Frequently displays poor posture. Physically active, but tires easily.

- *Provide reassurance and help in accepting changing body; parents need to reinforce positive qualities, seek professional help for health problems (e.g., skin eruptions, vaginal discharge, dental caries, drug use).*
- *Set realistic but firm limits that can be mutually agreed upon for security reasons; avoid threats.*
- *Exercise authority with tact.*

Leisure/play: enjoys activities centered around peer group (usually same sex, gradually mixing at social and sporting events). Enjoys school-related events (e.g., sports, dances, concerts, rallies, parties, plays, and various competitions). Likes shopping, talking on telephone, listening to music, spending time on grooming, sun bathing, watching soap operas and other TV, movies, cooking, sewing, reading popular magazines, and baby sitting, watching or participating in sports activities, working on bikes, cars, motorscooters, or other mechanical interests, watching/playing arcade/electronic games. Wants free time, unsupervised by adults, to "do my own thing." Shows interest in getting part-time jobs for extra spending money over regular allowances.

- *Provide opportunities for child to earn money and have some financial independence.*
- *Encourage independence and allow person to be an individual, to feel s/he has some control over what happens to him/her; however, be available and allow child to utilize parent, as s/he needs to do so.*
- *Provide honest answers to questions; repeat explanations as needed.*
- *Arrange for driver education prior to 16th birthday.*

Socialization: has an increasing interest in the opposite sex. "Going around" (liking each other but not really dating yet) progresses to group dates, then couple dating alone. Peer-group acceptance is strongest in early adolescence and the pressure to conform to group norms is nearly overwhelming to many teens. Strong friendship bonds are formed with 1 or 2 close peers. Age varies on dating, as some do not date a single person until late adolescence. Shows increasing hostility and alienation towards parents or authority figures. Expresses strong opinions and beliefs contrary to those of parents and school staff. Verbal conflicts over restrictions are common. Concerned with morality, ethics, religion, and social customs; is in the process of developing own values and standards, but peer group beliefs are strong influences. Idealism is prevalent. Reasoning is mature; thinking now includes abstract ideas. Wide variations in academic abilities and interests. Day-dreaming and sexual fantasies are common. Girls are more socially adept than boys; will take initiative to telephone boys and plan parties or other group activities. In early adolescence (age 12), girls have more interest than boys in physical appearance, physical development and attractiveness. By age 14, both sexes worry and fret over hair, skin, size of body parts, clothing, and physical details. As interest in opposite sex grows, so does the frequency of showers, shampoos, teeth brushing, and grooming habits.

- *Assist parents to provide gentle encouragement and guidance regarding dating; avoid strong pressures of either extreme.*
- *Continue to provide teenagers a warm, affectionate, loving, parental relationship (e.g., tell children you love them; tell them they are attractive, interesting, worthwhile, and special; encourage positive mental attitude; show them respect by*

helping to build their self-confidence and self-esteem; praise often, criticize less).
- *Explain that feelings do not have to be denied; that it is normal to have varied and changing moods and feelings (e.g., anger, irritability, tenderness, sensitivity, romantic longings, jealousy, guilt, anxiety, fear, embarrassment). Help adolescents to get in touch with feelings by talking about it with a trusted other, family member, or good friend. Parents need to understand child's conflicts as s/he attempts to deal with social, moral, political, and intellectual issues.*
- *Let the adolescent know it is OK to masturbate to avoid increasing the level of guilt and anxiety about it.*
- *Provide information and counseling regarding venereal disease, professional birth control resources.*
- *Encourage open discussion of problems, concerns, and questions.*
- *Assist to seek family counseling for coping with an adolescent who has problems of drug abuse, pregnancy, depression, learning handicaps, or other difficulties.*
- *Consider a parent support group to cope with parental feelings of guilt, fear, anger, and hopelessness.*

Sleep: approximately 7–9 hours/night.

Eating: prefers easy-to-obtain junk foods such as candy, carbonated drinks, potato chips. Concern over appearance may lead to crash diets, poor eating patterns, or serious eating disorders. Girls need approximately 1,500–3000 calories/day (average 2,200 cal/day). Boys need approximately 2,000–3,700 calories/day (average 2,700 cal/day)

- *Vitamin and iron supplements are often recommended.*

16 through 19 Years

Movement: has increased energy as growth spurt tapers. Muscular ability and coordination increase.

Leisure/play: enjoys working for altruistic causes. Sports activities (as both participant and observer) are well-attended. Likes beach and recreational activities like surfing, skiing, sailing, tennis, volleyball, hiking. Reading, TV, music, radio, and telephone are all still important. Likes challenging games (e.g., chess, bridge, poker, crossword puzzles). May explore new interests via volunteer work, summer jobs, high school occupational programs, part-time employment, and vacation trips. Dancing is popular; also enjoys attending concerts, plays, etc. Enjoys high-risk, competitive sports such as car racing.

- *Assist to set goals with adolescents and help them develop independence and competence in such things as grocery shopping, preparing nutritionally balanced meals, checkbook management, home and yard maintenance, first aid, health and safety measures.*

Socialization: continues to refine language, reasoning, thinking, and communicating skills. Begins to realize that inadequacies in these areas adversely affect job opportunities and limit career choices. Has achieved a more mature, interdependent relationship with parents. At 15 or 16, confides more in friends than in parents; at 18 or 19, parental advice and support is sought and the transition to adulthood is made. Dating in pairs and groups is common; romantic love affairs develop. Some look for permanence in a relationship; others decide to postpone permanent relationships until completion of college or establishment of job security. Has an increased ability to balance responsibility with pleasure. Develops an identity for self and an image of the kind of person s/he will become. Tries to develop characteristics thought to be desirable in a mate. Learns through satisfactions and frustrations of the problems living full time with peers, either in college or apartment settings. Peer group affiliation is not as rigid. Despite continuing peer influence, independent judgment emerges. Constantly seeks satisfactory part-time jobs to pay for car, dating, and other personal expenses. Effort is directed to become independent and self-supportive. Summers are spent working or getting extra course work for college. Plans more realistically for career. Assumes major responsibility for deciding on post-high school plans. More women are now seeking educational majors and careers that were formerly dominated by men (e.g., engineering, business, medicine).

- *Encourage parents to provide assistance as needed and desired (e.g., selecting a college, obtaining a scholarship and financial assistance, getting a job, planning a wedding, buying a car, getting insurance or a loan, using an acceptable, appropriate birth control method, resolving a health problem).*
- *Assist parents to adjust to the loss of their dependent child.*

Sleep: 6–8 hours/night.

Nutrition: Girls need approximately 1,200–3,000 cal/day (average 2,100 cal/day); boys need approximately 2,100–3,900 cal/day (average 2,800 cal/day).

- *Continue vitamin and iron supplements as recommended.*

APPENDIX 2
Nursing Diagnoses: Accepted List

Activity intolerance
Adjustment, impaired
Airway clearance, ineffective
Anxiety: mild, moderate, severe, panic
Body temperature, alteration in: potential
Bowel elimination, alteration in: constipation
Bowel elimination, alteration in: diarrhea
Bowel elimination, alteration in: incontinence
Breathing pattern, ineffective
Cardiac output, alteration in: decreased
Comfort, alteration in: pain
Comfort, alteration in: chronic pain
Communication, impaired: verbal
Coping, family: potential for growth
Coping, ineffective family: compromised
Coping, ineffective family: disabling
Coping, ineffective individual
Diversional activity, deficit
Family process, alteration in
Fear
Fluid volume, alteration in: excess
Fluid volume deficit
Gas exchange, impaired
Grieving, anticipatory
Grieving, dysfunctional
Growth and development, alteration in
Health maintenance, alteration in
Home maintenance management, impaired
Hopelessness
Hyperthermia
Hypothermia
Incontinence, functional
Incontinence, reflex
Incontinence, stress
Incontinence, total
Incontinence, urge

Infection, potential for
Injury, potential for: (poisoning, potential for; suffocation, potential for; trauma, potential for)
Knowledge deficit (specify)
Mobility, impaired physical
Noncompliance (specify)
Nutrition, alteration in: less than body requirements
Nutrition, alteration in: more than body requirements
Oral mucous membrane, alteration in
Parenting, alteration in
Post trauma response
Powerlessness
Rape trauma syndrome
Self-care deficit: feeding, bathing/hygiene, dressing/grooming, toileting
Self-concept, disturbance in: body image, self-esteem, role performance, personal identity
Sensory-perceptual alteration: visual, auditory, kinesthetic, gustatory, tactile, olfactory
Sexual dysfunction
Sexuality patterns, alteration in
Skin integrity, impairment of
Sleep pattern disturbance
Social interaction, impaired
Social isolation
Spiritual distress (distress of the human spirit)
Swallowing, impaired
Thermoregulation, ineffective
Thought processes, alteration in
Tissue integrity, impaired
Tissue perfusion, alteration in: cerebral, cardiopulmonary, renal, gastrointestinal, peripheral
Unilateral neglect
Urinary elimination, alteration in patterns of
Urinary retention
Violence, potential for: self-directed or directed at others

APPENDIX 3
Guidelines for Teaching Parents and Children

Definition/Discussion

Teaching is the process by which new information is presented so that learning may occur. The method used to teach information varies depending on the needs of the learner, the time necessary for the learner to grasp the information, and the methods of instruction most appropriate to the learner and the material being taught. Individuals learn, accept, and cope with new information/situations at different rates. Thus, the time each learner requires for each new learning experience will vary. Some will require more time, practice, and explanation than others. Be patient, and caution the learner to be likewise.

The learning/comprehension level will also vary among individuals and the level of the presentation will need adjustment accordingly. Use terms and words the learner will understand. Some individuals will benefit from audio/visual materials (e.g., reading pamphlets, viewing video tapes, listening to audio tapes, viewing pictures/drawings, handling equipment) explaining the content.

Three important basic learning conditions for teaching skills or procedures are

- *Contiguity*: The individual steps of the procedure must be taught in continuous order or sequence. Teaching may begin with the first step and work to the last one, or start with the last step and work backwards; it does not matter as long as the steps are in sequence.
- *Practice*: This permits the patient to rehearse the sequence until each step is learned satisfactorily. Practice will be most effective when the patient distributes it over a period of time (e.g., several times a day for several days) rather than trying to perfect the entire sequence all at once.
- *Feedback*: This provides the patient knowledge of progress. It is the most important variable in learning, and is highly motivating to the patient. A return demonstration of learning can be critiqued and corrected.

☐ GOAL

The learner (e.g., parent, guardian, child) will demonstrate the necessary skills, attitude, and knowledge for the effective control of the child's condition; will solve the problems of daily living; will meet the special learning needs of the child.

Nursing Actions

- Identify the learner(s)
- Assess the learner's ability to learn
  - age

- attention span, memory
- coordination (eye-hand, posture, balance)
- vision (color, focus, acuity)
- hearing
- reading and writing ability
- educational/cognitive level
- ability to communicate, seek, accept, and effectively use help
- language skills; cultural, ethnic, sexual, or racial influences
- beliefs/attitudes reagrding health, illness, medical treatment
- desire to learn about child's care; emotional acceptance of condition, psychologic adjustment, willingness to talk in personal terms
- motivation, willingness, and ability to modify life-style as indicated by disease/disability management or rehabilitation
- Involve the learner(s) in the planning, implementation, and evaluation of the teaching program
- Set teaching priorities according to the importance of child's need (i.e., for survival or for well-being) and the amount of time available.
- Identify the component steps of a learning task and work to achieve small goals that lead to larger goals; progress from simple to complex tasks.
- Use a relaxed, fairly informal manner; keep explanations simple and teaching sessions short (about 15-30 minutes); reduce distractions and interruptions; allow time for thinking, absorbing new information; encourage questions.
- Use visual aids (e.g., films, slides, pictures, models, charts); post charts and pictures on hallway walls or around a classroom for easy accessibility and frequent referral; use bulletin board displays with changing composition and educational themes.
- Use methods that are developmentally appropriate for the learner (e.g., puppets to teach the preschool child, peers to teach the adolescent); refer to *The Child Requiring Play Therapy*, page 226.
- Use the same equipment and supplies that will be used at home.
- Make use of your own hospital's resources, including booklets, leaflets, teaching sheets.
- Supervise return demonstrations and several successful practice sessions for skills taught.
- Provide a means for learner to review what has been taught

315

and to extend, share that knowledge with others at home who need to know; supply appropriate printed literature (bilingual if necessary), illustrations, diagrams, and written instructions.

- Make referrals to community agencies with education services, to an expatient/family/support group who is successfully rehabilitated and willing to help, to a community health agency.
- Record progress; chart all the areas taught, who was taught, their reactions, and an evaluation of what has been learned; use standard agency forms if available.
- Follow-up to determine if teaching was realistic, successful, and effective, contact the community health nurse or home care coordinator if a referral was made; consider calling patient/family to check progress.
- Share results of teaching experiences with other staff including nurse educators, clinical nurse specialists, and home care coordinator; consider possibilities of nursing research project, group teaching, or publishing booklets on commonly needed subjects.

EVALUATION OF TEACHING

A variety of techniques can be used to evaluate the effectiveness of teaching

- Return demonstration
- Verbal description of content in own words
- Verbal list of pertinent content
- Achievement of the goal for which teaching was instituted (e.g., weight loss achieved/maintained; blood pressure controlled within stated limits; remaining free from hypo/hyperglycemic episodes; selection of appropriate menu)

References

Acquired Immune Deficiency Syndrome

Boland, M., & Gaskill, T. (1984). Managing AIDS in children. *MCN: American Journal of Maternal/Child Nursing, 9,* 384–389.

Boland, M., & Klug, R. (1986). AIDS: The implications for home care. *MCN: American Journal of Maternal/Child Nursing, 11,* 404–411.

Epstein, L., et al. (1986). Neurologic manifestations of human immunodeficiency virus infection in children. *Pediatrics, 78,* 678–687.

Friedland, G., et al. (1986). Lack of transmission of HTLV-III/LAC infection to household contacts of patients with AIDS or AIDS-related complex with oral candidiasis. *New England Journal of Medicine, 314,* 344–349.

Gurevich, I. (1985). The competent internal immune system. *Nursing Clinics of North America, 20,* 151–161.

Iazzetti, L. (1986). Nursing management of the pediatric AIDS patient. *Issues in Comprehensive Pediatric Nursing, 9,* 119–129.

LaCamera, D., Masur, H., & Henderson, D. (1985). Symposium on infections in the compromised host. The acquired immunodeficiency syndrom. *Nursing Clinics of North America, 20,* 241–256.

Rogers, M. (1985). AIDS in children: A review of the clinical, epidemiologic and public health aspects. *Pediatric Infectious Disease, 4*(3), 230–236.

Rubinstein, A. (1986). Schooling for children with acquired immune deficiency syndrome. *Journal of Pediatrics, 109*(2), 242–244.

Rubinstein, A., et al. (1986). Pulmonary disease in children with acquired immune deficiency syndrome and AIDS-related complex. *Journal of Pediatrics, 108*(4), 498–503.

Sande, M. (1986). Transmission of AIDS: The case against casual contagion. *New England Journal of Medicine, 314,* 380–382.

Turner, J., & Williamson, K. (1986). AIDS: A challenge for contemporary nursing. *Focus on Critical Care, 13*(3), 53–61, Part I; (4), 41–50, Part II.

Weiss, S., et al. (1985). HTLV-III infection among health care workers: Association with needle-stick injuries. *Journal of the American Medical Association, 254,* 2089–2093.

Anxiety

Adams, R., & Passman, R. (1981). The effects of preparing two-year-olds for brief separations from their mothers. *Child Development, 52*(4), 1068–1070.

Calkin, J. (1979). Are hospitalized toddlers adapting to the experience as well as we think? *MCN: American Journal of Maternal/Child Nursing, 4,* 18–23.

Gohnsman, B. (1981). The hospitalized child and the need for mastery. *Issues in Comprehensive Pediatric Nursing, 5,* 67–76.

Hodapp, R. (1982). Effects of hospitalization on young children: Implications of two theories. *Children's Health Care, 10*(3), 83–86.

Kerr, N. (1979). The effect of hospitalization on the developmental tasks of childhood. *Nursing Forum, 18*(2), 108–130.

King, J., & Ziegler, S. (1981). The effects of hospitalization on children's behavior: A review of the literature. *Children's Health Care, 10*(1), 20–28.

Meissner, J. (1980). How can you improve care of the hospitalized child? . . . This assessment tool can help. *Nursing80, 10*(10), 50–51.

Passman, R., & Longaway, K. (1982). The role of vision in maternal attachment: Giving 2-year-olds a photograph of their mother during separation. *Developmental Psychology, 9,* 530–533.

Petrillo, M., & Sanger, S. (1980). *Emotional care of hospitalized children* (2nd ed.). Philadelphia: Lippincott.

Rey, M., & Rey, H. (1966). *Curious George goes to the hospital.* Boston: Houghton Mifflin.

Stevens, K. (1981). Humanistic nursing care for critically ill children. *Nursing Clinics of North America, 16,* 611–622.

Tresler, M., & Savedra, M. (1981). Coping with hospitalization: A study of school-age children. *Pediatric Nursing, 7,* 35–38.

Vipperman, J., & Rager, P. (1980). Childhood coping: How nurses can help. *Pediatric Nursing, 6,* 11–18.

Zurlinden, J. (1985). Minimizing the impact of hospitalization for children and their families. *MCN: American Journal of Maternal/Child Nursing, 10,* 178–182.

Appendectomy

Hatch, E. (1985). The acute abdomen in children. *Pediatric Clinics of North America, 32,* 48–49.

Powers, R., Andrassy, R., Brennan, L., & Weitzman, J. (1981). Alternate approach to the management of acute perforating appendicitis in children. *Surgery, Gynecology and Obstetrics, 152*(4), 473–475.

Rottenberg, R. (1985). RLQ pain: Is it what you think? *Patient Care, 19*(2), 70–78.

Savrin, R., & Clatworthy, H. (1979). Appendiceal rupture: A continuing diagnostic problem. *Pediatrics, 63,* 37–43.

Asthma

Hudgel, D., & Madsen, L. (1980). Acute and chronic asthma: A guide to intervention. *American Journal of Nursing, 80,* 1791–1795.

Kiriloff, L., & Tibbals, S. (1983). Drugs for asthma: A complete guide. *American Journal of Nursing, 83,* 55–61.

Landau, L. (1979). Outpatient evaluation and management of asthma. *Pediatric Clinics of North America, 26*(3), 581–600.

McCaully, H. (1980). Breathing exercises as play for asthmatic children. *MCN: American Journal of Maternal/Child Nursing, 5,* 340–344.

Simkins, R. (1981). Asthma: Reactive airways disease. *American Journal of Nursing, 81,* 522–524.

317

Simkins, R. (1981). The crisis of bronchiolitis. *American Journal of Nursing, 81,* 514–516.

Stempel, D., & Mellon, M. (1984). Management of acute severe asthma. *Pediatric Clinics of North America, 31,* 879–890.

Blood and Blood Product Transfusions

Blood transfusions today: What you should know and should do. (1978). *Nursing78, 8*(2), 68–72.

Committee on Transfusion Practices, American Association of Blood Banks. (1986). The latest protocols for blood transfusions. *Nursing86, 16*(11), 34–42.

Professional guide to drugs (2nd ed.). (1982). Horsham, PA: Intermed.

Putnam, R., et al. (1979). Blood therapy. *American Journal of Nursing, 79,* 926–948.

Smith, L. (1984). Protocols for handling transfusion reactions. *American Journal of Nursing, 84,* 1096–1101.

Burns

Hurt, R. (1985). More than skin deep: Guidelines for caring for the burn patient. *Nursing 85, 15*(6), 52–57.

Johnson, C., & Cain, V. (1985). CE burn care: The rehab guide. *American Journal of Nursing, 85,* 48–51.

Lushbaugh, M. (1981). Critical care of the child with burns. *Nursing Clinics of North America, 16,* 635–646.

Luterman, A., & Curreri, P. (1984). Emergency protocol for the severely burned patient. *Hospital Medicine, 20*(10), 131–146.

Robertson, K., et al. (1985). CE burn care: The crucial first days. *American Journal of Nursing, 85,* 29–45.

Rosequist, C., & Shepp, P. (1985). CE burn care: The nutrition factor. *American Journal of Nursing, 85,* 45–47.

Surveyor, J., & Cougherty, D. (1983). Burn scars: Fighting the effects. *American Journal of Nursing, 83,* 746–751.

Winkler, J. (Ed.). (1984). Burn care update. *Critical Care Quarterly, 7*(3), 1–84.

Cardiac Surgery

Bavin, R. (1983). Pediatric cardiac preoperative teaching—A family centered approach. *Focus on Critical Care, 10*(3), 36–43.

Fisk, R. (1986). Management of the pediatric cardiovascular patient after surgery. *Critical Care Quarterly, 9*(2), 75–82.

Gill, B., & Page-Goertz, S. (1986). Deep hypothermic arrest in children undergoing heart surgery. *Heart & Lung, 15,* 28–33.

Givens, L., & Ricks, J. (1985). Assessment of clinical manifestation of cyanotic and acyanotic heart disease in infants and children. *Heart & Lung, 14,* 200–204.

Hazinski, M. (1981). Critical care of the pediatric cardiovascular patient. *Nursing Clinics of North America, 16,* 671–698.

Oellrich, R. (1985). Pneumothorax, chest tubes, and the neonate. *MCN: American Journal of Maternal/Child Nursing, 10,* 29–35.

Page, G. (1985). Patent ductus arteriosus in the premature neonate. *Heart & Lung, 14,* 156–162.

Rushton, C. (1983). Preparing children and families for cardiac surgery: Nursing interventions. *Issues in Comprehensive Pediatric Nursing, 6,* 235–248.

Van Breda, A. (1985). Postoperative care of infants and children who require cardiac surgery. *Heart & Lung, 14,* 205–208.

Cast Care

Farrell, J. (1982). *Illustrated guide to orthopedic nursing* (2nd ed.). Philadelphia: Lippincott.

Holland, S. (1983). Up-to-date home care of a baby in a hip spica cast. *Pediatric Nursing, 9,* 114–115.

Lee, M. (1983). Special care for special casts. *Nursing83, 13*(7), 50–51.

Reid, H. (1984). Clinical forum: Plastering in the 80s. *Nursing Mirror, 159*(7), i–vii.

Wise, L. (1986). A comparison of orthopedic casts: Breaking the mold. *MCN: American Journal of Maternal/Child Nursing, 11,* 174–176.

Cerebral Palsy

Coffman, S. (1983). Parents' perceptions of needs for themselves and their children in a cerebral palsy clinic. *Issues in Comprehensive Pediatric Nursing, 6,* 67–77.

Davis, G., & Hill, P. (1980). Symposium of central nervous system disorders in children: Cerebral palsy. *Nursing Clinics of North America, 15,* 35–50.

Prensky, A., & Puldes, H. (1982). *Care of the neurologically handicapped child.* New York: Oxford University Press.

Steele, S. (1985). Young children with cerebral palsy: Practical guidelines for care. *Pediatric Nursing, 11,* 259–267.

Information from:

United Cerebral Palsy Associations, 66 East 34th Street, New York, NY 10016

National Easter Seal Society, 2023 West Ogden Avenue, Chicago, IL 60612

Chemotherapy

Beardslee, C., & Neff, E. (1982). Body related concerns of children with cancer as compared with the concerns of other children. *Maternal-Child Nursing Journal, 11*(3), 121–134.

Dodd, M. (1982). Cancer patient's knowledge of chemotherapy. Assessment and informational intervention. *Oncology Nursing Forum, 3*(4), 39–44.

Door, R., & Fritz, W. (1980). *Cancer chemotherapy handbook.* New York: Elsevier.

Mulne, A., & Koepke, J. (1985). Adverse effects of cancer therapy in children. *Pediatrics in Review, 6*(3), 259–268.

Pelton, S. (1984). Easing the complications of chemotherapy. *Nursing84, 14*(4), 39–44.

Spross, J. (1982). Issues in chemotherapy administration. *Oncology Nursing Forum, 9*(1), 50–54.

Veninga, K. (1985). Improving nutrition in children with cancer. *Pediatric Nursing, 11,* 18–20.

Vietti, T., & Bergamini, R. (1984). General aspects of chemotherapy. In W. Sutow, F. Fernback, & T. Vietti (Eds.), *Clinical pediatric oncology.* St. Louis: Mosby.

Waskerwitz, M. (1984). Special nursing care for children receiving chemotherapy. *Journal of Association of Pediatric Oncology Nurses, 1*(1), 16–25.

Chronic Illness

Balik, B., Broatch, H., & Moynihan, P. (1986). Diabetes and the school-aged child. *MCN: American Journal of Maternal/Child Nursing, 11,* 316–318.

Johnson, S. (1985). The family and the child with chronic illness. In D. Turk & R. Kerns (Eds.), *Health, illness and families, a life-span perspective.* New York: Wiley.

Kleinberg, S. (1982). *Educating the chronically ill child.* Rockville, MD: Aspen.

Larter, N. (1981). Cystic fibrosis. *American Journal of Nursing, 81,* 527–532.

McKeever, P. (1981). Fathering the chronically ill child. *MCN: American Journal of Maternal/Child Nursing, 6,* 124–128.

Monsen, R. (1986). Phases in the caring relationship. *MCN: American Journal of Maternal/Child Nursing, 11,* 316–318.

National Information Center for Handicapped Children and Youth. (1984). *Physical disabilities and special health problems.* Washington, DC: U.S. Department of Education.

Oremland, E. (1986). Communicating over chronic illness: Dilemmas of affected school-aged children. *Children's Health Care, 14*(4), 218–223.

Patton, A., Ventura, J., & Savedra, M. (1986). Stress and coping responses of adolescents with cystic fibrosis. *Children's Health Care, 14*(3), 153–156.

Robinson, C. (1985). Double bind: A dilemma for parents of chronically ill children. *Pediatric Nursing, 11,* 112–115.

Simpson, O., & Smith, M. (1979). Lightening the load for parents of children with diabetes. *MCN: American Journal of Maternal/Child Nursing, 4,* 293–296.

Cleft Lip/Palate

Albery, L. (1982). Speech and cleft palate—Bridging the gap. *Nursing Mirror, 154*(3), 34–35.

Davies, D. (1985). Cleft lip and palate. *British Medical Journal, 290,* 625–628.

Dorf, D., & Curtain, J. (1982). Early cleft palate repair and speech outcome. *Plastic and Reconstructive Surgery, 70*(1), 74–81.

Huskie, C. (1982). Speech and cleft palate—Working together. *Nursing Mirror, 154*(3), 36–41.

Romney, M. (1984). Congenital defects: Implications on family development and parenting. *Issues in Comprehensive Pediatric Nursing, 7,* 1–15.

Sanchez, C. (1980). Nursing care of the infant and child with cleft lip and palate. *Viewpoint, 17*(1), 14–15.

Styker, G., & Freeh, K. (1981). Feeding infants with cleft lip and/or palate. *Journal of Obstetric, Gynecologic, and Neonatal Nursing, 10*(5), 329–332.

Communicable Disease

American Public Health Association. (1983). *Control of communicable diseases in California.* California: California State Department of Public Health.

Child Day Care Infectious Disease Study Group. (1985). Considerations of infectious diseases in day care centers. *Pediatric Infectious Diseases, 4*(2), 124–136.

Committee on Infectious Diseases. (1986). *Report on the Committee on Infectious Diseases—1986 red book* (20th ed.). Evanston, IL: American Academy of Pediatrics.

Fulginiti, V. (1985). Current concepts in immunization. *Pediatric Consultant, Vol. 4.* New York: McNeil Consumer Products.

Smith, D. (1986). Common day care disease: Patterns and prevention. *Pediatric Nursing, 12,* 175–179.

Williams, L. (1982). Childhood immunizations. *Pediatric Nursing, 8*(1), 18–21, 53.

Congenital Heart Disease

Clare, M. (1985). Home care of infants and children with cardiac disease. *Heart & Lung, 14,* 218–222.

Cloutier, J., & Measel, C. (1982). Home care for the infant with congenital heart disease. *American Journal of Nursing, 82,* 100–103.

Dance, D., & Yates, M. (1985). Nursing assessment and care of children with complications of congenital heart disease. *Heart & Lung, 14* 209–213.

Kashani, I., & Higgins, S. (1986). The cyanotic child: Heart defects and parental learning needs. *MCN: American Journal of Maternal/Child Nursing, 11,* 259–263.

Loeffel, M. (1985). Developmental considerations of infants and children with congenital heart disease. *Heart & Lung, 14,* 214–217.

Slota, M. (1982). Pediatric cardiac catheterization: Complications and interventions. *Critical Care Nurse, 2*(3), 22–25.

Slota, M. (1982). Pediatric problems: Congestive heart failure (Part I). *Critical Care Nurse, 2*(5), 24–28.

Croup, Laryngotracheobronchitis, Epiglottitis

Barker, G. (1979). Current management of croup and epiglottitis. *Pediatric Clinics of North America, 26,* 565–579.

Simkins, R. (1981). Croup and epiglottitis. *American Journal of Nursing, 81,* 519–520.

Wilson, J. (1984). Pediatric emergency: Croup and epiglottitis. *Canadian Nurse, 80*(3), 25–29.

Cystic Fibrosis

Canam, C. (1986). Talking about cystic fibrosis within the family: What parents need to know. *Issues in Comprehensive Pediatric Nursing, 9,* 167–178.

Larter, N. (1981). Cystic fibrosis. *American Journal of Nursing, 81,* 527–532.

Matthews, L., & Drotar, D. (1984). Cystic fibrosis—A challenging long-term chronic disease. *Pediatric Clinics of North America, 31,* 133–152.

Rodgers, B., et al. (1981). Depression in the chronically ill or handicapped school-aged child. *MCN: American Journal of Maternal/Child Nursing, 6,* 266–273.

Selekman, J. (1977). Cystic fibrosis: What is involved in the home treatment program for these children, adolescents and young adults? *Pediatric Nursing, 3,* 32–35.

Depression

Aylward, G. (1985). Understanding and treatment of childhood depression. *Journal of Pediatrics, 107*(1), 1–9.

Brumback, R. (1985). Wechsler performance IQ deficit in depressed children. *Perceptual and Motor Skills, 61,* 331–335.

Digdon, N., & Gotlib, I. (1985). Developmental considerations in the study of childhood depression. *Developmental Review, 5,* 162–199.

Epstein, M., & Cullinan, D. (1986). Depression in children. *Journal of School Health, 56*(1), 10–12.

Goldstein, A. (1985). Depression and achievement in subgroups of children with learning disabilities. *Journal of Applied Developmental Psychology, 6,* 263–275.

Hodges, K., et al. (1985). Depressive symptoms in children with recurrent abdominal pain and in their families. *Journal of Pediatrics, 107*(4), 622–626.

Kashani, J., Shekim, W., & Reid, J. (1984). Amitriptyline in children with major depressive disorder: A double-blind crossover pilot study. *Journal of the American Academy of Child Psychiatry, 23*(3), 348–351.

Looff, D. (1983). Recognizing and treating primary affective disorders in children and adolescents. *Feelings and Their Medical Significance, 25*(5), 17–20.

Nelms, B., & Brady, M. (1980). Assessment and intervention: The depressed school-age child. *Pediatric Nursing, 6,* 15–19.

Nelms, B. (1986). Assessing childhood depression: Do parents and children agree? *Pediatric Nursing, 12*, 23–26.

Pfeffer, C. (1985). Clinical assessment of depression in children and adolescents. *Feelings and Their Medical Significance, 27*(1), 1–4.

Portner, E. (1982). Depressive themes in children's fantasies. *Journal of Childhood in Contemporary Society, 15*(2), 29–39.

Rotundo, N., & Hensley, V. (1985). The children's depression scale: A study of its validity. *Journal of Child Psychology and Psychiatry, 26*, 917–927.

Tishler, C. (1984). Depression in children and adolescents: Identification and intervention. *Public Health Currents, 24*(5), 19–22.

Developmental Disability

Beail, N. (1985). The nature of interactions between nursing staff and profoundly mentally handicapped children. *Child: Care, Health and Development, 11*(3), 113–129.

Bowness, S., & Zadik, T. (1981). Implementing the nursing process at a unit for mentally handicapped children. *Nursing Times, 77*(16), 695–696.

Childs, R. (1985). Maternal psychological conflicts associated with the birth of a retarded child. *Maternal-Child Nursing Journal, 14*(3), 175–182.

Curry, J., & Peppe, K. (1978). *Mental retardation: Nursing approaches to care.* St. Louis: Mosby.

Kosowski, M., & Sopczyk, D. (1985). Feeding hospitalized children with developmental disabilities. *MCN: American Journal of Maternal/Child Nursing, 10*, 190–194.

Krajicek, M. (1982). Developmental disability and human sexuality. *Nursing Clinics of North America, 17*, 377–386.

Nehring, W., & Engelhardt, K. (1985). Play behaviors and toy preferences of preschoolers with Down's syndrome. *MCN: American Journal of Maternal/Child Nursing, 10*, 166.

Pipes, P., & Carman, P. (1981). Nutrition and feeding of children with developmental delays and related problems. In P. Pipes (Ed.), *Nutrition in infancy and childhood* (2nd ed.). St. Louis: Mosby.

Powell, M. (1981). *Assessment and management of developmental changes and problems in children* (2nd ed.). St. Louis: Mosby.

Wasch, S. (1981). Hospitalization of profoundly and severely mentally retarded children. *Children's Health Care, 9*(4), 126–131.

White, J. (1983). Special nursing needs of hospitalized children with learning disabilities. *MCN: American Journal of Maternal/Child Nursing, 8*, 209–212.

Diabetes

Balik, B., Haig, B., & Moynihan, P. (1986). Diabetes and the school-aged child. *MCN: American Journal of Maternal/Child Nursing, 11*, 324–330.

Faro, B. (1983). Maintaining good control in children with diabetes. *Pediatric Nursing, 9*, 368–373.

Fow, S. (1983). Home blood glucose monitoring in children with insulin-dependent diabetes mellitus. *Pediatric Nursing, 9*, 439–442.

Lillo, R., & Masteller, D. (1982). Outpatient management of children in diabetic ketoacidosis. *Pediatric Nursing, 8*, 383–385.

Saucier, C. (1984). Self-concept and self-care management in school-age children with diabetes. *Pediatric Nursing, 10*, 135–138.

Simpson, O., & Smith, M. (1979). Lightening the load for parents of children with diabetes. *MCN: American Journal of Maternal/Child Nursing, 4*, 293–296.

Tauer, K. (1983). Physiologic mechanisms in childhood hypoglycemia. *Pediatric Nursing, 9*, 341–344.

Diarrhea/Gastroenteritis

Chaddha, B., Hansen, R., & Orosz, J. (1984). Disposing of diaper rash. *Patient Care, 18*(18), 57–69.

DeBenhem, B., Ellet, M., Perez, R., & Clark, J. (1985). Initial assessment and management of chronic diarrhea in toddlers. *Pediatric Nursing, 11*, 281–285.

Fitzgerald, J. (1985). Management of the infant with persistent diarrhea. *Pediatric Infectious Disease, 4*(1), 6–9.

Hamilton, J. (1985). Viral diarrhea. *Pediatric Annals, 14*(1), 25–28.

Levine, M. (1985). Infant diarrhea: Etiologies and newer treatment. *Pediatric Annals, 14*(1), 15–18.

Ling, L., & McCamman, S. (1978). Dietary treatment of diarrhea and constipation in infants and children. *Issues in Comprehensive Pediatric Nursing, 3*, 17–28.

Patient Education Aid. Diaper rash. (1984). *Patient Care, 18*(18), 93–94.

Death and Dying

Atwood, V. (1984). Children's concepts of death: A descriptive study. *Child Study Journal, 14*(1), 11–29.

Betz, C., & Poster, E. (1984). Children's concepts of death: Implications for pediatric practice. *Nursing Clinics of North America, 19*, 341–349.

Coody, D. (1985). High expectations: Nurses who work with children who might die. *Nursing Clinics of North America, 28*, 131–142.

Halpern, E., & Palic, L. (1984). Developmental changes in death anxiety in children. *Journal of Applied Developmental Psychology, 5*, 163–172.

Mills, G. (1979). Books to help children understand death. *American Journal of Nursing, 79*, 290–295.

Sahler, O. (Ed.). (1978). *The child and death.* St. Louis: Mosby.

Salladay, S., & Royal, M. (1981). Children and death: Guidelines for grief work. *Child Psychiatry and Human Development, 11*(4), 203–212.

Townley, K., & Thornberg, K. (1980). Maturation of the concept of death in elementary school children. *Educational Research Quarterly, 5*(2), 17–24.

Wass, H., & Cason, L. (1985). Fears and anxieties about death. *Issues in Comprehensive Pediatric Nursing, 8*, 25–45.

Wass, H., et al. (1983). Use of play for assessing children's death concepts: A re-examination. *Psychological Reports, 53*, 799–803.

Epilepsy

Chee, C. (1980). Seizure disorders. *Nursing Clinics of North America, 15*, 71–82.

McGrath, D. (1983). Video recording seizure activity in children. *MCN: American Journal of Maternal/Child Nursing, 8*, 218–220.

Mills, M. (1982). When a child has surgery for focal epilepsy. *MCN: American Journal of Maternal/Child Nursing, 7*, 304–308.

Ozuna, J., & Burchiel, R. (1985). Surgery for epilepsy. *AORN Journal, 42*(6), 879–885.

Parrish, M. (1984). A comparison of behavioral side effects related to commonly used anticonvulsants. *Pediatric Nursing, 10*, 149–152.

Vining E., & Freeman, J. (Eds.). (1985). Epilepsy and seizures. *Pediatric Annals, 14*(11), entire issue.

Literature from: Epilepsy Foundation of America, 1828 L Street, NW, Suite 406, Washington, DC 20036.

Failure to Thrive

Berwick, D. (1980). Nonorganic failure to thrive. *Pediatrics in Review, 1*(9), 265–270.

Hopwood, N. (1984). Failure to thrive: Investigating the nonorganic causes. *Consultant, 24*(6), 45–48, 51, 54.

Levine, M., et al. (1983). *Developmental-behavioral pediatrics.* Philadelphia: Saunders.

Steele, S. (1986). Nonorganic failure to thrive: A pediatric social illness. *Issues in Comprehensive Pediatric Nursing, 9,* 47–58.

Withrow, C., & Fleming, J. (1983). Pediatric social illness: A challenge to nurses. *Issues in Comprehensive Pediatric Nursing, 6,* 261–275.

Yoos, L. (1984). Taking another look at failure to thrive. *MCN: American Journal of Maternal/Child Nursing, 9,* 32–36.

Fever

Cushing, A. (1984). Fever diagnosis at your fingertips. *Emergency Medicine, 16*(20), 58–64, 66.

Donahue, A. (1983). Tepid sponging. *Journal of Emergency Nursing, 9*(2), 78–82.

Levi, M. (1984). On managing the febrile child. *Emergency Medicine, 16*(3), 166–168, 173–175, 178–180.

Press, S., & Fawcett, N. (1985). Association of temperatures greater than 41.1°C (106°F) with serious illness. *Clinical Pediatrics, 24*(1), 21–25.

Shaver, F. (1982). The basic mechanisms of fever: Considerations for therapy. *Nurse Practitioner, 7*(9), 15–16, 18–19.

Younger, J., & Brown, B. (1985). Fever management: Rational or ritual? *Pediatric Nursing, 11,* 26–29.

Gastroesophageal Reflux

Boyd, C. (1982). Postural therapy at home for infants with gastroesophageal reflux. *Pediatric Nursing, 8,* 395–398.

Herbst, J. (1983). Diagnosis and treatment of gastroesophageal reflux in children. *Pediatrics in Review, 5*(3), 75–79.

Johnson, D. (1985). Current thinking on the role of surgery in gastroesophageal reflux. *Pediatric Clinics of North America, 32,* 1165–1179.

Kurfiss-Daniels, D. (1982). Positioning as treatment for infant gastroesophageal reflux. *American Journal of Nursing, 82,* 1535–1537.

Orenstein, S., & Whitington, P. (1983). Position for prevention of infant gastroesophageal reflux. *Journal of Pediatrics, 103*(4), 534–537.

Orenstein, S., Whitington, P., & Orenstein, D. (1983). The infant seat as treatment of gastroesophageal reflux. *New England Journal of Medicine, 309,* 760–763.

Gastrostomy

Paarlberg, J., & Balint, J. (1985). Gastrostomy tubes: Practical guidelines for home care. *Pediatric Nursing, 11,* 99–102.

Perez, R., Beckom, L., Jebara, L., Lewis, M., & Patenaude, Y. (1984). Care of the child with a gastrostomy tube: Common and practical concerns. *Issues in Comprehensive Pediatric Nursing, 7,* 107–119.

Perry, S., Johnson, S., & Trump, D. (1983). Gastrostomy and the neonate. *American Journal of Nursing, 83,* 1030–1033.

Wink, D. (1983). The physical and emotional care of infants with gastrostomy tubes. *Issues in Comprehensive Pediatric Nursing, 6,* 195–203.

Grief and Loss

Mina, C. (1985). A program for helping grieving parents. *MCN: American Journal of Maternal/Child Nursing, 10,* 118–121.

Perilman, T. (1986). When that dying patient calls you Mommy. *RN, 49*(8), 24–27.

Romney, M. (1984). Congenital defects: Implications on family development and parenting. *Issues in Comprehensive Pediatric Nursing, 7,* 1–15.

Thomas, N., & Cordel, A. (1983). The dying infant: Aiding parents in the detachment process. *Pediatric Nursing, 9,* 355–357.

Videka-Sherman, L. (1982). Coping with the death of a child: A study over time. *American Journal of Orthopsychiatry, 52,* 688–698.

Waller, D., Todres, D., Cassem, N., & Anderten, A. (1979). Coping with poor prognosis in the pediatric intensive care unit. *American Journal of Diseases of Children, 133,* 1121–1125.

Williams, H., Frederick, P., & Rothenberg, M. (1981). The child is dying: Who helps the family? *MCN: American Journal of Maternal Child/Nursing, 5,* 261–265.

Wong, D. (1980). Bereavement, the empty-mother syndrome. *MCN: The American Journal of Maternal/Child Nursing, 5,* 384–389.

Wooten, B. (1981). Death of an infant. *MCN: American Journal of Maternal/Child Nursing, 6,* 257–260.

Guidelines for Teaching

Barnard, K., & Erikson, M. (1976). *Teaching Children with Developmental Problems.* St. Louis: Mosby.

Evans, M., & Hansen, B. (1981). Administering injections to different-aged children. *MCN: American Journal of Maternal/Child Nursing,* 194–199.

Hansen, B., & Evans, M. (1981). Preparing a child for procedure. *MCN: American Journal of Maternal/Child Nursing,* 392–397.

Wieczorek, R., & Natapoff, J. (1981). *A conceptual approach to the nursing of children—Health care from birth through adolescence.* Philadelphia: Lippincott.

Normal Growth and Development: Adolescent

Alan Guttmacher Institute (1982). *Teenage pregnancy: The problem that hasn't gone away.* New York: Author.

Babington, M. (1984). Adolescent use of oral contraceptives. *Pediatric Nursing, 10,* 111–114.

Barret, R., & Robinson, B. (1986). Adolescent fathers: Often forgotten parents. *Pediatric Nursing, 12,* 273–277.

Bradley, J. (1984). Do adolescents practice what they preach about health? *Pediatric Nursing, 10,* 285–289.

Elkind, D. (1984). Teenage thinking: Implications for health care. *Pediatric Nursing, 10,* 383–385.

Fullar, S. (1986). Care of postpartum adolescents. *MCN: American Journal of Maternal/Child Nursing, 11,* 398–403.

Narins, D., Belkengren, R., & Sapala, S. (1983). Nutrition and the growing athlete. *Pediatric Nursing, 9,* 163–168.

Nelms, B. (1981). What is a normal adolescent? *MCN: American Journal of Maternal/Child Nursing, 6,* 402–406.

Peach, E. (1980). Counseling sexually active very young adolescent girls. *MCN: American Journal of Maternal/Child Nursing, 5,* 191–195.

Planned Parenthood Federation of America. (1980). *How to talk to your teenagers about something that's not easy to talk about: Facts about the facts of life and what teens want to know but don't know how to ask.* New York: Author.

Sewall, K. (1983). Peer-group reality therapy for the pregnant adolescent. *MCN: American Journal of Maternal/Child Nursing, 8,* 67–69.

Sinkford, J. (1981). Dental health needs of children and adolescents. *Journal of the American Dental Association, 103,* 901–905.

Stone, A. (1982). Facing up to acne. *Pediatric Nursing, 8,* 229–234.

White, J. (1984). Initiating contraceptive use: How do young women decide? *Pediatric Nursing, 10,* 247–352.

Williams, J. (1986). Counseling adolescents about environmental teratogens. *Pediatric Nursing, 12,* 292–295.

Normal Growth and Development: Infant

Mones, R., & Asnes, R. (1986). The colicky baby: Helping parents cope. *Contemporary Pediatrics, 3*(4), 86–98.

Nelson, C., & Pescar, S. (1986). *Should I call the doctor? A comprehensive guide to understanding your child's illness and injuries.* New York: Warner.

Romanko, M., & Brost, B. (1982). Swaddling: An effective invention for pacifying infants. *Pediatric Nursing, 8,* 259–261.

Wagner, T., & Hindi-Alexander, M. (1984). Hazards of baby powder? *Pediatric Nursing, 10,* 124–126.

Winklestein, M. (1984). Overfeeding in infancy: The early introduction of solid foods. *Pediatric Nursing, 10,* 205–208.

Yoos, L. (1981). A developmental approach to physical assessment. *MCN: American Journal of Maternal/Child Nursing, 6,* 168–170.

Normal Growth and Development: Midchildhood

Betz, C. (1983). Bicycle safety: Opportunities for family education. *Pediatric Nursing, 9,* 109–111.

Denehy, J. (1984). What do school-age children know about their bodies? *Pediatric Nursing, 10,* 290–292.

Dorn, L. (1984). Children's concepts of illness: Clinical applications. *Pediatric Nursing, 10,* 325–327.

Elkind, D. (1986). David Elkind discusses parental pressures. *Pediatric Nursing, 12,* 417–418.

LaMontagne, L. (1984). Three coping strategies used by school-age children. *Pediatric Nursing, 10,* 25–28.

Luce, M., & Sande, D. (1983). Oral health in children: Prevention of dental caries. *Nurse Practitioner, 8*(1), 43–52.

McClellan, M. (1984). On their own: Latchkey children. *Pediatric Nursing, 10,* 198–201.

McCown, D. (1984). Moral development in children. *Pediatric Nursing, 10*(1), 42–44.

Millar, T. (1980). The reluctant learner: A strategy for intervention. *Children Today, 9*(5), 13–15.

Morgan, J. (1986). Prevention of childhood obesity. *Issues in Comprehensive Pediatric Nursing, 9,* 33–38.

Pacific Press Publishing Association. (1981). *Listen, a journal of better living* (Special Drug Issue). Mountain View, CA: Author.

Rowland, B., Robinson, B., & Coleman, M. (1986). A survey of parents' perceptions regarding latchkey children. *Pediatric Nursing, 12,* 278–283.

Weiss, R. (1981). Growing up a little faster—Children in single-parent households. *Children Today, 10*(3), 22–25, 36.

Wood, S. (1983). School aged children's perceptions of the causes of illness. *Pediatric Nursing, 9,* 101–104.

Normal Growth and Development: Toddler and Preschooler

Consumer's Guide to Dental Health. (1982). Caring for your children's teeth. *Journal of the American Dental Association, 104,* 19C–26C.

Edgil, A., Wood, K., & Smith, D. (1985). Sleep problems of older infants and preschool children. *Pediatric Nursing, 11,* 87–90.

Fish, L., & Burch, K. (1985). Identifying gifted preschoolers. *Pediatric Nursing, 11,* 125–127.

Goldberg, R. (1984). Identifying speech and language delays in children. *Pediatric Nursing, 10,* 252–259.

Gulick, E. (1986). The effects of breast-feeding on toddler health. *Pediatric Nursing, 12,* 51–55.

Hess, C., Kasprisin, C., Nix, K., Stevens, N., & Wong, D. (1984). Fluoride: Too much or too little? *Pediatric Nursing, 10,* 397–404.

Hitchens-Serota, J. (1986). Assessing parents' knowledge of pediatric dental disease. *Pediatric Nursing, 12,* 435–438.

Head Injury

Hausman, K. (1981). Critical care of the child with increased intracranial pressure. *Nursing Clinics of North America, 16,* 697.

Katkis, J. (1980). An introduction to monitoring intracranial pressure in critically ill children. *Critical Care Quarterly, 3,* 1–8.

Kunkel, J. (1981). Nursing management of the head injured child. *Critical Care Update, 8*(3), 22–24.

Maher, A. (1985). Dealing with head and neck injuries. *RN, 48*(3), 43–46.

Mauss-Clum, N. (1982). Bringing the unconscious patient back safely—Nursing makes the critical difference. *Nursing82, 12*(8), 34–42.

Mill, G. (1980). Preparing children and parents for cerebral computerized tomography. *MCN: American Journal of Maternal/Child Nursing, 5,* 403–407.

Parish, R., Woolf, A., Eichner, M., & Cauldwell, C. (1985). The significance of Babinski signs in children with head trauma. *Annals of Emergency Medicine, 14*(4), 329–330.

Rogers, P., & Kreutzer, J. (1984). Family crises following head injury: A network intervention strategy. *Journal of Neurosurgical Nursing, 16*(6), 343–346.

Sachs, P. (1985). Beyond support: Traumatic head injury as a growth experience for families. *Rehabilitation Nursing, 10*(1), 21–23.

Siegal, A. (1985). Head injuries: Emergency care tips. *Parents, 60*(6), 150, 153, 157–158.

Walleck, C. (1980). Head trauma in children. *Nursing Clinics of North America, 15,* 115–130.

Hydrocephalus

Aresenault, L. (1983). Delayed onset symptomatic hydrocephalus related to aqueductal stenosis. *Journal of Neurosurgical Nursing, 15*(10), 291–298.

Grant, L. (1984). Hydrocephalus: An overview and update. *Journal of Neurosurgical Nursing, 16*(6), 313–318.

Hausman, K. (1981). Nursing care of the patient with hydrocephalus. *Journal of Neurosurgical Nursing, 13*(6), 326–332.

Jackson, P. (1983). Peritoneal shunting for hydrocephalus. *Critical Care Update, 10*(4), 33–39.

Neveling, E., & Truex, R. (1983). External obstructive hydrocephalus: A study of clinical and developmental aspects in 10 children. *Journal of Neurosurgical Nursing, 13*(8), 256–260.

Hyperbilirubinemia

Brickley, J. (1982). How to keep an eye shield on a baby. *RN, 45*(11), 115.

Giving the green light to phototherapy. (1983). *American Journal of Nursing, 83,* 1376.

Perez, R. (Ed.). (1981). *Protocols for perinatal nursing practice.* St. Louis: Mosby.

Schreiner, R. (Ed.). (1982). *Care of the newborn.* New York: Raven Press.

Stoerner, J. (1981). Neonatal jaundice. *American Family Physician, 24*(5), 226–231.

Increased Intracranial Pressure

Coffey, R. (1984). Pediatric neurological emergencies. In J. Pierog & L. Pierog (Eds.), *Pediatric critical illness and injury.* Rockville, MD: Aspen.

Hausman, K. (1981). Critical care of the child with increased intracranial pressure. *Nursing Clinics of North America, 16,* 647–656.

Jackson, P. (1983). Assessing increased intracranial pressure in infants and young children. *Critical Care Update, 10*(9), 8–15.

James, H. (1986). Neurologic evaluation and support in the child with an acute brain insult. *Pediatric Annals, 15,* 16–22.

Kaktis, J. (1980). An introduction to monitoring intracranial pressure in critically ill children. *Critical Care Quarterly, 3*(1), 1–8.

McElroy, D., & David, G. (1986). SIADH and the acutely ill child. *MCN: American Journal of Maternal/Child Nursing, 11,* 193–196.

Mitchell, P., Habermann-Little, B., Johnson, F., van Inwegen-Scott, D., & Tyler, D. (1985). Critically ill children: The importance of touch in a high-technology environment. *Nursing Administration Quarterly, 9*(4), 38–46.

Slota, M. (1983). Neurological assessment of the infant and toddler. *Critical Care Nurse, 3*(5), 87–92.

Slota, M. (1983). Pediatric neurological assessment. *Critical Care Nurse, 3*(6), 106–112.

Infectious Mononucleosis

Alpert, G., & Fleisher, G. (1984). Complications of infection with Epstein-Barr virus during childhood: A study of children admitted to the hospital. *Pediatric Infectious Disease, 3*(4), 304–307.

Burr, L. (1983). When symptoms point to mononucleosis. *Patient Care, 17*(12), 58–68.

McSherry, J. (1983). Myths about infectious mononucleosis. *Canadian Medical Association Journal, 128*(6), 645–646.

Sabetta, J. (1984). Diagnosis: infectious mononucleosis. *Hospital Medicine, 20*(3), 109.

Shurin, S. (1979). Infectious mononucleosis. *Pediatric Clinics of North America, 26,* 315–326.

Intravenous Catheter

Abbott, P., & Schlacht, K. (1984). Pediatric IVs: A special challenge. *Canadian Nurse, 80*(10), 24–26.

Arthur, G. (1984). When your littlest patients need IVs. *RN, 47*(7), 30–35.

Feldstein, A. (1986). Detect phlebitis and infiltration before they harm your patient. *Nursing86, 16*(1), 44–47.

Frey, A. (1985). Pediatric dosage calculations—IV medications. *NITA, 8,* 373–379.

McGowan, D., & Parks, B. (1985). Pediatric drug information. *Pediatric Nursing, 11,* 298.

McGrath, B. (1980). Fluids, electrolytes, and replacement therapy in pediatric nursing. *MCN: American Journal of Maternal/Child Nursing, 5,* 58–62.

Rimar, J. (1982). Guidelines for the intravenous administration of medications used in pediatrics. *MCN: American Journal of Maternal/Child Nursing, 7,* 184–197.

Streckfuss, B. (1985). Pediatric I.V. care. *NITA, 8*(1), 75–82.

Teitell, B. (1984). Considerations for neonatal IV therapy. *NITA, 7,* 521–526.

Leukemia

Adams, J., & Guido, G. (1984). The adolescent coping with cancer. *Dimensions of Critical Care Nursing, 3*(2), 70–75.

Armstrong, G., Wirt, R., Nesbit, M., & Martinson, I. (1982). Multidimensional assessment of psychological problems in children with cancer. *Research in Nursing and Health, 5,* 205–211.

Beardslee, C., & Neff, E. (1982). Body related concerns of children with cancer as compared with the concerns of other children. *MCN: American Journal of Maternal/Child Nursing, 11,* 121–134.

Koocher, G. (1985). Psychosocial care of the child cured of cancer. *Pediatric Nursing, 11,* 91–93.

Kramer, R., & Perin, G. (1985). Patient education and pediatric oncology. *Nursing Clinics of North America, 20,* 31–47.

Lovejoy, N. (1983). The leukemic child's perceptions of family behavior. *Oncology Nursing Forum, 10*(4), 20–25.

Mulne, A., & Koepke, J. (1985). Adverse effects of cancer therapy in children. *Pediatrics in Review, 6*(3), 259–268.

Poplack, D. (1985). Acute lymphoblastic leukemia in childhood. *Pediatric Clinics of North America, 32,* 669–698.

Ross, D., & Ross, S. (1984). Stress reduction procedures for the school-aged hospitalized leukemic child. *Pediatric Nursing, 10,* 393–395.

Ross, D., & Ross, S. (1984). Teaching the child with leukemia to cope with teasing. *Issues in Comprehensive Pediatric Nursing, 7,* 59–66.

Ruccione, K. (1983). Acute leukemia in children: Current perspectives. *Issues in Comprehensive Pediatric Nursing, 6,* 329–362.

Spinetta, J., & Spinetta, J. (1981). *Living with childhood cancer.* St. Louis: Mosby.

Stutzman, H. (1985). Explaining leukemia to classmates. *Journal of the Association of Pediatric Oncology Nurses, 2*(1), 15.

Veninga, K. (1985). Improving nutrition in children with cancer. *Pediatric Nursing, 11,* 18–19.

Wallace, M., Bakke, K., Hubbard, A., & Pendergrass, T. (1984). Coping with childhood cancer: An educational program for parents of children with cancer. *Oncology Nursing Forum, 11*(4), 30–35.

Waskerwitz, M., & Ruccione, K. (1985). An overview of cancer in children in the late 1980s. *Nursing Clinics of North America, 20,* 5–29.

Meningitis

Edwards, M., & Baker, C. (1981). Complications and sequelae of meningococcal infections in children. *Journal of Pediatrics, 99,* 540–545.

Gaddy, D. (1980). Meningitis in the pediatric population. *Nursing Clinics of North America, 15*, 83–97.

Jadavji, T., Humphreys, R., & Prober, C. (1985). Brain abscesses in infants and children. *Pediatric Infectious Diseases, 4*, 394–398.

Medical staff conference. (1984). Meningitis. *The Western Journal of Medicine, 140*, 433–436.

Muwaswes, M. (1985). Increased intracranial pressure and its systemic effects. *Journal of Neurosurgical Nursing, 17*, 238–243.

Nebens, I., & Jackson, B. (1982). A case of acute fulminating meningococcemia. *American Journal of Nursing, 82*, 1390–1393.

Sell, S. (1983). Long-term sequelae of bacterial meningitis in children. *Pediatric Infectious Diseases, 2*, 90–93.

Wing, S. (1981). Brain abscess. *Journal of Neurosurgical Nursing, 13*, 123–126.

Wink, D. (1984). Bacterial meningitis in children. *American Journal of Nursing, 84*(4), 456–460.

Yoshikawa, T., & Norma, D. (1981). Bacterial meningitis—disease of young and old. *Consultant, 21*(11), 219–231.

Meningocele/Myelomeningocele

Clarkson, J. (1982). Self-catheterization training of a child with myelomeningocele. *Journal of Occupational Therapy, 36*(2), 95–98.

Coffman, S. (1986). Description of a nursing diagnosis: Alteration in bowel elimination related to neurogenic bowel in children with myelomeningocele. *Issues in Comprehensive Pediatric Nursing, 9*, 179–191.

Hill, M. (1978). Meningomyelocele: The child and the family. *Issues in Comprehensive Pediatric Nursing, 2*, 51–63.

Jeffries, J. (1982). Behavioral management of fecal incontinence in a child with myelomeningocele. *Pediatric Nursing, 8*, 267–270.

Myers, G. (1984). Myelomeningocele: The medical aspects. *Pediatric Clinics of North America, 31*, 165–175.

Passo, S. (1980). Malformations of the neural tube. *Nursing Clinics of North America, 15*, 5–21.

Richardson, K., et al. (1985). Biofeedback therapy for managing bowel incontinence caused by meningomyelocele. *MCN: American Journal of Maternal/Child Nursing, 10*, 388–392.

Nasogastric Intubation

Strange, J. (1983). An expert's guide to tubes and drains. *RN, 46*(4), 35–42.

Yolden, C., Grindle, J., & Carl, D. (1980). Taking the trauma out of nasogastric intubation. *Nursing80, 10*(9), 64–67.

The Normal Neonate

Danforth, D. (1986). La Leche League discusses crying babies. *Baby Talk, 51*(12), 32–33.

Gibbons, M. (1984). Circumcision: The controversy continues. *Pediatric Nursing, 10*, 103–110.

Haddock, N. (1980). Blood pressure monitoring in neonates. *MCN: The American Journal of Maternal/Child Nursing, 5*, 131–135.

Hazuka, B. (1980). Prevention of infection in the nursery. *Nursing Clinics of North America, 15*, 825–831.

Klaus, M., & Kennell, J. (1982). *Parent-infant bonding.* St. Louis: Mosby.

Ludington-Hoe, S. (1983). What can newborns really see? *American Journal of Nursing, 83*, 1286–1289.

Marmet, C., & Shell, E. (1984). Training neonates to suck correctly. *MCN: American Journal of Maternal/Child Nursing, 9*, 401–407.

Moore, M. (1981). *Newborn family and nurse* (2nd ed.). Philadelphia: Saunders.

Sardana, R. (1985). Examining for defects ... the newborn. *Nursing Mirror, 160*(2), 38–42.

Scanlon, J., et al. (1981). *A system of newborn physical examination.* Baltimore: University Park Press.

Schreiner, R. (1982). *Care of the newborn.* New York: Raven Press.

Shipman, S., & Robinson, D. (1981). Normal newborn care. In R. Perez (Ed.), *Protocols for perinatal nursing practice.* St. Louis: Mosby.

Taylor, L. (1981). Newborn feeding behaviors and attaching. *MCN: American Journal of Maternal/Child Nursing, 6*, 210–212.

Nephrotic Syndrome

Ford, B. (1983). Nephrotic syndrome. *Nursing Times, 79*(31), 58–60.

McEnery, P., & Strife, F. (1982). Nephrotic syndrome in childhood. *Pediatric Clinics of North America, 29*, 875–894.

Workman, B. (1984). Nephrotic syndrome. *Nursing Times, 80*(24), 32–36.

Neuroblastoma

Pizzo, P. (1986). Management of pediatric cancer. *Hospital Practice, 21*(3), 111–116.

Wallace, M., Bakke, K., Hubbard, A., & Pendergrass, T. (1984). Coping with childhood cancer: An educational program for parents of children with cancer. *Oncology Nursing Forum, 11*(4), 30–35.

Waskerwitz, M., & Ruccione, K. (1985). An overview of cancer in children in the 1980s. *Nursing Clinics of North America, 20*, 5–29.

Nonaccidental Trauma

Christensen, M., Schommer, B., & Velasquez, J. (1984). An interdisciplinary approach to preventing child abuse. *MCN: American Journal of Maternal/Child Nursing, 9*, 108–112, 113–117.

Elvik, S., Berkowitz, C., & Greenberg, C. (1986). Child sexual abuse—The role of the nurse practitioner. *Nurse Practitioner, 11*(1), 15–22.

Kelley, S. (1985). Drawings: Critical communications for sexually abused children. *Pediatric Nursing, 11*, 421–436.

Kempe, C., & Helfer, R. (1980). *The battered child* (3rd ed.). Chicago: University of Chicago Press.

Manciaux, M. (1984). Battered, ill-treated, abandoned. *World Health Forum, 5*, 21–23.

Newberger, E. (Ed.). (1982). *Child abuse.* Boston: Little, Brown.

Oates, R., et al. (1985). Mothers of abused children: A comparison study. *Clinical Pediatrics, 24*(1), 9–13.

Ryan, M. (1984). Identifying the sexually abused child. *Pediatric Nursing, 10*, 419–423.

Sasserath, V. (Ed.). (1983). *Minimizing high-risk parenting.* Skillman, NJ: Johnson and Johnson.

Sink, F. (1986). Child sexual abuse: Comprehensive assessment in the pediatric health care setting. *Children's Health Care, 15*(2), 108–113.

Wailes, J. (1983). Nonaccidental injury—Battered baby syndrome. *Nursing Mirror, 157*(16), 20–22.

Osteogenic Sarcoma

Battista, E. (1986). Educational needs of the adolescent with cancer and his family. *Seminars in Oncology Nursing, 2*(2), 123–125.

Boren, H. (1985). Adolescent adjustment to amputation necessitated by bone cancer. *Orthopaedic Nursing, 4*(5), 30–32.

Gregorcic, N. (1985). Functional abilities following limb-salvage procedures. *Orthopaedic Nursing, 4*(5), 24–28.

Hall, M. (1983). Using relaxation imagery with children with malignancies: A developmental perspective. *American Journal of Clinical Hypnosis, 25*(2–3), 143–149.

Nirenberg, A. (1985). The adolescent with osteogenic sarcoma. *Orthopaedic Nursing, 4*(5), 11–16.

Novotny, M. (1986). Body image changes in amputee children: How nursing theory can make a difference. *Journal of Association of Pediatric Oncology Nurses, 3*(2), 8–13.

Olson, R. (1986). Compliance with treatment regimens ... adolescent cancer patients. *Seminars in Oncology Nursing, 2*(2), 104–111.

Spross, J., & Hope, A. (1985). Alterations in comfort: Pain related to cancer. *Orthopaedic Nursing, 4*(5), 48–52.

Pain

Abu-Saad, M. (1984). Assessing children's response to pain. *Pain, 19*, 163–171.

Abu-Saad, M., Holzemer, W. (1981). Measuring children's self-assessment of pain. *Issues in Comprehensive Pediatric Nursing, 5*, 337–349.

Beyer, J., & Byers, M. (1985). Knowledge of pediatric pain: The state of the art. *Children's Health Care, 13*(4), 150–159.

Broome, M. (1985). The child in pain: A model for assessment and intervention. *Critical Care Quarterly, 8*(1), 47–55.

Burokas, L. (1985). Factors affecting nurses' decisions to medicate pediatric patients after surgery. *Heart & Lung, 14*, 373–378.

Dale, J. (1986). A multidimensional study of infant's responses to painful stimuli. *Pediatric Nursing, 12*, 27–31.

Eland, J. (1985). The child who is hurting. *Seminars in Oncology Nursing, 1*(2), 116–122.

Hawley, D. (1984). Postoperative pain in children: Misconceptions, descriptions and interventions. *Pediatric Nursing, 10*, 20–23.

Jerrett, M. (1985). Children and their pain experience. *Children's Health Care, 14*(2), 83–89.

Mather, L., & Mackie, J. (1983). The incidence of postoperative pain in children. *Pain, 15*, 271–282.

McCaffery, M. (1977). Pain relief for the child. *Pediatric Nursing, 3*(4), 11–16.

Play Therapy

Axline, V. (1969). *Play therapy* (rev. ed.). New York: Ballantine.

Betz, C. (1983). Teaching children through play therapy. *AORN Journal, 38*(4), 709, 712–713, 716–717.

Bolig, R., Fernie, D., & Klein, E. (1986). Unstructured play in hospital settings: An internal locus of control rationale. *Children's Health Care, 15*(2), 101–107.

Burson, J., & Brannigan, C. (1984). Use of play in nutritional support of hospitalized children. *Issues in Comprehensive Pediatric Nursing, 7*, 283–289.

D'Antonio, I. (1984). Therapeutic use of play in hospitalized children. *Nursing Clinics of North America, 19*, 351–359.

Darbyshire, P. (1985). Happiness is an old blanket ... children's comfort toys, Part I. *Nursing Times, 6–12, 81*(10), 40–41.

Dasen, P. (1984). The value of play. *World Health Forum, 5*, 11–13.

Kielhofner, G., et al. (1983). A comparison of play behavior in nonhospitalized versus hospitalized children. *American Journal of Occupational Therapy, 37*(5), 305–312.

LaMontagne, L. (1984). Three coping strategies used by school-age children. *Pediatric Nursing, 10*, 25–28.

Meer, P. (1985). Using play therapy in outpatient settings. *MCN: American Journal of Maternal/Child Nursing, 10*(6), 378–380.

Poston, L. (1982). Finding time to play. *MCN: American Journal of Maternal/Child Nursing, 7*, 19–20.

Poster, E., & Betz, C. (1983). Allaying the anxiety of hospitalized children using stress immunization techniques. *Issues in Comprehensive Pediatric Nursing, 6*, 227–233.

Sesame Street Hospital Admission Kit. Milwaukee: Will Ross, Inc. (Dept. AJN, P.O. Box 372, 4285 N. Port Washington Road, 53201).

Sparling, J., et al. (1984). Play techniques with neurologically impaired preschoolers. *American Journal of Occupational Therapy, 38*(9), 603–612.

Verzemnieks, I. (1984). Developmental stimulation for infants and toddlers. *American Journal of Nursing, 84*, 748–752.

Pneumonia

Pinney, M. (1981). Pneumonia. *American Journal of Nursing, 81*, 517–518.

Rokosky, J. (1981). Assessment of the individual with altered respiratory function. *Nursing Clinics of North America, 16*, 195–209.

Pyloric Stenosis

Rockenhaus, J. (1985). Ingestion, digestion and elimination. In S. Mott, et al. (Eds.), *Nursing care of children and families, a holistic approach*. Menlo Park, CA: Addison Wesley.

Spenner, D. (1980). When the baby is sick and the mother's concerns are ignored. *American Journal of Nursing, 80*, 2222–2224.

Radiation Therapy

Delly, P. (1981). Planning care for the patient receiving external radiation. *American Journal of Nursing, 81*, 338–342.

Pizzo, P. (1986). Management of pediatric cancer. *Hospital Practice, 21*(3), 111–116.

Snyder, C. (1986). *Oncology nursing*. Boston: Little, Brown.

Varricchio, C. (1981). The patient on radiation therapy. *American Journal of Nursing, 81*, 334–447.

Range-of-Motion Exercises

Cuica, R., Bradish, J., & Trombly, S. (1978). Active range-of-motion exercises: A handbook. *Nursing78, 8*(8), 45–49.

Cuica, R., Bradish, J., & Trombly, S. (1978). Passive range-of-motion exercises: A handbook. *Nursing78, 8*(7), 59–65.

Ellis, J., Nowlis, E., & Bentz, P. (1980). *Modules for basic nursing skills* (2nd ed.). Boston: Houghton Mifflin.

Renal Conditions

Bauer, D. (1980). Preventing the spread of hepatitis B in dialysis units. *American Journal of Nursing, 80,* 260–261.

Binkley, L. (1984). Keeping up with peritoneal dialysis. *American Journal of Nursing, 84,* 729–733.

Binkley, L. (Ed.). (1981). Transplantation. *Nephrology Nurse, 3(6),* whole issue.

Cairoli, O., & Voyce, P. (1982). *Memory bank for hemodialysis.* Baltimore: Williams & Wilkins.

Chambers, J. (1981). Assessing the dialysis patient at home. *American Journal of Nursing, 81,* 750–754.

Cianci, J., Lamp, J., & Ryan, R. (1981). Renal transplantation. *American Journal of Nursing, 81,* 354–355.

David-Kasdan, J. (1984). Alteration in body image in the hemodialysis population. *Journal of Nephrology Nursing, 1,* 25–28.

Davis, V., & Lavandero, R. (1980). Caring for the catheter carefully, Part I. *Nursing 80, 10(12),* 67–71.

Faris, M. (1980). *When your kidneys fail.* San Diego: National Kidney Foundation.

Fleming, L. (1984). Step by step guide to safe peritoneal dialysis. *RN, 47(2),* 44–47.

Hekleman, F. (1985). A framework for organizing a CAPD training program. *Journal of Nephrology Nursing, 2,* 56–60.

Hughes, C. (1985). Stabilizing catheters—Tenckhoff catheter placement. *American Nephrology Nurses Association Journal, 12(3),* 204.

Irwin, B. (1981). Now—Peritoneal dialysis for chronic patients, too. *RN, 44(6),* 49–52.

Lane, T. (1983). Standards of care for the CAPD patient. *Home Health Care Nurse, 4(5),* 34, 36, 41–45.

Levi, M. (1984). Learning to live with dialysis. *Journal of Nephrology Nursing, 1,* 153–154.

Levi, M. (1985). Learning to live with dialysis—Dialysis or transplant. *Journal of Nephrology Nursing, 2,* 27.

Moncrief, J., & Popovich, R. (1981). *CAPD update.* New York: Masson.

Montefusco, C. (1984). Cyclosporin immunosuppression in organ transplant recipients—Nursing complications. *Critical Care Nursing, 4(2),* 117–119.

Payne, G. (1984). Reducing stress in renal patients and their families. *Journal of Nephrology Nursing, 1,* 138–140.

Peterson, L. (1984). Home dialysis training. *American Nephrology Nurses Association Journal, 11(4),* 27–29.

Pitman, N. (1982). *Nephrology nursing standards of clinical practice.* American Association of Nephrology Nurses and Technicians.

Plaweski, H. (1985). Counseling the sexually dysfunctioning hemodialysis patient. *Journal of Nephrology Nursing, 2,* 166–168.

Powers, A. (1981). Renal transplantation: The patient's choice. *Nursing Clinics of North America, 16,* 551–564.

Rambaks, I. (1985). Post-transplant hypertension and the renal transplant. *Journal of Nephrology Nursing, 2,* 115–118.

Rhodes, V. (1985). Monthly home patient checklist—A dialysis assessment tool. *Journal of Nephrology Nursing, 2,* 28–29.

Richard, A. (1985). Renal transplantation—Nursing management of the recipient. *JOARN, 41,* 1022–1036, 1038, 1040, 1041.

Sandeval, M., & Parks, C. (1981). The evolution to CAPD. *Nephrology Nurse, 3(5),* 27–30, 32.

Sorrels, P. (1981). Peritoneal dialysis: A rediscovery. *Nursing Clinics of North America, 16,* 515–530.

Stevenson, J. (1984). Health related problems of patients on hemodialysis. *Journal of Nephrology Nursing, 1,* 101–105.

Topor, M. (1981). Chronic renal disease in children. *Nursing Clinics of North America, 16,* 587–598.

Weiss, M. (1981). Evaluation of a home hemodialysis instruction program. *Nephrology Nurse, 3(4),* 8, 10–12, 42–43.

Reye's Syndrome

Budd, R., & Rothwell, R. (1983). Spotting Reye's syndrome while there's still time. *RN, 46(12),* 39–42.

Dalgas, P. (1983). Reye's syndrome update. *MCN: American Journal of Maternal/Child Nursing, 3,* 345–349.

Feaster, S. (1984). Intracranial hypertension: A Reye's syndrome complication. *Dimensions of Critical Care Nursing, 3(1),* 24–29.

Haller, J. (1980). Intracranial pressure monitoring in Reye's syndrome. *Hospital Practice, 15(2),* 101–108.

Jemison-Smith, P., & Hamm, P. (1983). Infection control update: Reye's syndrome. *Critical Care Update, 10(7),* 54–55.

Martelli, M. (1982). Teaching parents about Reye's syndrome. *American Journal of Nursing, 82,* 260–263.

Miller, J., & Arsenault, L. (1983). Reye's syndrome. *Journal of Neurosurgical Nursing, 15(3),* 154–164.

Scoliosis

Allard, J., & Dibble, S. (1984). Scolosis surgery: A look at Luque rods. *American Journal of Nursing, 84,* 609–611.

Davis, S., & Lewis, S. (1984). Managing scoliosis: Fashions for the body and mind. *MCN: American Journal of Maternal/Child Nursing, 9,* 186–187.

Faro, B. (1980). By losing control of herself, Linda controlled her parents . . . and us. *Nursing80, 10(4),* 62–64.

Halladay, J. (1984). Update on scoliosis. *Canadian Nurse, 80(8),* 44–45.

Holt de Toledo, C. (1979). The patient with scoliosis: The defect—Classification and detection; the orthoplastic jacket. *American Journal of Nursing, 79,* 1589–1598.

Jones, M. (1985). Clinical approach to the child with scoliosis. *Pediatrics in Review, 6(7),* 219–223.

Kaarn, M., & Crawford, A. (1984). Postoperative nursing management of the patient following posterior spinal fusion. *Orthopedic Nursing, 3(2),* 21–25.

Micheli, L., Magin, M., & Rouvales, R. (1979). The patient with scoliosis—surgical management and nursing care. *American Journal of Nursing, 79,* 1599–1607.

Miller, D., & Lever, D. (1982). Scoliosis screening: An approach used in the school. *Journal of School Health, 52(2),* 98–101.

Schatziner, L., Brower, E., & Nash, C. (1979). Spinal fusion: Emotional stress and adjustment. *American Journal of Nursing, 79,* 1608–1612.

Thomas, P. (1983). Nursing care of patients undergoing posterior fusion with segmental (Luque) spinal instrumentation. *Orthopedic Nursing, 2(3),* 13–20.

Thomassen, P. (1984). Helping your scoliosis patient walk tall. *RN, 47(2),* 34–37.

Tibbits, C. (1980). Adolescent idiopathic scoliosis. *Nurse Practitioner, 5(2),* 11–20.

Watkins, P. (1985). Straightening up—Scoliosis surgery. *Nursing Times, 81*(8), 40–43.

You can help children with scoliosis. (1981). *Patient Care, 15*(8), 111–127.

Siblings

Abidin, R. (1982). Parenting stress and the utilization of pediatric services. *Children's Health Care, 11*(2), 70–73.

Craft, M. (1986). Validation of responses reported by school-aged siblings of hospitalized children. *Children's Health Care, 15*(1), 6–13.

Dorn, L. (1984). Children's concepts of illness: Clinical applications. *Pediatric Nursing, 10*, 325–327.

Harder, L., & Bowditch, B. (1982). Siblings of children with cystic fibrosis: Perceptions of the impact of the disease. *Children's Health Care, 10*(4), 116–120.

Knafl, K., & Dixon, D. (1983). The role of siblings during pediatric hospitalization. *Issues in Comprehensive Pediatric Nursing, 6*, 13–22.

LaMontagne, L. (1984). Three coping strategies used by school-age children. *Pediatric Nursing, 10*, 25–28.

Shonkwiler, M. (1985). Sibling visits in the pediatric intensive care unit. *Critical Care Quarterly, 8*(1), 67–72.

Siemon, M. (1984). Siblings of the chronically ill or disabled child: Meeting their needs. *Nursing Clinics of North America, 19*, 295–307.

Trahd, G. (1986). Siblings of chronically ill children: Helping them cope. *Pediatric Nursing, 12*, 191–193.

Zelaukas, B. (1981). Siblings: The forgotten grievers. *Issues in Comprehensive Pediatric Nursing, 5*, 45–52.

Literature from: The Sibling Project, SSSH/PCC, 124 Franklin Place, Woodmere, NY 11598.

Sickle Cell Anemia

Flanagan, C. (1980). Home management of sickle cell anemia. *Pediatric Nursing, 6*, 29–33 (B-D).

Gradolf, B. (1983). Sickle cell anemia in children. *Issues in Comprehensive Pediatric Nursing, 6*, 295–306.

Hathaway, G. (1984). The child with sickle cell anemia: Implications and management. *Nurse Practitioner, 9*(10), 16–22.

Pack, B. (Ed.). (1983). Symposium on sickle cell disease. *Nursing Clinics of North America, 18*, 129–229.

Reindorf, C. (1980). Sickle cell anemia: Current concepts. *Pediatric Nursing, 6*, 34–39 (E-G).

Suicide

Adams, B. (1983). Adolescent health care: Needs, priorities, and services. *Nursing Clinics of North America, 18*, 237–248.

Denholm, C. (1985). Hospitalization and the adolescent patient: A review and some critical questions. *Children's Health Care, 13*(3), 109–116.

Eisenberg, L. (1984). Depression and suicide in children and adolescents. *Pediatric Annals, 13*(1), 21–61.

Elkind, D. (1984). Teenage thinking: Implications for health care. *Pediatric Nursing, 10*, 383–385.

Finigan, J. (1986). Assessment of childhood and adolescent depression and suicide potential. *Journal of Emergency Nursing, 12*(1), 35–38.

Fletcher, B., & Johnson, C. (1982). The myth of formal operations: Rethinking adolescent cognition in clinical contexts. *Children's Health Care, 11*(1), 17–21.

Hals, E. (1985). Suicide prevention . . . What should be included in a curriculum. *Health Education, 16*(4), 45–47.

Miller, D. (1986). Affective disorders and violence in adolescents. *Hospital and Community Psychiatry, 37*(6), 591–596.

Moss, N. (1984). Child therapy groups: In the real world. *Journal of Psychosocial Nursing, 22*(3), 43–48.

Niven, R. (1986). Adolescent drug abuse. *Hospital and Community Psychiatry, 37*(6), 596–607.

Rice, M. (1983). Review: Identifying the adolescent substance abuser. *MCN: American Journal of Maternal/Child Nursing, 8*, 139–142.

Shamoo, T. (1985). Suicide intervention strategies for the adolescent. *Techniques, 1*, 297–303.

Shulman, V. (1985). Suicidal behavior at school: A systematic perspective. *Journal of Adolescence, 8*, 263–269.

Valente, S. (1985). The suicidal teenager. *Nursing85, 15*(12), 47–49.

Tonsillectomy and Adenoidectomy

Bradoff, A. (1979). T&A controversy—When should tonsils and/or adenoids go? *Patient Care, 13*, 116–117.

Farnsworth, S. (1985). Susan's sore throat. *Nursing Mirror, 161*(7), 36–39.

Paradise, J. (1981). Tonsillectomy and adenoidectomy. *Pediatric Clinics of North America, 28*, 881–891.

Sharman, W. (1985). Tonsillectomy through a child's eyes. *Nursing Times, 81*(49), 48–52.

Total Parenteral Nutrition

Barfoot, K. (1986). Home care of the child receiving nutritional support: A global approach. *Journal of the National Intravenous Therapy Association, 9*(3), 226–229.

Bender, J., & Faubion, W. (1985). Parenteral nutrition for the pediatric patient. *Home Healthcare Nurse, 3*(6), 32–39.

Coran, A. (1981). Parenteral nutrition in infants and children. *Surgical Clinics of North America, 61*, 1089–1099.

Haas-Beckert, B. (1987). Removing the mysteries of parenteral nutrition. *Pediatric Nursing, 13*, 37–41.

Kerner, J. (1983). *Manual of pediatric parenteral nutrition*. New York: Wiley.

Zlotkin, S., Stallings, V., & Pencharz, P. (1985). Total parenteral nutrition in children. *Pediatric Clinics of North America, 32*, 381–400.

Tracheostomy

Fuchs, P. (1984). Streamlining your suctioning technique—tracheostomy suctioning. *Nursing84, 14*(7), 39–43.

Nursing photobook: providing respiratory care. (1980). Horsham, Pa: Intermed.

Traction

Cohen, S. (1979). Nursing care of a patient in traction. *American Journal of Nursing, 79*, 1771–1778.

Tube Feedings

Bayer, L., Scholl, D., & Ford, E. (1983). Tube feeding at home. *American Journal of Nursing, 83*, 1321–1324.

Blackman, J., & Nelson, C. (1985). Reinstituting oral feedings in children fed by gastrostomy tube. *Clinical Pediatrics, 24*(8), 434–438.

Konstantinides, N., & Shronts, E. (1983). Tube feeding: Managing the basics. *American Journal of Nursing, 83*, 1312–1320.

Moore, M., & Green, H. (1985). Tube feeding of infants and children. *Pediatric Clinics of North America, 32*, 401–417.

Paine, J. (1985). Practical aspects of nasogastric feeding in pediatric patients from a ward nursing perspective. *Nutritional Support Services, 5*(10), 10, 12, 14, 25.

Zimmaro, D. (1986). Diarrhea associated with enteral nutrition. *Focus on Critical Care, 13*(5), 58–63.

Ulcerative Colitis

Joachim, G. (1983). Getting the right information: a data collection tool for patients with inflammatory bowel disease. *Society of Gastrointestinal Assistants Journal, 6*(2), 42–49.

Kraft, S. (1982). Ulcerative colitis. *Society of Gastrointestinal Assistants Journal, 5*(2), 3–6.

Lewicki, L., & Leeson, M. (1984). The multisystem impact on physiologic processes of inflammatory bowel disease. *Nursing Clinics of North America, 19,* 71–80.

Metz, G. (1984). Medical management of inflammatory bowel disease. *Journal of Enterostomal Therapy, 11*(3), 114–115.

Myer, S. (1984). Overview of inflammatory bowel disease. *Nursing Clinics of North America, 19,* 3–9.

Nemer, F., & Rolstad, B. (1985). The role of the ileoanal reservoir in patients with ulcerative colitis and familial polyposis. *Journal of Enterostomal Therapy, 12*(3), 74–83.

Phillips, S. (1982). Research in inflammatory bowel disease. *Society of Gastrointestinal Assistants Journal, 5*(2), 15–19.

Postier, R., O'Malley, V., & Pruitt, L. (1984). Continence-preserving operations for ulcerative colitis and multiple polyposis. *Journal of Enterostomal Therapy, 11*(6), 237–239.

Simons, M. (1984). Using the nursing process in treating inflammatory bowel disease. *Nursing Clinics of North America, 19,* 11–25.

Stotts, N., Fitzgerald, K., & Williams, K. (1984). Care of the patient critically ill with inflammatory bowel disease. *Nursing Clinics of North America, 19,* 61–70.

Wilson, C. (1984). The diagnostic workup for the patient with inflammatory bowel disease. *Nursing Clinics of North America, 19,* 51–59.

Wilms' Tumor

Armstrong, G., Wirt, R., Nesbit, M., & Martinson, I. (1982). Multidimensional assessment of psychological problems in children with cancer. *Research in Nursing and Health, 5,* 205–211.

Gibbons, M., & Boren, H. (1985). Stress reduction: A spectrum of strategies in pediatric oncology nursing. *Nursing Clinics of North America, 20,* 83–103.

Kramer, R., & Perin, G. (1985). Patient education and pediatric oncology. *Nursing Clinics of North America, 20,* 31–47.

Tringali, C. (1986). The needs of family members of cancer patients. *Oncology Nursing Forum, 13*(4), 65–70.

Index